THE NEW
FAMILY
HERB DOCTOR

THE NEW ZEALAND
❦ FAMILY ❦
HERB DOCTOR

A Guide to Recipes
and Herbal Remedies

James Neil

SENATE

The New Zealand Family Herb Doctor

First published in 1891 by Mills, Dick & Company,
Dunedin, New Zealand

This edition published in 1998 by Senate,
an imprint of Tiger Books International plc,
26A York Street, Twickenham,
Middlesex TW1 3LJ, United Kingdom

Cover design © 1998 Tiger Books International

1 3 5 7 9 10 8 6 4 2

ISBN 1 85958 540 X

Printed and bound in the UK by
Cox & Wyman, Reading, England

IMPORTANT NOTE

The recipies, remedies, and treatments in this book are
not intended to replace treatment from health
professionals. Do not under any circumstances undertake
any of the suggested treatments without first seeking
advice from a suitably qualified person.

INTRODUCTION.

NOW that the earth is, so to speak, flooded with medical books, it is almost needful to make an apology for adding another to the long list. But there are several reasons why we feel it incumbent upon us to produce the "Family Herb Doctor": (1) Most medical works are written for the profession in such language as ordinary people cannot understand. (2) That the remedies recommended are, as they have been termed, "edge tools," requiring a skilful hand to use with safety. (3) Their price is beyond the means of many to procure. (4) They are most of them out of date with this progressive age; and, lastly, all are, as far as we know, unacquainted with some of the valuable herbs found in Australia and New Zealand. These reasons, we think, are sufficient to warrant us in offering to the public of New Zealand and Australia the valuable information which will be found in the succeeding pages. The illustrations of the plants, as well as the entire work of the book, are local, and show that we are advancing in our self-reliant progressive industry. It will be our aim to give our readers in plain, simple words the benefit of our experience and knowledge gathered during the last twenty years we have been in the study and practice of herbal medicine. Although it is not our intention to discuss theology in our pages, yet as we believe that human happiness and even health are largely dependent on the fear of the Lord, which is the beginning of wisdom, we shall write in such a way as we trust will prove our conviction that Christians ought to do all things for the glory of God and the good of their fellow-beings.

We do not propose to follow the questionable example of many herbal book writers, who deal largely in abuse of the regular doctor and his drugs; while we cannot (even apart from our training as herbalist) endorse many of the doctors methods and medicines, so-called, yet we cannot deny that they as a body are honestly endeavouring to do their best for the benefit of suffering humanity. The cause of bitterness against them found in some of the herbal books arose from the fact that the old-school doctors, filled with professional pride, not only looked down on all irregulars, especially herbalists, but persecuted them with great severity. But happily for us, the age of narrow bigotry is passing away. It is our happiness to know many of the regular school who are just men and true, so broad in their liberality that they would not prevent people choosing their medical attendant from any school or system. As it says in Scripture "A humble spirit is of great price in the sight of God," so is it in that of good men; it will prevent its possessor losing much useful information, for it is an acknowledged fact that very many of the valuable remedies which have blessed humanity have come from the non-professional, which the proud M.D. would not receive for a time, as they did not come to him backed by scholastic authority. As an illustration of this unreasonable folly we may mention a case that occurred in connection with ourselves. A Mrs. —— had very badly ulcerated breasts; one of them had three deep sores, the other two, from which a constant discharge of humour was issuing. Her relations called in three medical men, who simply advised the routine treatment of linseed poulticing. A female friend called to see her, and advised her to send to our shop for a quarter of a pound of slippery elm powder, telling her how to prepare it by mixing it with milk into a paste and laying it on the sores. After it was put on she fell asleep and slept for twelve hours—(she had not slept for three nights and days before). When it was changed it showed a marked improvement. Ten more poultices of this valuable medicine effected the cure. Here is the point: Two of the doctors (regulars) seeing the remarkable cure, would not humble themselves to take note of an old woman's remedy but to the credit of the third (a homœopath), he carefully noted down the name of this valuable medicine, and said he would use it in similar cases.

Some of our readers may call in question our ability to write a creditable work on medicine, doubtless comparing us unfavourably with the master minds of the past, who may be said to stand as giants in front of us, who are but dwarfs beside them. Granted that this is true, still as dwarfs on the shoulders of giants can see further and more than the giants, so we, having their experience, together with what we have been able to glean ourselves, can take our position along with them as disseminators of useful knowledge for the benefit of our race. We have one serious fault to find with most medical books, both botanic and regular, namely, that the great source of blessing and healing is almost ignored, namely God, who gives us all things richly to enjoy and employ to the benefit of one another. It is but right for us to use the means, but we should never forget that life and death are in the hands of our Creator. We cannot close our introduction better than by reminding all that our faculties, means of knowledge, experience, food, medicine, and all that we have and are comes from our Divine Benefactor, who, concerning the destiny of our race has declared that in the age to come sickness and all unhappiness, even death itself shall be abolished for ever. Amen.

We are indebted to the following authors for some of the valuable information that will be found in our pages; (we have now their works in stock and can highly recommend them):—Dr. Coffin's Botanic Guide to Health, Dr Fox's Working Man's do., Dr. Skelton's do., Dr. Stevens's, Prof. Brown's, Dr. Beach's, Dr. Gunn's, Dr. Robinson's, and others. Our motto is to learn from every writer truth that may be useful to us in doing good to suffering humanity.

A BRIEF HISTORY OF MEDICINE.

To those who reject the Bible account of man's creation, the necessity of medicine must be an enigma. Why, if man is now in the condition that God made him, did He make him subject to disease and death? The Bible alone explains what would be to us an inscrutable mystery. It tells us that God formed man out of the dust of the ground, and breathed into his nostrils the breath of life, and man became a living soul; then he had the perfection of innocence, and enjoyed the blessedness of walking with his Maker, who is the true source of happiness. How long he continued in this primeval state we do not know, but in an evil hour he disobeyed God, who expelled him from Eden's happy bowers. Just here a disputed point of theology comes up, namely, was man made mortal or immortal, or has he an immortal soul. We believe, from a careful study of the Scriptures, that he was created mortal, that the tree of life would have constantly renewed his life if he had not sinned. Our reason for not believing in the popular doctrine of the immortality of the soul, is because it is not said in any part of the Bible that the soul is immortal, but it very distinctly says in several parts that the soul can and will die. We do not intend to discuss the point further, but if any of our readers desire it, we shall be happy to supply abundant proof for our belief in the mortality of the soul. One thing is certain, that sin and suffering came into our world; this being so, we have reason to thank God for giving us the means of cure. It may be affirmed that, notwithstanding man's fallen condition in the primitive times, sickness was seldom felt; the reason why is because he lived closer to nature and was free from hereditary taint. Previous to the deluge human life averaged ten times its present limits, but the written doom came at last and man returned to the dust out of which he was taken. A sad and gloomy prospect indeed if we had not the Divine assurance that though "a man die yet shall he live again. The doctrine of a resurrection to an

eternal life of happiness is the true hope of the Christian. In
Genesis i. 29, God says: "Behold I have given you
every herb-bearing seed which is upon the face of all the
earth, and every tree in which is the fruit of a tree yielding
seed, to you it shall be for meat." From these words and
several others of a like import, the herbalist derives scriptural
authority for his system of medicine. It must be a matter of
conjecture as to how man got to know that by eating or
drinking the juice of certain herbs his sickness would be
cured. We may imagine one of the primitives striking his
leg against anything; knocking the skin off, he would look
for something to cover it, and the first thing coming to his hand
would be a broad leaf, most likely the plantain which grows
everywhere and is generally known as healing leaves:
one of these leaves bound on the sore would soon heal it.
Probably a severe fall might cause this same individual a bleeding
from the internal organs, and reasoning from the effect of the
leaves he applied to stop the bleeding and heal the sore on the
leg, he would eat some of the same leaves; and if unpleasant to
eat he might boil them and drink the tea; or he might feel the
discomfort of indigestion, and, after trying several, would
find the herb that relieved him best, and giving it a name,
would use it again, and doubtless tell his children about it;
and so after this manner the adage that necessity is the mother
of invention, many of the medicinal plants were discovered.
It is a matter of faith with some and doubt with others that
every plant has one or more medicinal properties. In Ayer's
Almanac for 1884 there is the best definition of what gardeners
consider their greatest enemy—weeds. It says: "A weed is
a plant the virtues of which we have not yet found out. We
are ready to admit that in the early ages of our race before
artificial living was introduced, man had little or no need of
physic, but as time rolled on and man step by step departed
from God and nature in his manner of living, the various
diseases which now desolate our homes and fill our hearts with
sorrow, were added, to teach him that sin must bring suffering."
The first intimation that medicine was practised as an art

or profession is in connection with the ancient Egyptians, who had a most wonderful skill in preserving the dead, and we might suppose that they also had some knowledge as to how to keep the living in health. The works of these men can be seen to this day in the mummies to be found in almost all museums. The first medicinal plant we read of is the Balm of Gilead. There is a plant found in many countries bearing this name, but it cannot be accurately determined that it is identical with the scriptural one. Hyssop is an example in point, for while the scriptural plant bearing this name had an aperient property, our modern one has not. In Solomon's time, who was contemporary with Homer, the first profane writer and historian, the business of an apothecary is first mentioned. We suppose that this included the doctor as well as the medicine vendor. Then Jeremiah, the prophet, asks in plantive tones if there is no balm in Gilead and no physician there. Passing on to the time of our Saviour we find Him in His answer to the self-righteous Pharisees saying : "They that are whole need not a physician, but they that are sick"; and when that notable miracle was wrought on the woman with the bloody issue the writer himself (a doctor) said that she had spent all her living with physicians who did not then practice on the no cure no pay principle, which would not be a paying one for most doctors now-a-days. In the apostle's time we read of Celsus, a doctor and one of the earliest and bitterest opponents of Christianity, having just before reading his words discussed with some infidel student of medicine, and knowing that many of the profession are unbelievers and scoffers, we thought that Celsus was a worthy progenitor of such, and we almost concluded that the medical body was wholly tainted with this poison; but when we thought of Luke, the beloved physician and evangelist of our Lord, and the matchless purity seen in his justly termed Immortal Gospel, and Book of Acts, which will live when all the learned writings of scientific infidels have been forgotten for millions of years, we concluded that doctors as a class can show as many devout Christians as other professions. Before Christ,

history tells us of a truly great medical man, named
Hippocrates, a Grecian. He was the first to give a detailed
account of man's wonderful mechanism. He also classified
the symptoms and stages of fever and other diseases. An
interesting story is told of his skill: After he had retired from
busy life to a quiet farm, a terrible plague broke out in
Athens. The people were dying in numbers. The king or
governor sent for him, and as he was doubtful of his prompt
obedience, an armed band carried with it orders to bring him
at once. He came and carefully examined some of the stricken
ones, then gave orders for immense bonfires to be kindled in
the city, so as to purify the atmosphere. He ordered the
patients hot baths and hot medicated wines. It is said that
in a few days the plague was stayed. This man is now called
the Father of Medicine, although his title may well be
disputed, as there were doubtless many wise and successful
physicians before him. After him came Esculapius, Galen,
and others, men who were successful in their calling, as their
remedial agents were of a simple botanic or organic nature.
We read that one of the physicians of Julius Cæsar wrote
an article extolling the virtues of a plant named Wood Betony,
which we find an excellent remedy in headaches of the chronic
form. With the decline of the Roman Empire and the unholy
alliance between church and state, inaugurated by the great
Constantine, came the dominion of priestcraft, which gradually
took into its own unskilful hands the healing of the sick.
The scientific treatment, if it ever was worthy of the name,
gave place to the empirical; charms, incantations, and holy relics,
were principal in their *materia medica;* then came holy water from
wells consecrated to holy virgins and saints, some simple herbs,
and prayer concluded their stock in trade. With the dawn of the
Reformation this priestly monopoly was invaded and broken up
in England. For a long time the art of surgery was practised
by the barbers in London. Some of these became noted
experts, and prompted by selfish motives, and perhaps by
better ones, they petitioned Henry VIII. for a monopoly,
which he, with the consent of Parliament, granted; giving the

barbers of London a monopoly of eight miles in and around the capital in which to practise the art of Chirurgery, as it was then termed. Some time after, the first college for the training of students was founded ; then the surgeons united medication to their practice, and from this it may be termed modern beginning, there sprang the numerous halls of learning that flourish in every civilised land. It is interesting to follow this history step by step down the stream of time, but space forbids us to do more than note the important changes as they were introduced. The one which may be regarded as the greatest and in its pernicious effects the most to be lamented of all changes, ancient or modern, was the introduction of minerals and poisonous acids prepared from them by a noted empiric named Paracelsus, who has been justly termed the "Prince of Quacks." This man (or arrogant fool) burned the books of his medical predecessors, declaring that he would follow no man, as he counted himself wiser than them all. It would have been a blessing for humanity if the doctors had treated his mischievous teachings in the same manner by burning them. The many thousands whose systems have been ruined by mercury, falsely termed medicine, will rise in judgment against him, for it was this man that caused the faculty at first to introduce into the human stomach that slow but sure poison, promising health and long life to all his followers. He himself only lived about 40 years, his own early death denying his false system of mineralisation. Notwithstanding the inroads of mineral medication the common people, and even some of the doctors, had not lost faith in simple botanic remedies. Reading an old medical dictionary of over 100 years ago, it is pleasing to see that three-fourths of all it recommends is from the vegetable kingdom. In country districts the old and experienced mothers were the family physicians, whose stores were replenished from the fields around. Except in cases of extreme sickness and approaching death, a doctor was seldom seen in the villages. At the beginning of our present century two new schools of medicine were started, which have proved thorns in the side of the allopathists (whose creed means we cure by contraries), *i.e.*, the homœopathic school (whose creed means we cure by similars), and the school we own as ours, viz., the botanic eclectic, having no creed unless it be a preference for vegetable agents instead of mineral. As everything that is human will advance (or it may be retrograde) the eclectic system, which as its name indicates, chooses from every source agents that will assist in relieving or curing disease. It had its beginning in America, by Samuel Thompson, a New England farmer, whose life teaches us the fact that wisdom does not always come through the recognised channels of human learning. In fact, most of our valuable medicines have been found by such children of nature as Thompson and others who studied in the fields and by the bedsides of suffering friends. This man was born in the backwoods of America, and from youth to manhood was engaged in clearing the forest. As a youth he took an interest in medicine, and this natural taste was encouraged and improved by an old lady termed an herbalist, who took young Thompson to the meadows with her as she gathered her store of herbs and roots. One day, while felling timber he had the misfortune to almost sever his foot with a misguided blow. There was a root doctor several miles from the settlement; thither his father drew him on a rough sledge. By good treatment he recovered, and for a number of years enjoyed such good health that he thought little about medicine; he married and settled on his own frontier homestead. The neighbourhood soon became populated. As an encouragement to a young doctor to settle Thompson gave him a piece of ground whereon to put his house. Several young Thompsons came home, and not being very robust, the doctor had a good many visits to make and charge Thompson with. It happened that the eldest child, a girl, took ill with what was then termed canker rash, a very bad eruptive fever. One of her eyes was lost, and the doctor gave her up as lost; he said she could not live till the morning. Thompson told him he would try and save the child himself. He first made a tea of bayberry bark, which he thought contained a purifying or anti-canker property. He then got two hot bricks, put them in a bucket of hot water, directing his wife to cover him with blankets round the neck. He stripped the child and held her between his knees over the steam, her head like his own being uncovered. He steamed her for 20 minutes, giving her some of the bayberry tea every few minutes; by this means a great perspiration was induced. After sponging her carefully they put her in warm clothes to bed, and sat watching her. From the first they were encouraged by improving signs, and ere morn had come there was a great improvement. The doctor was surprised to see the child, and was not over pleased at the success of a lay-man. Thompson told him he intended to doctor his own family in future, and afterwards gave him a hint to shift, which he soon did. For a long time the family did not want any doctoring; but the neighbours soon learnt of Thompson's skill in herbs, and applied to him when in need of medical aid. His fame grew apace, and the doctors began to persecute him and by this means advertise him. About this time an epidemic of fever broke out in a town not far from him. Many had died and many were dying; eight out of ten of the patients were lost by the doctors. Some of the leading men heard of Thompson, and called a meeting at which it was resolved that a postchaise be sent at once for him. He returned with it, taking a friend as an assistant. They began at once and gave the same treatment in every case, and did not lose one patient. The treatment was what is now known (see index) as the Thompsonian course. The many calls on his time prevented him from giving due regard to his family and farm; so that, after consulting with his friends on the subject, he determined to sell out and devote himself to healing the sick. In his visits to the woods to collect his remedies he found out a way to test the virtue of plants. Chewing some of the leaves, he learned to detect their virtue by the taste and impression left in his mouth. If bitter, he concluded them tonic; if sour and leaving a roughened feeling on the tongue, they were rightly judged astringent; if nauseating, then he classed them emetics; and first in this class he discovered that most potent of vegetable medicines,

Lobelia Inflata. If he had done nothing more than introduce this to the world his name ought to be honoured. It is a lamentable evidence of our fallen nature that a man should be persecuted by his fellows for doing good. The fact that it has always been so is proved by the life of Thompson and other benefactors. The nearest doctor to Thompson was a Dr. French, who did his utmost to crush him. And why? Because Thompson had succeeded in curing a lady whom Dr. French had given up to die. This, and many other splendid cures wrought by him caused the doctor to speak evil of him, and wish him out of the way, for he (Thompson) had proved how little value the college training of some doctors was when compared with one whose nature had been endowed with true genius and a love for the healing of the sick. Dr. French had been watching an opportunity to accuse his supposed enemy of mal-practice. At last one of Thompson's patients died. The doctor had learned that *lobelia* had been given to the young man that had succumbed. This was all that was wanted. He laid and swore to an information charging Samuel Thompson, the self-styled herb doctor, with manslaughter. Upon this charge Thompson was apprehended, lodged in gaol, and kept there until the sittings of the Supreme Court, which were only held once in six months. Poor Thompson had to lie in prison for four months.

The case referred to was that of a young man with fever, whom Thompson had cured, but having to leave before complete recovery, Thompson told him to keep in-doors for a week. Before the week was on a beautiful spring day, the young man went out and sat down on a damp grassy bank till he felt a chill. He returned home, took to his bed, and alarming symptoms set in. Then Dr. French was sent for, who said he had been poisoned by *lobelia*, given him by Thompson. This is the origin of the same falsehood published now in most of the old school medical books. It is a strange poison that of which a man can take any quantity from a grain up to an ounce! We have taken a tablespoonful, with the result of a thorough emetic, which seemed to chase away our fever and make us feel renewed in health.

Thompson's trial came on at last. To their credit, numerous friends who had been cured rallied round him, so much so that the prosecutor lost heart, and would have given almost anything to have got out of it; but there were more doctors than himself in it now, and it had to go to the jury. The first witness called proved the facts of the case. A specimen of the dreaded poison, procured by the doctors, was handed to another witness, who looked it over, picked off a spray, and commenced chewing it. The learned judge, amid the silence of the court, sternly asked the witness if he intended to poison himself in their presence. The witness replied, "Your Honor, I could not poison myself with this herb. It is not *lobelia* at all, it is *marsh rosemary*." This created quite a sensation, and was a great crusher for the doctors. When the instigator of this iniquitous suit was put in the box he was terror-stricken, for he knew that his ignorance and perjury had caused the innocent man to be kept four months in a cold and poisonous dungeon. He knew also that damages, exceeding his estate, could be recovered from him. In the witness-box, when questioned, he did not, he said, know much about the prisoner. He had heard evil things about him, was sorry he believed them, and was sorry that he had instituted this suit. The judge characterised the case as a most malicious one, and directed the jury to acquit the prisoner, which they instantly did. Dr. French found it to his advantage to clear out very soon after.

After this Thompson had rest from his enemies, who now began to use his method of treatment and medicines, taking care not to give him the honour. To prevent this and save himself from further molestation he went to Washington and took out a patent for his course of medicine. He had the satisfaction of living to a good old age and witnessing the good done by himself and some of his agents. When dying he said to his friends : "I have tried to help my fellow-men in their sickness by what remedies I could find. They have not been pleasant, I admit, but it is for you, my survivors, to carry on the good work." Four years ago, while in Boston, the grave of this great but little known man was shown to us. The principal charges that Thompson brought against the doctors were the then almost uniform treatment or maltreatment of bleeding. This inhuman practice was carried out to such an extent that it is said by eye-witnesses that the floors of the free dispensaries were sometimes covered with blood resembling a battle-field. Acting on the principle and teaching of Thompson, some of the doctors started the new school, which they termed the eclectic or reformed practice of medicine. One of the leaders was Dr. Beach, who was not manly enough to give Thompson the honour of his discoveries, but instead ridiculed and abused him. Thompson never claimed to be an educated man, and it makes Dr. Beach rather small in the eyes of honest herbalists to vaunt over a mistake of Thompson's in reference to anatomy. Thompson had said that the gall-duct emptied into the stomach, when it in fact emptied into the duodenum, sometimes called the second or smaller stomach. About fifty years ago Dr. Coffin came over to England and introduced the botanic system, pure and simple. His Botanic Guide to Health has passed through some 60 editions. It is a good work, but is sold at a price above its commercial value. For seeing its author and family have made princely fortunes out of it, we fail to see that its price should be so high, namely 6/- in England, where books of a similar kind are sold at 2/6. Dr. Coffin was a fine specimen of man, not only physically, as his portrait shows, but in manner. We are often told by some of our customers who have consulted him, that he was a gentleman. In one of his lectures he tells how he was converted to herbalism. He was a bound apprentice to an old-school doctor, and having a natural taste for the medical calling, was prospering, and would doubtless have shone, even as a regular, but, to the grief of his parents, he took ill and rapidly developed consumptive symptoms. A terrible cough, emaciation and bleeding, from the lungs led to the conclusion of galloping consumption.

As he lay in a dying state one day, an Indian woman presented herself at the door and begged a drink of cider. She happened to catch a look at the wan face of young Coffin, and asked his mother if that was her son. She replied in the affirmative. The Indian asked if the white man could not cure him. The mother said, "No." "Well," she said, "if you give me a gallon of cider I will cure him." Mrs. Coffin said, "You will get a hogshead if you do." The bargain was struck. The woman went out to the bush and gathered her apronful of herbs; returning she put some of them into a saucepan and boiled them and gave him the first wineglassful, which he said sent a warm glow over him, and caused him to say, "Mother, I think that woman will cure me." In a short time a manifest improvement was seen. The cough was relieved, the expectoration was lessened, and in a few weeks he was cured. During his sickness his master, the doctor, (who took the deepest interest in his case) had dosed him with physic to no purpose. While taking the herbs they did not let on to the doctor, who was jubliant at the supposed success of his treatment. He brought other doctors to see the case, who were also delighted at the prospect of successfully coping with this human scourge. The doctor asked the young man when he intended to resume his duties. "Never," he said, "with you or your school. I will follow a better system of medicine, the one to which I owe my life." He then showed him in a cupboard the medicine he had sent during the time of the herbal treatment, told him of the Indian woman's cure, and said, "I am going to learn from these children of the prairie how to heal the sick." This he did, and spent three years in what to him was the true college of Nature. Commencing practice in America he was very successful, as a list of the cases treated, and recorded in his book will show. This might not be considered evidence, but there are numerous witnesses now living, whose cases were parallel. During the visitation of cholera in 1848 his medicine and method (the steaming process of Samuel Thompson), was instrumental in rescuing thousands from death. A gentleman in this city, a Mr.

Calverly, whose father was an agent of the doctor's for Wakefield, in Yorkshire, tells us that he accompanied his father in treating his cholera patients, and that, if called before the last stage, they never lost a case. They had one medicine—Dr. Coffin's Anti-cholera Powder (see list of compounds)—and heat applied externally. Coffin had a hard fight with the regulars, who dubbed him a quack, but as he was a powerful and eloquent speaker on the platform, to which he invited them, they found him too many for them, and left him alone. The good work begun by him was taken up by others, who in their turn met the opposition and refuted the false accusations of bigoted opponents. Dr. John Skelton (not skeleton) as some have put it with Coffin's name, and said, "What a terrible system, beginning with a coffin and ending with a skeleton!" But it is not so, as it did not begin nor end with these gentlemen. Coffin certainly kept many out of their coffins for a time, and Skelton helped him in the same good work. Many others are now following them, the effect of their labour being seen in the medical liberalism of the present time.

Before closing this brief sketch of medical history I trust the reader will not consider it out of place to give a few facts regarding medical botany in New Zealand, and the honour we had in being its first public exponent. In the early days of the goldfields, there was an old gentleman named Westwood who gave himself out as an herbalist. His tent or canvas store could be seen and will be remembered by some who visited Wetherstones, Tuapeka, the Dunstan, and other localities. In the early days we did not then think of medicine, so never took any care to look at his stock; but we were told by a gentleman in Dunedin that one day he was amongst a crowd at the shop of Westwood, who was descanting on the power and potency of herbal medicine, and maledicting mineral drugs, when a knowing digger lifted up a piece of bluestone from Westwood's stall, and asked him, amid the laughter of the crowd, what kind of herb was that. According to the gentleman that told us, he was bowled out. What became of this old party we don't know, we are certain he did not do much in making herbalism known in New Zealand. In 1862 we met on the West Coast (South Island), a gentleman well known in Dunedin, Captain Stewart, who informed us of the wonderful cures that had been effected by the use of simple herbs. His mate, a Mr. George Balshill, had recently come out from Glasgow, where he had in a private way, practised medical botany, as taught by Dr. Coffin in his "Guide to Health." Soon after we left the coast, intending to return to Scotland, the land of our birth. While *en route*, in Melbourne the lady we stayed with was an enthusiastic herbalist. She gave us a reading of Dr. Foxe's book, which we read with much interest, and a conviction that herbs were the true medicine of nature. This lady counselled us strongly to begin the practice if we returned to New Zealand, affirming with much confidence that we would make our pile by so doing. We are glad that we took her advice. Nor was she far out in her prediction. While in Glasgow we served for a short time with an herbalist and dentist, named Clark, in London street, who was a decided expert in tooth-pulling. There is no exaggeration in saying that he had a bushel of teeth which he had extracted. In dressing his dentist's window he used to cover the bottom of it with them, as grocers spread theirs with currants, nuts, peas, &c. He did a considerable trade in herbs too, and like most steady young men was fairly prosperous. From this time we determined to make medical botany our life work, and before returning ordered our first stock from a wholesale house in London. We arrived in Dunedin in the end of 1872, and anxiously awaited the arrival of our goods, which being long delayed, we found employment in the meantime with a confectioner, running his cart into the country. One day while thus engaged, the horse, which seemed to have a large share of the evil spirit in it, had his blinder torn off by trampling on the reins and giving his head a jerk. Seeing him preparing for a bolt, we sprang and caught him by the nose and held on to him, calling or pleading with some men working in an adjoining brickyard, to come to our help. But these selfish men would not help us, but cried out, "Let him rip!" Seeing no help, and feeling the want of strength to hold on, we let go, but in doing so were knocked down by the wheel, which passed over our chest and broke three ribs, one of which perforated the lung tissue, causing what is termed emphysema, rupturing the lung with the concussion. Blood rushed into our mouth, and we verily thought our end was come. One who saw the accident, a cabman, drove in haste to town for a doctor, who when he came made a very superficial examination, and said no bones were broken. He applied a poultice and prescribed Port wine. He paid three visits, but as our condition got worse, we determined to call in other aid. The second doctor made a thorough examination, found three ribs fractured, and put on a strait-jacket of sticking-plaster. About six weeks after, the abscess forming in the right lung broke with a violent fit of coughing, which continued for one month, during which we coughed night and day. Just at this time our stock of herbal medicines came to hand. As soon as they were unpacked we directed a mixture of them to be put on and boiled. We commenced taking it, and also an emetic of Lobelia every week, and in a month the doctor, who had shaken his head in doubt as to our recovery, now pronounced us convalescent. It was a long time before we were able to do much, but some kind friends who believed in our system of medicine, knowing that we had a stock, bought and recommended the herbs to their friends. Getting stronger, we were asked to see some who could not leave their homes. These we visited with a friend—the late Mr. Yates—who was an experienced herbalist from Yorkshire, where the system is well known and trusted. To this friend we owe much, as he gave us the benefit of his knowledge, and how he examined and treated patients. With him we treated a patient given up by the doctors of consumption. To our delight this patient recovered, and was for the time he remained here a walking advertisement of our business. Carrying on this style of visitation for a while, we determined at last to take a shop. In 1876 we opened our Botanical Dispensary in George street. In one year we found the shop too small, and removed into the large double one, where we continued for over ten years— an astonishment to many of our friends at the success which followed us.

Ten years ago, seeing the disadvantage we were under in not having an education in general medicine, we determined to take advantage of our local University ; so we attended three sessions at the Otago Medical School, after which we visited the United States and entered as a student at the Bennett Eclectic College in Chicago, where we graduated in 1883. Returning home we were not satisfied, and the following year we visited New York and attended the Polyclinic College of that city. The Polyclinic, as its name indicates, is an institution for post-graduates or doctors. It is largely taken advantage of by doctors from the country, who wish to be posted in the latest improvements in medicine and surgery. Since our return we have extended our business to Auckland, Timaru, and Invercargill, where we have branches established. At the beginning we had to import all our herbs, but now we grow at our nursery in Caversham some that need cultivating, and gather more which we can find growing wild. In Wellington, Christchurch, and Auckland, others, since our establishing the cause, have adopted it and are now doing good work; showing beyond doubt that in the despised (by some) herbs of the field there is virtue stored up for the relief and cure of man's ailments. In justice to the regular system of medicine we must admit that great improvement has taken place of late. The introduction of chloroform and ether as anæsthetics, saving the terrible torture attendant on operations, and the abolition of bleeding and much of blistering, also the disuse of mercury, antimony, and some of the old-fashioned misnamed remedies, is cause for thankfulness. It is our earnest prayer that men may gain more knowledge, and find out better means for the cure of human suffering. In closing this chapter let us express our joy at the hopeful signs

of the times.   Many are running to and fro, and knowledge
is being increased on the earth.   May the progress continue
till the great Physician comes, who will abolish suffering and
death, and give life and immortality to all that love and obey
Him, to whom be the glory for ever and ever.   Amen.

MEDICAL BOTANY.

" He causeth the grass to grow for the cattle, and the herbs for the
  service of man."—Psalm civ. 14.

It seems strange that anyone should need to be informed that
Herbal Medicine is, as Sir John Hill, M.D., affirms, "the
true medicine of nature."   An observer of the animals can see
how their instinct leads them, when not in perfect health, to the
herbs for relief.   This fact has given names to certain plants,
for example, Dog Grass, Swine's Grass, Catnip, Bird Pepper,
Goose Grass, &c., &c.   The time is past when men of the
regular school ridiculed the idea of there being any virtue in
the herbs of the field unless they had been named and appro-
priated by the faculty.   Conversing with an M.D. of the old school
some time ago, he admitted that they got the best of their medicine
from the vegetable kingdom.   It is surprising to see the
number of new remedies that are being noticed in the
medical journals, and almost all from the same rational source.
The reason why this is so can be accounted for by the fact
that men are turning their attention to the true source of
supply, as indicated in the portion of Scripture quoted above.
Also that the chief objections to herbal medicine are
nearly overcome by the improved methods of preparation.   At
the beginning of our present century doctors were dreaded for
their cruel tactics, principally bleeding and blistering; also

for their nasty medicine. For instance, rhubarb in powder, blue pills, black drafts, &c. The herbalist, with his big doses of decoctions, some of them as bitter as gall, was not much in favour either, especially with children; but now some art has been introduced, and medicines formerly considered disgusting are now rendered comparatively pleasant, and the big doses are concentrated from a wineglassful to a teaspoonful. While in most cases this can be done without impairing the efficiency of the agent, still there are some that experience proves are best taken in large doses and as near their natural condition as possible. Infusions or decoctions are the simplest way of extracting the virtues of herbs or roots.

In this division of our work we will describe the principal herbs, roots, barks, seeds, &c., used in the Botanic System, and such as are also common to the Allopath and Homœopath. As we intend to fill our pages only with useful matter, we will not notice the almost innumerable variety that are set forth in some botanical books, nor will we give them more credit for virtue than we believe they merit; for it has occurred to us, as it must have to others, that it was a wonder anybody died if the descriptions which some writers gave of the medicinal virtues of herbs were true. Some people think that there is a kind of mysterious charm in some medicines. For instance, a person came to our shop and asked for 6d worth of sarsaparilla, to take the pimples and blotches off his face. We told him we did not think that such an amount would do him much good, but he thought it would be quite enough to cure him. This class of people are the extreme of another, who scoff at all medicine, and dub it all quackery. We have heard the boastings of such while in good health, but have seen them, when ill, take the very nastiest drugs. Moderation in all things good is the golden mean.

The order we intend to follow in this division of our book is to arrange in groups or classes, according to the virtue possessed by each. The vegetable *Materia Medica* is divided thus:—Alteratives, Antacids, Anthelmintics, Antiseptics, Antispasmodics, Astringents, Carminatives, Cathartics, Demulcents,

Diaphoretics, Diuretics, Emmenagogues, Errhines, Expectorants, Lithontriptics, Narcotics, Nervines, Sialagogues, Stimulants, Styptics, Tonics.

ANTHELMINTICS

(That is, Worm Destroying and Expelling.)

The foremost in this class is Spigelia or Pink Root, (Carolina Pink.) This perennial plant is a native of America; it grows from 12 to 20 inches high, the stems are square, its leaves lance shaped, its flowers are a rich carmine colour, externally paler at the base and orange yellow within each stem; terminates in a spike which leans to one side and supports from four to twelve flowers with short foot stalks; when ripe it has a double capsule containing many seeds. The whole plant may be used, or the root alone, as it is stronger and more certain in its results. The dose of the powdered root is from 10 to 30 grains, or the sixth part of a teaspoonful, the spoon being level; this may be given night and morning from four to six times, then a brisk purge to remove from the bowels the dead worms. It also enters into combination with other ingredients to form various worm-medicines. (See list of compounds).

CHENOPODIUM ANTHELMINTICUM (AMERICAN WORM-SEED, A PERENNIAL).

Also known in America as Jerusalem Oak. It grows wild amongst rubbish, along fences, vacant sections, &c. It flowers from July to September, and ripens its seeds through the autumn. The whole herb has a strong, peculiar, offensive, aromatic smell, and retains it when dried. It has green yellowish leaves dotted on their under surface; the flowers are small of

the same colour as the leaves; the stem grows from two to five
feet high. Its medical properties are similar to the Spigelia;
but it is better for the destruction of the round stomach worm,
as they are sometimes called. The dose for a child from two
to five years is one-third of a teaspoonful of the powdered
seeds in jam, treacle, or any way suitable, given the first thing
in the morning for a few times, then followed by an opening
medicine. An adult dose is from a half to a teaspoonful, given
in a similar way. The oil distilled from the seeds is called
chenopodium, or oil of worm seeds; it has the same properties,
and may be given in doses of five to twenty drops in an
emulsion of gum arabic.

WORMWOOD (Artemisia Absinthium).

This is one of the most ancient known plants. It is
mentioned several times in the Bible as well as in the earliest
medical books. It was formerly supposed to have vermifuge
properties; but experience has proved that it is weak in this
respect. It makes a very good injection in seat or pin worms,
which infest the lower bowels. It is so well known that a
description is not required. For a tonic and appetiser it is
far-famed, in biliousness and indigestion it is also good.
While in Chicago we visited the office of a very wise old
eclectic doctor, who was getting a dollar a head from quite a
stream of patients. We noticed a stock of wormwood pressed
into 1 oz. packets. Remarking that it was a good old herb,
he said, "Yes, I give it in every case of impaired appetite;
it makes them eat well." We asked him if he told them
what it was. "Not likely," he replied; "that would never do,
at least not for the dollars." Some time ago a person from
Oamaru was troubled with indigestion, so badly that he lost
flesh and became very weak. He was recommended an
infusion of this plant with horehound; the effect was a return
of health. The infusion is made by pouring a pint of boiling
water on an ounce, keep in the steam, and take a wineglassful
cold one to three times a day. Very large doses or long
continued will weaken the stomach, cause headaches, &c.

MALE FERN (Aspidium Filx mas).

This variety of the fern grows almost everywhere, and as it is not generally known we will give it a place in our illustrations, so that our readers may be able to recognise it. Its properties are contained in the roots dried and powdered. Dose : from a tea- to a table-spoonful fasting, three or four mornings, then an aperient (it will be noticed that we recommend the same course in those vermifuges that do not contain an opening quality). The species of worms over which the male fern has the most power is the tape. It is the largest of all—sometimes measuring 100 feet. Some of our readers will hardly believe this ; but it is true. We can show some specimens that we were instrumental in expelling with the oil of the male fern, the dose of which is from half to one tea-spoonful in capsule or emulsion. When dealing with this form of worm trouble we will give the most successful means for its cure.

COWHAGE (Dolechos Pruriens).

This is the hair off fruit of the abovenamed plant. It is very useful in expelling the round worms, which are like the earth ones. The hairs taken in treacle or honey from five to ten grains for four doses, each night, then followed by a purge, will dislodge the enemy. There is one peculiarity about these hairs, which many will not forget, that is the torment which they cause if they get on the skin ; it feels as if a swarm of bees had stung it. This is rather remarkable, seeing that they have no effect on the mucous membrane of the mouth and intestines. The cowhage may also be taken for taps-worm.

POMEGRANATE RIND.

This tree grows in Africa and most hot countries. The fruit is pleasant acidulous, somewhat similar to the orange, and used for the same purpose. The flowers, the rind, and the bark of the root have been used in medicine as as ringents ; it is in the rind that the vermifuge property is found. A Dr. Christian says that it seldom fails to expel the tape-worm if properly administered. The directions are : Steep two ounces of the fresh rind or bark (if you can get it) or one ounce of the dry broken rind, in two pints of water all night, then simmer down to one pint. Give a wineglassful every two hours till the whole is taken. Sometimes the effect will be seen in pieces of the worm coming away in the motions; if not it must be repeated for several mornings. The difficulty with most people is to know whether they have a tape-worm. This matter will be fully dealt with in our treatment of worms. (See index). The pomagranate may also be used as a remedy for diarrhœa, as a gargle for sore throats, and as a wash in leucorrhœa.

ARECA NUT (BETEL NUT).

This nut is a valuable vermifuge medicine. It grows on a tree in India named Areca Catechu, one of the palm family. The fruit is about the size and shape of a small egg of an orange colour, in which the nut is found. It somewhat resembles a nutmeg, only it is a little larger and smooth; it is also much harder. The natives of India have great faith in it, a number of them having come to our city lately have bought large quantities of them from us. Besides its worm destroying properties it is also a valuable astrigent. It is largely used in America as a toothpowder and paste; being first burnt, then powdered, and mixed with other ingredients. In England and in the colonies it is principally given to dogs and horses for worms. The dose for a horse is a tablespoonful of the powder with a soft mash or in a drink (given in a lemonade bottle); for a dog a teaspoonful for a medium sized one. When taken two or three times it is needful to follow it with a purge. It can be taken by the human family as well; dose, from a half to a teaspoonful in combination with or followed by a cathartic; but we would not advise it in preference to any of the fore-going as a vermifuge, on account of its strong astringency.

ASTRINGENTS.

This class of remedies abounds in the vegetable world. They are highly valuable, especially in hot countries, and during the hot seasons of more temperate ones, when diarrhœa, dysentery, and bowel complaints are common. The first on the list is our famous New Zealand

KOROMIKA (NATIVE VERONICA).

Its virtue has long been known to the Maoris, who speedily cured the early settlers with it. As we intend to give it in our illustrations, a description of its appearance will not be needed. It is found growing in almost every native bush. The simplest, and as good as any other way to use it is to take three or four of the leaves and eat them, and their effect will soon be manifest; or an infusion made of an ounce of the leaves chopped up, to a pint of boiling water. Steep one hour; strain, and give a wineglassful every one, two, or three hours, according to the urgency of the case. The dose for children will be according to age, from a teaspoonful up. We find that the dried leaves do not act so well, as they seem to lose their power by being kept. A fluid extract can be made in two ways: 1st. Infuse in the above proportion, strain, and evaporate slowly till you have the same weight as that of the leaves you used; let it cool, then add one-tenth of spirits of wine, to keep it from fermenting or souring. 2nd. Take a given quantity of the plant, chop it up, then pour on it the same weight of spirits of wine; let it steep two or three days or a week; then press it out, strain through a fine cloth; bottle, and give, for an adult, a teaspoonful less or more, according to age and urgency of case.

STRINGY BARK (EUCALYPTUS OBLIQUA).

This tree is a native of Australasia, (called Red Gum); it is well known to bushmen, and can be found in most of our forests. It is a very valuable astringent in diarrhœa, as the following case will show :—

A Mr. McGregor, of the Peninsula, then living in Canterbury, had a neighbour who was so hopelessly ill that the attending doctors gave him up. McGregor went to the bush, pulled off some stringy bark, cut it in pieces, and boiled two ounces in a quart of water with an ounce of ginger down to one pint. This he strained and sweetened and gave him a wineglassful of it. Shortly after taking it he began to mend, and was well in a couple of days. Those in the bush who are subject to this complaint should try this remedy.

The bark of the wattle tree is another good astringent, having succeeded when other means have failed. In using these simple nature's remedies you need not be afraid of a handful, as there is no fear of poisoning. They all may be prepared similarly to above, and given in doses suitable to age and condition of patient.

GUM CATECHU.

This is said to be the strongest vegetable astringent that we have. It is an extract of the wood of a small tree that grows in India, called the Acacia Catechu. The wood is cut into chips, boiled, the liquor reduced to a thickness, then evaporated in the sun till it is solid and dry. Its only medicinal property lies in its astringency. It may be given in several ways : first, in powder, the dose being from a fourth to a teaspoonful; in water, a decoction of one ounce to the pint; dose from a teaspoonful to a tablespoonful for fluxes of all kinds. A piece kept in the mouth and sucked is good for swelling of the uvula and curing the tickling cough caused by the enlargement; spongy gums and sore throat will also be relieved by its use. The tincture is a very good form in which to administer it, especially the compound tincture. It is thus prepared :—

Catechu Gum	1½ ounce
Stick Cinnamon	½ ounce
Proof Spirit	1 pint

Let it stand eight days, strain and bottle. Dose : half to two teaspoonfuls. As it enters into various compounds it is not needful to speak further of it at present.

BISTORT ROOT (POLYGONUM BISTORTA).

(Also called Sapentary, Dragonwort, Osterick, and Passions).

It is a wild plant, growing in most places in the old country; it flowers in northern latitudes about May; it grows about a foot and a half high, the leaves are large like the dock, of a blush green colour, the flowers are of a bright red colour and grow on the top of the stalk, the bottom part of which is round, with little leaves on it; the spike on which the flower grows is about the size of a man's thumb, its roots are short and knobbed, outwardly black, but when dried and broken it has a pale colour between a pink and brown. We have not seen it in the colonies, but no doubt it will soon be introduced here, as it is a valuable plant, and most useful as a tanning agent on account of its great astringency. Dr. Robertson says it is the most powerful astringent in the world, and has a powerful faculty to resist poison. It is useful in all discharges and bleedings; like the others of this class it can be used in powder, decoction, and tincture, in similar doses; it is also good in whites in females. As a gargle in sore and ulcerated throats it will be found in our compounds, and as one in our family medicine chest.

RASPBERRY LEAVES (RUBUS STRIGOSUS).

The foregoing are powerful astringents, too strong for some cases, but we have an abundant supply of milder ones. One of the best and most common is the raspberry leaf. Nearly all Herbal authors describe it as the red variety, but the pale is now so uncommon that it it is hardly needful to point this out. The delicious fruit which this shrub yields makes it a favourite with housewives and jam-makers, and we might add jam-eaters. It is a question which is the more valuable—the fruit or the leaves. We are inclined to vote for the latter, but it is safe to set them down as both being good. Simple as this old wife's remedy may seem, yet it has been a blessing to many, which we can easily prove. It is valuable in sore mouths of infants; combined with gum myrrh it has a beneficial effect on scald heads, and running from the ears; it is also good for relaxation in infants and adults, having a cleansing effect on the mucous membrane of the whole digestive tract; it is one of the ingredients of Dr. Coffin's famous consumption mixture; and to those about to become mothers it should take the place of ordinary tea, as it seldom fails to make a difference in easing the labour. It is not too much to say that we have gathered and sold hundreds of pounds of these healing leaves. To make a tea of the fresh leaves steep a good handful in a quart of boiling water; sweeten, and drink freely. Of the dried leaves an ounce to the same quantity of water as above. Its other uses will be found further on, in our treatment division.

BURNET HERB (Pimpinella Sanguisorba),

Is another mild astringent. An old herb doctor writes of it thus: "It is a most precious herb, little inferior to betony. The continual use of it preserves the body in health and the mind in vigour. It is a friend to the heart, the liver, and the principal parts of man's body. Two or three of the stalks with leaves put into wine, especially claret, are known to quicken the spirits and drive away melancholy. It is a special herb against infection, the juice being taken in some drink, and the party laid to sweat. It has also astringent properties, and will stop flows of blood or humours, staunch bleeding inward or outward, women's too abundant courses, the whites, and chlorotic belchings of the stomach. It is a good herb for all sorts of wounds both of the head and the body, either inward or outward, used either in juice or decoction, or by powder of the root, or distilled, or made into an ointment." We cannot endorse all that, especially as, while reading over the book from which we quote (Robinson's Family Herbal), we see the same sanguine descriptions given of most of the plants. But that it is a valuable medicine other and more recent writers affirm. It grows in gardens and wild —the latter is the best. It can be identified by its large wing-shaped leaves, notched at the edges, of a brownish-green colour on the upper side, and greyish under. The stalks are mounted by small dark purple flowers, the root is black and long, having little taste or smell. But we must curtail our descriptions, as we have so many to enumerate.

BLACKBERRY LEAVES AND ROOT

Form a pleasant drink with condiments, for looseness of the bowels in children and adults in good quantities, prepared like raspberry leaves.

CRANE'S-BILL OR HERB-ROBERT (GERANIUM MACULATUM),

The root is a valuable moderate astringent. Combined with other remedies it makes a good medicine for the whites and gleety discharge.

OAK BARK (QUERCUS ALBA).

Is a favourite with some of the faculty as an injection in uterine troubles. It is a good tonic as well as an astringent; makes a capital wash for inflammation of the eyes, in combination with raspberry leaves: one ounce each to a quart of water. Simmer half an hour; cool, clear, and with a soft rag bathe the eyes three times a day. The decoction may be used as a tonic and astringent where these qualities are required.

BLOODWORT (LAPATHUM SANGUINEUM).

This is a variety of the dock. It may be distinguished by its leaves being striped with red lines in the centre and veins; they are long and pointed, with smooth red stem, and the root, which has a reddish smooth skin, not unlike the rhubarb when cut. For spitting of blood we know it is good. A person who broke a blood vessel was taken to our hospital, and was there for six weeks, spitting blood daily; at last he came out, took a decoction of bloodwort for four days and was cured, two ounces of the green root or leaves, sliced, and simmered in a pint of water. Dose: a wineglass three or four times a day, will do good each time. We will close this list with

BAYBERRY BARK (Myrica Cerifera).

One of our chief remedies and principal ingredients in the world-renowned composition powder. It is the bark of the root that is chiefly used in medicine; besides its mild astringent qualities it is a valuable antiscorbutic, curing scurvy and similar disorders. The stomach, digestive organs, and bowels are benefited, and their nucous coats cleansed by it. Used in diarrhœa and dysentery it will be found a good remedy; in scrofula and ulcers it is valuable. Another notice of this valuable agent will be found in our list of antiseptics.

ANTISPASMODICS.

This is a class of medicine that removes or moderates spasms by soothing and relaxing the nerves. The principal in this list is

LOBELIA INFLATA.

(It is sometimes called Indian Tobacco.)

Grows about a foot high, has but one stem, very hairy and angular, branches thick about the middle, the stem rising above them; the leaves are irregular, toothed, and of a pale green colour, with small blue flowers, which are followed with capsules bearing seeds. The whole plant is medicinal, but the greatest strength is in the seeds. To Samuel Thompson belongs the honour of introducing this most valuable medicine to the world. It is certainly not a pleasant medicine to take, and its action is very depressing in emetic doses. Just before it operates you feel as if you were going to die, but after (it is almost the universal experience) the feeling is one of great relief. Some of the Yankees to whom Thompson administered it called it the stomach screw. There is nothing like it for emptying the stomach, but there is no danger with it notwithstanding what doctors and their books say. Had it been the poison that text-books declare it, we and others would have been in our graves long ago. We have given a man one or two ounces of the powder at one time and yet he lived. How is it then that this false rumour has got abroad? This is how: 1st. Thompson's trial. (See page 15). 2nd. Some have rather unwisely given it to people in the flickering out of life. They have died, and thinking that none but doctors could give a certificate of death, the friends of the dead have sent for the doctor, who, when he had learned the facts of the case, refused to certify to the cause of death. The coronor then held an inquest, ordered very likely the same doctor to make a post-mortem examination, who found lobelia in the stomach, the unlucky herbalist would then be prosecuted, and as it happened last year in England, fully acquitted, it being proved by other doctors that lobelia was not a poison, nor did the patient die from its effects. It is a mercy for us that doctors sometimes differ. No, Lobelia cannot poison a healthy person, for as soon as the stomach has too much of it, up it comes; it is like pouring water into a full vessel. There is one class of sufferers to whom it has proved a blessing, namely asthmatics. Here is the testimony of an M.D., (Dr. Butler), who had the misfortune to be an asthmatic, his attacks sometimes lasting six or eight weeks. During one of these he took a tablespoonful of the acid tincture, and in a few minutes his breathing was as free as ever. He took three or four doses more, which he says he felt all over his system. After this he was completely cured. We could quote several such testimonies, where lobelia had a marvellous effect, but we are sorry to say it is not always so successful; still it stands first as a remedy in spasmodic, and also in humid asthma; it is also a valuable relaxant in infantile convulsions. Dr. Whitford of Chicago told us of a sample case. He was called to a child in very bad convulsions. The doctor who had been attending before him had prescribed heroic doses of bromide of potassium, but to no purpose. He took out his pocket case and gave the child 12 drops fluid extract of lobelia. Its convulsions relaxed in a minute, and the child was well soon after. The same gentleman told us of a neighbouring doctor of the old school, who was carrying about with him for a month or so a very bad jaundice. Dr Whitford met him several times, till he felt the shame of a doctor plainly telling people by his looks that he could not cure himself of what is usually a simple trouble; and so he said to him, "Doctor, when you are tired of that little trouble come round to my office and I will cure you." Pocketing his prejudice, he came and was cured with a few doses of lobelia. A good emetic of it will send off a bilious attack almost at once. Time and space prevent our dwelling further at present on this valuable herb, but in our part on the treatment of diseases, and as an ingredient in many of our compounds, we shall show our faith in its merits. It can be taken, first in an infusion of one ounce of the dried herb to a pint of water, dose, from a tablespoonful to a teacupful; as an emetic, of the powdered herb, a teaspoonful to a cup of boiling water, or in weak Composition Tea; cover, let cool, strain, sweeten, and drink if for an emetic till it has its effect. Spoonful doses of this make a good cough mixture.

The powdered seeds. as we stated, are about four times the strength, and should be used accordingly. Lobelia will be found among the illustrations.

ASSAFŒTIDA.

This valuable gum is the juice of a tree named Ferula Narthax Assafœtida. It is imported from Persia, Afghanistan, and neighbouring countries. It was reckoned one of the best in the old practice for spasms of all kinds. The smell of it being so unpleasant renders it repugnant to most people. The general opinion expressed about its flavour is a comparison to rotten onions. On this account it is seldom given in the crude state; pills and tincture being the usual way it is administered. The complaints in which it has been found beneficial are, asthma, hysteria, melancholia, nervous debility, accompanied with flatulency. The dose of the powder is 5 to 10 grains three times a day; tincture, one to two teaspoonfuls three or four times a day.

SKUNK CABBAGE (Ictodes Fœtida).

This is a wild plant, a native of America. It grows in boggy places, and flowers early in Spring. It has a resemblance to the cabbage, hence its name. (It seems a curious fact that some of the antispasmodics should smell so bad, while they are so good). The root is the part used, and it forms a valuable ingredient in many of our mixtures. It is seldom taken by itself, but there can be no harm in trying it. Dose of the powder, half to a teaspoonful for asthma, spasms, cough, &c.

AMERICAN HELLEBORE (Veratrum Viride).

The green hellebore root is a medicine of much repute in America and Canada, where it grows in the swamps and moist places. It is described as a plant with a round stem, rising from three to six feet high, with long oval leaves which lessen in size as they get higher on the stem. The flowers are of a greenish yellow colour, and are in bloom from May to July. The root alone contains the medicinal principle. We can scarcely recommend its use in domestic practice, as it is very powerful and an overdose is dangerous; it is, however, a good antispasmodic, and in small doses lessens the heart's action very perceptibly. Its use in fevers accompanied with a bounding pulse is appreciated by all schools of medicine. Americans mostly use it in the fluid extract; dose, 1 to 3 drops not oftener than every hour, till its characteristic effects are felt in the nausea it occasions; it should then be discontinued. The tincture may be given in doses of from 3 to 6 drops, as above. In all cases of arterial excitement where there is a strong constitution this remedy will act well.* In case of poisoning with this agent the antidote will be found in our chapter on Poisons and their Antidotes.

---

* The white variety of Hellebore has similar properties.

YELLOW JESSAMINE (Gelseminum Sempervirens),

Is said to be one of the most beautiful plants in the Southern States of America. It has a climbing habit, ascending lofty trees and forming festoons from one tree to another, and in its flowering season scenting the atmosphere with its sweet odour. The stem is smooth and shining; it twines round the article it grows upon; the leaves are dark-green on the upper surface, pale under; the flowers are yellow; they are said to be poisonous. The root is the part used in medicine. We can say from our many years' experience of the use of this medicine that it is all its most ardent admirers claim for it, that is, when it is in good condition, not having lost its strength through age. Professor Davis of Chicago, while speaking of Gelsemine, said that the most of what was found in the shops was about as good as a decoction of the straw out of a last year's hen's nest. The tincture of Gelsemine is, we think, the best preparation. We have found it an excellent medicine in neuralgia, curing after all others tried had failed. A lady in this city had the complaint for about two years, trying all, even a voyage to the old country. She came back with her old enemy. Consulting us, we gave her a 2-ounce bottle, directing her to take half a teaspoonful three times a day. We see her occasionally, but she has never complained of the neuralgia since, that is four years ago.

Dr King in the American Dispensatory writes: "It is said by some to be the only agent yet discovered that will subdue in from 2 to 20 hours, and with the least possible injury to the patient, the most formidable and the most complicated, as well as the most simple fevers incident to our country and climate, quieting all nervous irritability and excitement, equalising the circulation, and promoting perspiration, rectifying the various secretions without causing nausea, vomiting, or purging, and is also adapted to any stage of the disease. It may follow any preceding treatment with safety. Its effects are clouded vision, double-sightedness, or even complete prostration, with inability to open the eyes. This gradually passes off in a few

hours, leaving the patient refreshed and restored. As soon as
the heaviness or partial closing of the eyes has been induced,
no more of the remedy is necessary, even if this should occur
after the first dose. If carried to such an extent that the
patient cannot open his eyes, the reaction may be too great
for the system to recover from, hence its use should cease as
soon as the above symptoms appear." We have heard it
asserted, however, that no one ever was poisoned with it.
The dose of the simple tincture is from five drops for a child to
one teaspoonful. We shall speak further of it in treating
diseases.

MOTHERWORT (Leonurus Cardiaca).

This plant is known to possess antispasmodic properties,
as well as others, which prove its value as high amongst
medicinal herbs. Its chief use is in hysteria, and to
promote the menses; given in a strong infusion warm and
sweetened, it relieves painful menstruation. In feebleness of
the heart it is also excellent. The solid extract, formed into 5
grain pills, and one or two taken three times a day, has been
found to do much good in heart affections. As its name,
" mother's herb " indicates, it is a friend to women generally.
The ancients called it Cardiaca, because it strengthens the
heart and cures palpitation.

THE MISTLETOE (Viscum Album).

We will close this list with the above old remedy mentioned by
Pliny and others. The powdered leaves are given in epilepsy.
A patient continuance of the infusion has effected a cure in some
bad cases. The juice of the plant evaporated makes bird-
lime. Applied to tumours it softens and heals them; while
mixed with rosin it is said to make a good ointment in ulcers.
It can be seen growing in clusters on the branches of trees. It
is a parasite, and will only grow on them. The leaves are
small, of a pale green colour. In season it has small white
berries which some aver are of a poisonous nature. A case is

mentioned of a child, who, having eaten a quantity, was completely prostrated ; but after an emetic, by which a great quantity was thrown out, she recovered. This medicine is not much used now, others having superseded it.

ALTERATIVES.

This variety of remedies acts on the blood, changing its character principally through the organs of nutrition. They are a very numerous class, and are needed in all scorbutic, scrofulous, syphilitic, and skin diseases.

In order of merit they are put thus in Dr. Skelton's "Science and Practice of Medicine." He gives only their botanical names, we will give their English.

Mandrake Root.	American Sarsaparilla.
Black Root.	Poke Root.
Sarsaparilla.	Mezereon Root.
Clivers.	Burdock Root.
Red Clover Tops.	Bitter Sweet Bark or Root.
Stillingia.	Fumitory.
Yellow Dock.	Guaiacum Chips.
Great Water Dock.	

As we describe the two first in our chapter on Cathartics, it is only needful to remind our readers that like many others they have more than one virtue ; their Alterative power acting in harmony with their Cathartic.

SARSAPARILLA (Similax Radix)

Is the world renowned blood purifier. Honesty compels us, however, to say that it has a better name than it really merits. One reason for this is that nearly every compound

mixture for the blood is called by its name, when, in fact, most
of them have only a small amount, and some none at all of it in
them.   Experience has proved that alone the Sarsaparilla does
not do much good.   Notwithstanding the great esteem in which
it is held, it is ridiculous for persons with faces covered with
blotches and black-heads to expect a handful of this
root to cure them; and some have such a high opinion of it—no
wonder they are disappointed in it.   Having thrown out this
hint to guard people from being dissatisfied with a short trial of
it, we do not for a moment wish it to be understood that we have
no faith in it, for we have witnessed some splendid cures effected
with it in combination.   There is a man now in this city who had
an ulcerated leg for over sixteen years.   He was in several
hospitals, getting a little better, but never well.   He saw our
compound decoction advertised, came, got a bottle, which he
repeated every week for fourteen months; at the end of that
time he had taken 60 bottles, and from then, 11 years ago,
his leg has been whole.   Some of our readers will stand
aghast at a medicine that has to be taken in such quantities
and so long; but seeing the time that the disease had lasted,
the time was not unreasonable.   Patience is a virtue of much
benefit to the possessor.   There are thousands now in their
graves who would have been alive if they had persevered
with one remedy; but instead they tried so many, not giving
any of them a fair chance.   Time fails us to tell of the many
such instances we have met with in our practice.

The Sarsaparilla is a family plant, having relatives in
almost every land.   There is the famous Jamaica variety
which stands highest in favour.   It is described as a prickly vine,
climbing and clinging to trees; its leaves are dark-green, small,
oval, and pointed; the seed-producing parts, scarcely deserving
to be called flowers, are six-leaved, and have in the centre
two seed cells.   The roots are the only part used, they are long
and slender, about the thickness of a goose quill; as sold in
the shops the roots are split and cut up in pieces about an inch
long.   The outer coat is of a light reddish brown, the inner
white.

The variety growing in Australia is very similar to the Jamaica, but the roots are larger. It is to be found at the Melbourne and Sydney heads as well as on the diggings. The supple jack is our New Zealand Sarsaparilla, not unlike it in outward appearance; the root, however, is very dissimilar, the supple jack being round and knotty. We have made an extract of it, but it is not rich in extractive matter. We doubt not but that it is as good as the imported, and we can recommend it to those living in the vicinity where it grows. For the blood the compound decoction is the best form.

There are two ways of preparing it where it is wanted as a tonic as well at an alterative. The mixture is :—

Sarsaparilla	2 ounces
Sassafras	1 ounce
Guaiacum	1 ounce
Liquorice Root	1 ounce
Snake Root	½ ounce

Simmer one hour in two quarts of water, strain, and take one to two wineglassfuls three times a day. In cases where there is a syphilitic taint, one to two drachms of the iodide of potassium should be added. In the blood form alone the snake root is omitted. The American Sarsaparilla or Bambo Briar has similar qualities.

CLIVERS (Galium Aparine).

(Goose Grass, Hay Riff, &c).

This creeping tendril grows very abundantly in all countries. It is to be found under hedges, covering stones, old fences, &c. It has long branching square stalks with small leaves like a mouse's ear. When you feel it it is like a sharp, fine-toothed saw, being covered with innumerable hair-like prickles. The flowers are small and white; the roots are hair-like and red, making, it is affirmed by some, a good dye. The whole plant is medicinal; the expressed juice in tablespoonful doses has been known to cure bad cases of blood-poisoning, scurvy, pimples, and disease of the skin, in general. The dried herb is infused an ounce to the pint, dose, a wine glassful four times a day. Dr Skelton says, it is best steeped all night in cold water, as hot water, he affirms, takes some of its virtue away. We gather several hundred of pounds of this valuable herb every season. Dr. Smith, in the Reformed Practice, says, "It is a most valuable diaphoretic." He found it also excellent in suppression of urine and gravelly disorders. The juice mixed with oatmeal applied to tumors will disperse them in a short time. A teaspoonful of it should be taken in the morning, and the bowels kept open with castor oil. In stone and gravel it is an excellent solvent.

RED CLOVER TOPS (Trifolium Pratense.)

Samuel Thompson found out that the extract of Red Clover flowers made a good plaster in cancerous ulcers. Since his time it has been proved good as an inward medicine in impurity of the blood. It is largely used in America by the eclectics and some of the regulars. While in Chicago we saw an establishment devoted entirely to the manufacture and sale of Red Clover preparations. Thompson's plan of making the extract was as follows: Fill a copper, tin, or enamel vessel with fresh tops, cover with water, let it simmer one hour, take out the tops, drain them, put in the same water another lot, do the same three times, then strain the liquor through a fine cloth and evaporate slowly till it is the consistency of treacle; spread on cloth or white leather. The decoction is made by boiling an ounce in a pint of soft water. A wineglassful or two three or four times a day.

STILLINGIA ROOT (Stillingia Sylvatica.)
Queen's Root—Queen's Delight.)

This is a native of America, growing from two to three feet high, the flowers are yellow. Scientific botanists say there are male and female flowers found on the same plant. The root is the part used, and is good in all cases of long-standing blood diseases. To make a good decoction, simmer one ounce in a quart of water down to a pint. Dose, a wineglassful three times a day. The tincture is prepared by steeping two ounces of the bruised root in a pint of proof-spirit.

Dose, a teaspoonful in water three times a day. Like most other medicines of this class it is generally compounded in mixtures for the blood.

YELLOW DOCK (RUMEX CRISPUS).

If there is one plant hated by amateur gardeners, it is this dock. It comes uninvited, and comes to stay, unless very great diligence is used to oust it. While it is much despised on this account, yet it is a good blood purifier, also a laxative. A decoction of the fresh roots, cut or scraped, 2 ounces to the pint ; a wineglassful 2 to 4 times a day, will prove our assertion. Some families, when other vegetables were scarce, have tried the leaves as a substitute for cabbage, and found a marked benefit from them. They make a good ointment, for the itch, with sulphur and lard. A valuable wash is made by boiling 3 ounces in a quart of water. After washing the skin with healing soap and water, bathe with the dock decoction ; do this every night in eruptions of the skin till well. For chronic erysiplas, or an inflamed puffiness of the skin, boil an ounce of the dry crushed root in a pint of water, strain through a fine cloth, and take a wineglassful 3 times a day. A lady in this city got this recipe from a brother in America, and testifies to its efficacy. The great water dock has similar properties. It is like the sharp-pointed dock, but much larger. It grows near water, and attains a height of about 6 feet, with large round roots.

BURDOCK (ARCTIUM LAPPA).

This species of the dock is not so common as the others. It differs in most respects from them. The leaf is much larger, and when full-grown resembles a small tree branching out from the stems. Growing from the top of the branches are the burrs, which, in shape, resemble prickly balls, the size of a walnut ; at first green, then a pinkish brown, and, when ripe, grayish. These balls are filled with seeds at the bottom of the prickles. This short description, with our illustration of this undoubted blood purifier, will enable our readers to identify it, as it is found growing in many parts of the colonies. We cultivate it in our Nursery at Caversham. The preparation recommended for the other class of docks will do for this. The burdock seeds, however, have valuable properties in addition to their alterative; they are nervine and diuretic. The leaves chopped up and simmered in lard make a good healing ointment for sores and inflammations; also wet with spirits of hartshorn and vinegar they are fine for sprains and bruises. A tincture of the seeds, 2 ounces, bruised and steeped in a pint of proof spirit, makes an excellent blood cleanser, if persevered with.

Dr Skelton strongly recommends the decoction of the Burdock as a wash in skin diseases, &c.

POKE ROOT (PHYTOLACCA DECANDRA).

A native of America, growing abundantly all over the States. It is described as a beautiful wild plant, attaining the height of eight feet. It has branching stems, broad green leaves, white flowers, green in the centre, which in autumn ripen into dark purple shining berries. The largest plants have often flowers and green and purple berries growing at the same time. In the spring the young shoots are boiled and eaten like spinach. The juice of the berries is said to be beneficial in chronic rheumatism. The root, however, is the part exported, as it is considered the medicinal part.

As a blood medicine its virtue lies in reducing tumours, glandular swellings, &c. For these purposes it is not only taken inwardly, but the boiled root is mashed up and put on the swelling. The powdered root mixed with warm water will answer the same purpose. The decoction is made in the usual way, 1 ounce to the pint; a wineglassful 3 to 6 times a day. As this useful plant has been acclimatised in Europe, there is no reason why it should not be in the colonies. We intend to get some of the seeds this season and try them. Since writing the above we have seen in a reliable medical journal that the juice of the poke berry is a good anti-fat. A teaspoonful taken three times a day is recommended for this purpose, also for swelling of the glands.

MEZEREON ROOT (Daphne Mezereum).

This is a hardy shrub 3 to 4 feet high, with high, branching stem, smooth bark which peels off easily from the wood. The leaves are lance-shaped, pale green, and toothed. The flowers precede the leaves, coming early in the spring and sometimes blooming amid snow. They are of a pale rose colour, and have a fragrant odour. The berries are oval, fleshy, and of a bright red colour.

It is the bark of the root wherein its medicinal qualities are found. Being very acrid, it is seldom used alone. The sarsaparilla, said to be old Dr Townsend's, most of which is manufactured by the cordial makers, has the Mezereon as one of its ingredients. In some countries it is used as an irritant to blister the skin with. The fresh bark laid on will raise a blister in 24 hours, and continued, will keep it an open sore. "The United States Pharmacopœia" gives the compound decoction of Sarsaco into which mezerion enters, thus :—

Sarsaparilla (cut and bruised),	6 ounces.
Sassafras (coarse powdered),	1 ,,
Guaiacum chips,	1 ,,
Liquorice root (bruised),	1 ,,
Mezereon (cut),	½ ounce.
Water,	3 pints

Direction.—Simmer the sarsaparilla and guaiacum half an hour, then add the other ingredients, cover and keep it hot for two hours; strain through the strainer enough cold water to make up to three pints. The dose is from one to two wineglassfuls two to six times a day. During the use of this decoction the patient is recommended to wear flannel next the skin and avoid exposure.

FUMITORY (Fumaria Officinalis).

This is a small plant which grows in corn and other fields in almost every country. We have seen it, and are now selling what was gathered growing wild near Auckland city. Although a weed, it is a beautiful one, and possesses undoubted virtue in skin diseases of an eruptive character.

The following description will give the reader an idea of its appearance. It shoots forth from one square, slender stalk, the small branches leaning downward; all round on the branch are long leaves, finely cut and jagged, of a green, sea-blue, pale colour, becoming whiter as the autumn comes on; at the end of the branches stand many flowers in a long spike, as Dr Robinson remarks, like little birds, of a reddish, purple colour with white centres; after the flowers come small brown husks having small black seeds. The root is yellow, small, and not long.

The medicinal properties of this plant are not confined to its alterative quality, it is recommended as a tonic. The expressed juice, a deobstruent, that is, clearing obstructions from the internal organs; also as a remedy in inflammation of the eye, dropped into it first causing pain, after, taking out redness, swelling, and clearing the sight. Mixed with the juice of dock and vinegar, it is good as an outward application in pimples, blotches, scabs, &c. The infusion of the dried herb is an ounce to the pint, of which one or two wineglassfuls may be taken three to six times a day.

BITTERSWEET (Solanum Dulcamara).

(Woody Night Shade.)

This is another climbing shrub, with a round, slender-branching stem, rising sometimes six to eight feet high. The leaves are soft and smooth, of a dark green colour. The flowers are arranged in clusters of a violet blue and purple colour, with a green spot at their base, and a yellow tinge at the top. The berries are oval, and of a bright scarlet. They continue to hang in beautiful clusters after the leaves are gone. The Bittersweet is common in America and Europe. The twigs and bark are the parts used in medicine, and should be gathered in autumn. The strongest and best is the bark of the root, which may be known by the red colour of the middle layer of its coating. It possesses but feeble narcotic properties, although it belongs to a family of plants some of which, like the deadly night-shade, are highly poisonous. The Bittersweet was used by the American doctors for various complaints, but, at present, its use is almost confined to skin diseases, those of a scaly nature, psoriasis, ptyriasis, lepra, &c. The usual way in which it is administered is a decoction of one ounce of the bark to a pint of water; boil in a covered vessel 15 to 20 minutes ; strain through a cloth, and take a wineglassful three or four times a day. It is sometimes beneficial in skin diseases to bathe the parts affected with the same medicine. There cannot be any harm in so doing ; in fact we would advise it in some forms. The Bittersweet enters into some of our compounds.

GUAIACUM (Lignum Vitæ).

This is the wood of a West Indian tree, of considerable size at maturity. It is forty to sixty feet high. The branches are knotted, and covered with a striped bark, of an ash-gray colour. The stem is of the same colour, variegated with green or purple spots. The leaves are sharp, and in pairs, of which there are sometimes three or four in a bunch ; small, smooth, and dark green. The flowers are of a rich blue colour, eight or ten growing together. Near the upper leaves there is one seed. It is hard, and of an oblong shape. The Lignum Vitæ is a very dense wood : it sinks in water. The chips, which is the form usually seen, are of a yellow colour. The name was given to the wood on account of its supposed great remedial power. During the 15th and 16th centuries it was thought a specific in venereal, but lately it is discarded, to a great extent, in the treatment of that disease. It is, however, useful in combination with other alteratives in chronic affections of the blood. It enters into the compound decoction of sarsaparilla. In powder it is an ingredient in our purifying mixture for skin complaints. The gum of the same tree has a great reputation in rheumatics. The compound tincture is the best form of its administration. We must close this list, although there are many good herbs besides those mentioned, as our treatment of complaints will shew.

ANTISEPTICS AND DISINFECTANTS.

These medicines act in arresting putrefactions, covering the unpleasant smell arising from ulcers, gangrene, &c., and in preventing contagion. In this list we are compelled to acknowledge some of the mineral class, for they have been proved good antiseptics; it will be seen, however, that their use is external.

VEGETABLE CHARCOAL (Carbo Ligna)

Is foremost in this list. It is prepared from any kind of wood, however, the acacia and poplar trees are said to yield the best. It has been known for ages that charcoal had a purifying effect on animal matters. Boiled with tainted meat it will remove the taint, coarsely powdered and packed in a filter, it will purify and sweeten water It has a wonderful capacity to absorb gases, on this account it is valuable in certain kinds of indigestion. where gas forms in the stomach and bowels. it is also valuable in cholera and some bowel complaints. During the last visitation of that plague in Russia there was a firm that insisted upon all their employés taking a spoonful of the powdered charcoal in a glass of water every time they came to work in the factory, where a large number of hands were employed. It was affirmed that not one who took this valuable antiseptic became a victim, or even had the cholera.

For fetid breath a teaspoonful should be taken occasionally. Mixed with slippery elm and yeast it is a splendid poultice for foul ulcers and gangrene. It is also good as a tooth powder. The shell of cocoa or the areca nut and bread, when burnt and powdered, make a good sample for this purpose. For preparing it on a small scale an iron vessel with a close fitting lid, such as a camp oven, must be had. The article to be charred is cut up in ordinary pieces and placed in the vessel, which, being covered, is put on a good fire, the fire surrounding it kept at a red heat for an hour; it is allowed to cool, then powdered and kept from the air. The dose of the powder is from one to two teaspoonfuls three times a day.

CHLORIDE OF LIME (Calax Chlorinate.)

This article of commerce is well known. It is manufactured in large chemical works by slacking common lime, putting it in a close chamber, and passing chlorine gas through it as long as it will be absorbed. It is then dried, and should be kept air-tight, and when sprinkled about cesspools, closets, and similar places, it checks the effluvia. Two ounces of it stirred in a pint of water makes a disinfectant solution, also a bleaching one, removing mildew and stains from white cloth. A solution half this strength is recommended as a wash for putrid sores, and an injection in chronic inflammation of the womb. There is another good use for chloride of lime, it is said to drive rats away. Put it into their holes and they will clear, which would be a blessing, as they are certainly destructive vermin.

WILD INDIGO ROOT (Baptisia Tinctoria).

This is a perennial plant, growing wild in America, on the dry uplands and woods. It has a smooth very branching stem and small blue green leaves, and yellow flowers, which appear at the end of summer. The whole plant becomes almost black when it is dried. The root is the portion used, which, when broken, is of a dark brown colour. In large doses it is said to act as an emetic and cathartic; in small it is a mild laxative. It is a great remedy with homœopaths in typhoid and similar fevers; both the regulars and eclectics use it for the same class of diseases; also an antiseptic in gangrene, for which purpose it is given in decoction, one ounce of the root simmered in a pint of water, one tablespoonful every four to six hours, care being taken to check its purging qualities. If needful give an astringent, as tincture of Bistort, Catechu, Cranesbill or Koromika. A good poultice may also be applied to gangrenous sores by mixing three parts of the powdered root with one part of slippery elm. Apply warm and renew every two to four hours.

BAYBERRY BARK (Myrica Cerefera).

This is a very valuable medicine, having besides its antiseptic quality, astringent, antiscorbutic, and another peculiar one, an errhinge, that is a snuff, which gives relief in some forms of headache, earache, pains in the eyes, and catarrh of the nostrils. This tree belongs to the family of laurels, and grows all over the North American states within a radius of twenty miles from the sea. The bark is of a greyish colour. The roots from which it is taken should be dug up early in spring or autumn. The powdered bark is famous for diarrhœa, dysentery, and as a general astringent, especially in those cases where there is foulness of breath, heavy coated tongue, or ulcers in the mouth, gums, or throat. It makes one of the best gargles, also a valuable wash in discharges from the womb. Sprinkled on indolent ulcers and covered with an elm poultice it has been found excellent. The bark may be taken in decoction, 1 oz. to the pint three to six times a day; or an infusion of the powder, a teaspoonful to a cup of boiling water, stir, let it cool, pour off, and drink the clear. The berries of the bayberry have around their seeds a wax which is much used in America. It makes an ointment mixed with some softer material, as it is very hard. We will give a form for its preparation in our list of compounds.

GOLDEN SEAL (Hydrastis Canadensis).

The root of this plant is now one of the most popular drugs in America, where it is employed by all schools of medicine. Like others, its virtue is not confined to one class. Although it stands high as an antiseptic, it is no less celebrated as a tonic and stomachic. The plant is described as a small perennial herb, with a thick fleshy yellow root, from which many fibres proceed. The stem is erect, from six inches to a foot in height; and there are usually but two leaves, which are different in size, springing from foot stalks; they seem like the stem dividing into two heads. The leaves are covered with a soft downy covering (called in Botany pubescent); are roundish heart-shaped; there are generally five to seven lobes to each leaf, which is unequally nicked at the edge. There is but one flower, which rises from the foot stalk of the upper leaf; it is of a whitish rose colour or purple; it falls soon after it has opened. The berry is a red or purple shade, and contains granules enclosing the seed. The berry is not unlike the rasp, but is not eatable. The root is the medicinal part, which is generally used in powder form. An ounce infused in one and a half pints of boiling water; dose, from a tablespoonful to a wineglassful. This same strength makes an excellent injection in whites and catarrhal discharges of the mucous membrane; in some forms of dyspepsia it is best to take the powder in the crude form, as much as will lie on a shilling, swallowed with water; as an ingredient in a decoction it is best to use the crushed root. Simple preparations are tincture and fluid extract, the dose of which is from half to two teaspoonfuls of the former and from five to thirty drops of the latter.

GUM MYRRH.

This gum is known all over the civilized world for its antiseptic qualities; it is also tonic and stimulant. It is the juice got by incising the bark of a small tree growing in Arabia, from whence, after hardening, it is exported in large quantities. There are three ways in which it is used: first little pieces of the gum the size of a pea may be swallowed, in this way it is good for fetid breath and sweetening the stomach. When it is used with other things in a decoction it may be used in the crude form. 2. Powdered, it may be swallowed in water. Dose: about as much as will lie on a sixpence. Sprinkled on sores it is an antiseptic; and with other ingredients it makes a good toothpowder. 3. Probably the best preparation is the tincture; it being of a resinous substance, spirits dissolve it best. For a tonic medicine, a teaspoonful in water is good. In this form it makes an excellent gargle and mouth wash. Dr. Dale, of Glasgow, recommends it as a consumptive food, equal parts of powdered myrrh, ginger, and slippery elm one tea-spoonful taken in milk. We have prescribed this with good results. One of our customers declares that he has recommended many to come for our tincture of myrrh, and that it has cured them of liver complaints. There can be no question but it is a good medicine.

AUSTRALIAN BLUE GUM (Eucalyptus Globulus).

Although not put down in the text-books as an antiseptic, yet it has this property. A doctor in one of the London hospitals reports the case of a man with gangrene of the lungs. His breath was simply horrible. Various remedies were tried in vain. The fluid extract of the leaves was given him in 30 drop doses four times a day. The improvement was soon manifest, and recovery complete. It has been successfully used in typhoid and other fevers of a putrid nature. It is also an astringent. Many are the cures related to us by old colonials of diarrhoea and fluxes of the bowels. The leaves, chopped and simmered in lard, make an ointment for sores, also rubbed in for rheumatic pains; although for this purpose, the best way is to bruise, boil, and apply the leaves hot as a poultice to the parts affected. The essential oil is an excellent rubificant (liniment). In the last-named complaint it is largely used as such. The redistilled oil is now used as a cure for colds, five to ten drops on sugar three or four times a day is the best way to take it. Inhaling it is also good for colds in the head; put 10 to 20 drops in a cup, fill up with hot water, hold the head over the steam and draw it into the mouth and nose, about twice a day will be sufficient. Mixed with linseed meal the powdered leaves make a good poultice for bad-smelling sores; proportion, three of the linseed meal to one of the powdered leaves. Happy for us we are not troubled with malarial fevers as they are in America and other places, but in any infected district it is reasonably asserted the blue-gum, if largely cultivated, would prevent this trouble. Altogether it is a valuable tree, not only as a medicine, but also for its enduring timber. Experiments may further develop its medicinal value. We have already noted Bistort and Cranesbill, which, although principally astringent, are also antiseptic. There are several good antiseptics in the regular medicine list. However, we believe we have given the best of them, but the scriptural injunction stands good here: "Prove all things, and hold fast that which is good."

ANTACIDS.

There is but one medicine that comes under this head in the vegetable list, that is charcoal. One teaspoonful three times a day is a valuable remedy in acidity; but while herbal medicines have little power to relieve this unpleasant symptom, many can prevent it or put the stomach in such a condition of health that acid will not generate in it. The other antacids are the carbonates of soda, potash, and ammonia; none of them can be claimed as a cure, they only relieve. If our readers are troubled with it let them take stomach bitters as a preventive; we have known it to work wonders. Rhubarb and magnesia is also a good mixture to relieve acidity and correct the stomach. The dose of the carbonate of soda as an antacid is 10 to 60 grains in water when urgently needed; we would not advise it often as it is rough on the stomach if continued long. The carbonate of ammonia is 3 to 10 grains dissolved in water; the bicarb. of potash 10 to 40 grains taken similarly.

Another remedy that works well with some people is

SPANISH JUICE.

A little piece chewed and swallowed occasionally gives the desired relief. We need hardly remind our readers that prevention is better than cure; therefore, avoid anything that you find causes acidity; but, properly medicated, the stomach ought to tolerate and digest the usual run of food.

CATHARTICS.

The remedies belonging to this class are very numerous. They act on the stomach and bowels in two distinct ways; 1st, by passing out of the stomach quickly, and causing a secretion of the watery elements of the blood along the course of the intestines. This is the class called Salines. Epsom Salts stand first in efficacy. A solution taken warm on an empty stomach causes a very quick and watery motion. We will speak more fully of salines in our chapter on the medicines of the faculty. Vegetable cathartics as a rule produce their effects through the blood, liver, and bile. Some of them have other properties, which we will name in this chapter, as it would take up valuable space to mention them often.

The first on this list is the old and world-renowned

ALOE,

Mentioned in Scripture and in the earliest books of medicine. It grows in various parts of the world; there are several species of it named after the country where it is grown. Socotrine is the kind held in highest favour. The plant is described as growing about 18 inches in height, woody and leafless below, where it is very rough from the remains of former leaves. It is surrounded at the top by several sharp-pointed spear-leaves curved inward at the point, with numerous small white lines at the edges. Its flowers are scarlet at the base, pale and green at the top. The medicinal part is the juice of the plant, dried and powdered. The dose is from three to ten grains if taken alone, but, on account of its extreme bitterness and griping tendency, it is best given with stimulants and carminatives. In the making of pills aloe is almost universally employed, as its effects are chiefly on the lower bowel; it is not advisable to take it if troubled with piles. It is said to have a beneficial effect in indigestion, lowness of spirits, female obstruction, &c., &c.

The other kinds of aloes are very similar to the above.

RHUBARB (Rheum.)

This is the same domestic garden plant that everybody knows. The root is used alone in medicine, although the stalks have also an effect on some people, causing looseness. While it cannot be doubted that the rhubarb known as turkey is superior to ours in strength, still the prejudices of people have a good deal to do with the neglect of our own, which has undoubted medicinal properties.

Rhubarb is a good medicine for indigestion. It is often carried in the pocket. A small bit the size of a pea is chewed and swallowed as often as is desirable to gently open the bowels, or it may be taken in powder from a quarter to a teaspoonful if it is desired to act on the bowels quickly; the powdered form is the best. 10 grains of bicarbonate of potash will make it more effective and partially cover its taste. Rhubarb in the fresh roots may be made into a decoction by scraping and slicing an ounce in a pint and a half of water to a pint; drink a wineglassful of the cold strained decoction two to four times a day. A favourite mixture with mothers is a quarter ounce of the powder with one ounce of magnesia. Dose for a child, a small teaspoonful in water.

Rhubarb enters into many of our compounds.

MANDRAKE (Podophyllum Peltatum.)

This plant is a native of America, growing throughout the States. The stem is about one foot high, round and smooth, divided into two, and bearing at the junction a solitary flower, which is white and hanging to the side. The flowers appear at the end of May and the beginning of June in America, but December and February here. We mention this as we hope it will yet be cultivated in the colonies. In passing through Kansas on our way to San Francisco we saw it growing in abundance along the line; digging some of the roots we kept them carefully in their native earth till we transplanted them in Dunedin, where they grew well, but in removing them to another garden they were lost. The root is the medicinal part and has quite a number of properties: purgative, antibilious, anthelmintic, hydragogue, antidyspeptic. It is now the substitute for the chief drug of the old school, (mercury), having all its supposed virtues and none of its evils. It is a sure and active purge, and is used in constipation, biliousness, indigestion, chronic liver complaints, venereal diseases, dropsy, &c. The dose of the powdered root is from 10 to 30 grains; but it is not so much used in the crude form as in the active principle or resin, known as podophyllin, a yellow powder prepared by precipitating the soluble matter of the decoction and drying it. The dose of this is from one half to two grains carefully taken, as large doses are dangerous, causing severe purging and vomiting. Mixing it with cayenne pepper, in the proportion of one part to two of the cayenne keeps it from griping, and increases its virtue in indigestion. It enters into several compounds. As it is an important medicine we will represent it in our illustrations.

BLACKROOT (Leptandria Virginica.)

(Also Culver's Root, Indian Physic, &c.)

It might be called the sister of the former, as it has similar properties, but much milder. It is an herbacous perennial with a simple erect stem, terminating in a long spike of white flowers; the leaves are in clusters of from four to seven, are lance-shaped and finely toothed at the edge; it flowers in July and August. The root contains the properties. As it is only imported in the roots it may be useful to give a description of them. They are round, smooth, generally broken, but when not they are about 6 inches long, black outside, dark within; very brittle when dry, no smell, slightly bitter taste. When used alone it is best taken in an infusion of the powder; from half to a teaspoonful in a cup of boiling water, strained and sweetened, will cleanse the intestines; if it does not operate in three or four hours it may be repeated. In fevers, typhoid and bilious, it acts favourably. In regular practice the concentrated powder, obtained in the same way as podophyllin, is often prescribed in doses from one to four grains. The compound powder in our compounds will be found a good medicine for the liver, &c.

SENNA (Cassia).

This is an old and popular medicine. It grows in Upper Egypt and India. It is described as a small under-scrub, two or three feet in height, with a straight woody branching stem; the leaves are sharp-pointed and small, of a yellowish colour; the flowers are yellow. The leaves are the part used. Senna tea is familiar to us from childhood. It is not held in much favour by most juveniles, who think it is often prescribed by their mothers as a punishment more than for any good it does them; this, however, is a mistake, although it must be admitted that sometimes mothers may overdose their children. Senna has a tendency to gripe. This, with its sickly, nauseous flavour, accounts for its abhorrence by young people and some older ones. To prevent both of these properties, (1), never boil it; (2) use some aromatic, such as cardamons, corianders, or ginger. A comparatively pleasant tea may be made thus:—

Take senna, 1 oz.; cardamon seeds, ½ oz.; sugar, 4 ozs.; ginger, ½ oz. Infuse in 1½ pints of hot water till cold or all night. Strain and press through a cloth, and take from one to four wineglassfuls morning or morning and night. Where it is desirable to thoroughly cleanse the alimentary canal, drink freely of warm water or some simple warm liquid, The fluid extract in teaspoonful doses is a good and easy way to take it.

MOUNTAIN FLAX (Linum Catharticum).

(Purging Flax).

Dr. Robinson describes it as a pretty little herb, growing on hilly pastures and in the fields. The stalk is about 8 inches high, round form, divided at the top into small branches. The leaves are small, oblong, two at each joint. The flowers are small and white. The plant resembles the chickweed, but on examination it is seen to be of the flax kind. The root is small and thready. It makes a strong but safe purge, owing to the drastic principle in it called *binin* in the old country. The country folk boil it in beer as a remedy for rheumatic pains, and for coughs, dropsy, &c. It is a good antibilious physic where a good cleansing of the bowels is wanted. It may be taken in extract or pills, 4 to 8 grains, two or three times a day; or in infusion, a wineglass three to four times a day. It is a good thing to put into other mixtures when a relaxing effect is desired, or when a binding effect is not.

NEW ZEALAND FLAX (Phormium Tenax).

There is no need to describe this plant to our New Zealand readers, as it grows in most parts of the colony. It is becoming a valuable article of commerce, and is not now likely to be cut down and destroyed, as it was at one time. It has been found to contain medicinal principles. The root, washed, cut into pieces, and boiled, is aperient, although not markedly better than any of the previously described; yet if people in the bush are out of the ordinary opening medicines, it may be tried. Prepare it as above; cover the roots with water, let them simmer half an hour, strain through a cloth or fine wire-strainer, and if desired sweeten. Take a tablespoonful one to three times a day; if not sufficient take more, if too much take less. The same decoction is good to bathe chilblains with, while it is warm. We are told by a gentleman

that it acts like a charm when used on unbroken chilblains.
We prepare a fluid extract of it.

CASTOR OIL (Olium Ricini).

This is the old time-honoured laxative. It is doubtless
valuable in its way, but it is only a cathartic pure and simple,
and many complain of its binding tendency after it has
operated. As it is defined in the list of regular medicines,
we will not dwell upon it further here.

JALAP,

Another old cathartic, will also be found amongst the regulars.

MANNA

Is a mild laxative, the concrete saccharine exudation of the
tree known in scientific botany as Frascinus Ornus. The
variety known as flake manna is the best. It comes in the
form of prisms or stalactites, several inches long, of a
yellow-white colour, brittle, light, and soft. The taste is sweet
and mild. Some people think that this substance is the same
or in some way resembles the manna given from Heaven to
the Israelites. This idea is no doubt inferred from the name
being the same; but while manna is a pleasant and good
medicine, it would not do for people to live upon. We heard a
Jew once, who thought himself a poet, speaking of the manna
which his ancestors received from above, give rather more
credit to Moses than he deserved. "Moses," said he, "gave
them bread from Heaven which was not baked in a pan or an
oven." A higher authority said, "Moses did not give you
that bread, but my Father." We are all too apt to forget the
First Cause of our mercies, while looking to the medium
through which they come. Manna, however, is a mild and
most agreeable laxative for children, some of whom are terrors
when medicine is forced upon them. This they will consider
in the light of a sugar-plum. It is also suitable for pregnant
women and such as are troubled with piles. The dose for an

adult is from one to two ounces; children one to four drachms.
It may be eaten or dissolved in water. It enters into several
worm mixtures.

CASCARA SEGRADA (RHAMNUS PURSHANA).

The California buckthorn. A small tree growing on the
Pacific slope, called by the early Spanish settlers Sacred Bark.
It is reasonable to suppose that they must have known of its
virtues, notwithstanding the fact that it is only a few years
since it was introduced to the faculty and the general public.
Being so comparatively unknown we cannot find a picture of it,
or we should like to give it a place amongst our illustrations.
However, we hope to acclimatise it soon, as it is one of the
very best cathartics yet discovered; also a first-class tonic. For
these purposes it has been used with great success during
the last six years by the American doctors, and during the last
three or four years by the physicians and others in all parts of
the world. While its virtues may be said to be beyond praise
in its abovenamed properties, it has lately been found to be
a specific in rheumatism. This latter virtue was discovered
by a doctor in the U. S. army, who, while troubled with rheumatism took a good dose of the Cascara as an aperient, it
surprised him to find that his rheumatic pain was gone soon
after. He had occasion to prescribe for the same painful
affection the following day. Cascara was given and the same
effect was noticed; the pains were relieved very soon, and in
a couple of days a cure was effected. The doctor had charge
of a division of a large hospital in which were some 25 cases
of rheumatism. He resolved before making known his discovery to test it well; so he gave it to all these patients with
the most gratifying results, nearly all were relieved and cured.
The iodide of potassium, which is the sheet-anchor of the
regulars, was almost superseded by the new remedy, although
the doctor found that in some cases the combination was
advantageous. The above facts have been set forth in most
of the medical journals. After noticing the above we tried
the same remedy and found it correct. It is now the chief

medicine in our rheumatic cure, which we have not yet known to fail. The form in which the doctor above referred to prescribed Cascara Segrada was the fluid extract; the dose 30 drops three times a day; if too severe on the bowels omit a dose or two, or take an astringent. The bark in decoction is one ounce to the pint; simmer an hour; cool and strain, and in order to correct its griping tendency and very bitter taste, an ounce of tincture of cardamons, ginger, peppermint, or other aromatics, may be added, with sugar if desired.

We close this list with

BUTTERNUT BARK (Juglans Cinerea).
(Sometimes called Oil Nut, or White Walnut.)

This is a mild aperient, opening without griping. The tree from which the bark is obtained belongs to the walnut family, this kind growing plentifully in the United States and Canada. Its action on the stomach resembles rhubarb, mild and non-irritating. The inner bark is the part used. The virtue is extracted with boiling water. It may be made into a decoction with others to meet indications, or by itself, but as it is not strong an extract is the best form for ordinary use. The solid extract is simply made by evaporating the decoction of 2 ozs. to the pint to the proper consistency. In addition to the above quality it is also a blood purifier which is of great value in skin eruptions of a recent character. Dr. Fox recommends it as the best aperient after or in itself as a worm expeller. Dr. Dawson says that in his experience 2 ounces of the bark in a pint of proof spirits will act as a purge in doses of one or two teaspoonfuls. The dose of the solid extract is from 20 to 30 grains (half to a teaspoonful) for a brisk purge. These doses are for adults. Children in proportion to age.

AROMATICS AND CARMINATIVES.

This class of remedies expels wind from the stomach and bowels. It will be seen that they principally consist of aromatics, which nearly all have this property.

PEPPERMINT (MENTHA PEPERITA).

This plant grows almost anywhere. A root of it introduced into a garden will spread all over it in time. Those who have seen the spearmint will not fail to identify the peppermint, as it is almost identical, the only difference being that it has darker leaves and flowers, and a little different smell. With these distinctions the two plants may be described together as being perennial herbs, with creeping roots. The lower stems of the peppermint shoot out along the ground, growing leaves which strike independent roots, and spread in all directions. The leaves are about two inches long; light green in the spearmint, and dark green in the peppermint. The flowers in the former are white, tinged with purple; in the latter, they are purple. It grows about a foot high. Although it is the essential oil and essence that are used as carminatives, which, no doubt, is the best form, still the herb may be used for the same purpose. A handful of the leaves, infused in a cupful of water, will relieve a windy stomach. Small doses may be given to babies; a teaspoonful or so for very young ones. The essence of peppermint is also good to rub on as a liniment for headaches. Painted on burns it soothes and removes the pain. The essence of spearmint is a valuable remedy when applied to external piles. Altogether the family of mints, of which there are several members, are highly beneficial as carminatives; also in colds and as gentle stimulants.

CARRAWAY SEEDS (CARUM CARUI.)

A good many of our readers will remember, with a certain amount of pleasure, the small comfits prepared by covering the seeds with sugar in the revolving pan of the confectioner. It may be thought that these only pleased the taste. This they did, but without doubt they also acted as carminatives. These seeds are a wholesome spice added to biscuits, gingerbread, &c.; powdered we use them in some of our compounds. The essential oil is the strongest, of which 5 drops may be taken 3 times a day on sugar as a carminative.

DILL SEED (Anethum Graveolens).

The essential oil is used in medicine. Fifteen drops rubbed up in a mortar with magnesia ½ an ounce, and water one pint, filtered through blotting-paper or French filtering-paper, make the dill water which may be termed the babies' comforter. Crying babies are generally dosed with it. The quantity varies with the age of infants. While we cannot say it is the best, it is good and safe for babies. There is nothing better than the Mother's Friend. (See compounds.) A decoction of the dried herb is good to stop vomiting and sickness of the stomach; also to assist in bringing on the monthly term in females.

FENNEL SEED (Fœniculum Vulgare.)

This plant has a tall erect round smooth stem, from which many branches spread out. It can hardly be said to have leaves, as they are more like small branches ending in small yellow flowers, looking much like a wild parsnip. It grows abundantly in broken ground, especially on the reclamations at Wellington, Napier, and Auckland, where we have seen it covering acres about the railway stations. The seeds powdered make a good carminative. A teaspoonful infused in a cup of boiling water will expel wind and ease griping pains. Of late the compound liquorice powder has come into favour as a mild aperient; fennel seed powder is an important ingredient in it. The essential oil, which can be seen under the microscope when the seed is cut across, is the active principle; the dose of which is from one drop for an infant to five or even ten in extreme cases for adults. The water is prepared in the same way as dill water. In taking rhubarb or senna it is advisable to use the fennel, as it not only helps to disguise the taste, but prevents griping, especially in the senna. About half as much of the fennel as the others will be sufficient.

ANISEED (Pimpinella Anisum.)

The anise plant is a native of Egypt; it was brought to Europe early in history. It is mentioned in holy scripture as one of the offerings of the Pharisee. (See Matt. xxiii. 23.) In secular history we learn that it was cultivated in the gardens of Charlemagne, the founder of the German Empire. Besides its carminative qualities (which are very similar to the last and may be taken the same way and in similar doses), it has a beneficial effect on the organs of the throat and chest. In the cough of infants a few drops of the essence has been found to answer well. The celebrated paregoric owes its peculiar smell and much of its virtue to the oil of aniseed. The essence is simply one part oil and nine parts rectified spirits; the dose of which is from five drops to a teaspoonful. It is also used in blend for flavouring liquor and comfits. In this list may be mentioned the following as having a carminative quality: Cardamon Seed, Cinnamon, Cloves, Coriander Seed, &c. They have all been found useful and may be tried when the other fails, or when they are at hand. The doses, &c., will be found given in the regular medicine. We will close this list with

CALAMUS ROOT (Acorus Calamus),
(Or Sweet Flag.)

This is a carminative, aromatic, and stomachic. It is a native of Europe and America, it is found growing in low swampy ground and along the sides of ditches and streams. It flowers early in summer. The leaves as well as the root have an aromatic odour. The plant is described as having long sword-shaped, smooth green leaves above, but near their origin from the root, of a red colour, variegated with green and white. The flowers are of a green yellowish colour; the fruit is an oblong capsule divided into three cells containing numerous seeds. The root is one of the best medicines known for a stomach tonic; we have heard people say that this alone cured them of terrible pains in that organ. It is very bitter, and on this account is a good tonic and appetiser, causing an activity in the secretions of the stomach. Those who are trying to leave off tobacco find it a help to ward off the craving for the pipe to chew a piece of the root occasionally. The powder in combination with marsh mallow is Dr. Fox's Colic Mixture, and a valuable one it is. In bitters calamus will be found a most useful ingredient.

DEMULCENTS.

This group of medicines has more or less nutrient qualities. Their work is to soothe the parts they come in contact with, and shield the stomach and intestines, and the mucous membrane. As poultices and lotions they are also good.

The inner bark of the

SLIPPERY ELM (Ulmus Fulva),

Deserves the highest place in this useful list. The tree itself is thus described in the American Dispensatory: "This species of Elm is indigenous, growing in all parts of the United States north of the Carolinas, but most abundantly west of the Alleghany Mountains. It flourishes in open, elevated situations, and requires a firm dry soil. From the white elm it is distinguished by its rough branches, its larger, thicker, and rougher leaves, its downy buds, and the character of its flowers and seeds. Its period of flowering is in April. The inner bark is the part used, and is brought to the shops

separated from the epidermis.   Large quantities are collected
in the lower peninsula of Michigan.   It is in long, nearly flat
pieces, 12 to 60 inches long and from 1 to 2 lines thick, of a
fibrous texture and a tawny colour, which is reddish on the
inner surface, and a peculiar, sweetish, and not unpleasant
odour and a highly mucilaginous taste when chewed.   The
inner surface finely ridged, fracture fibrous and mealy.   The
tranverse section delicately checquered.   By grinding it is
reduced to a light grey fawn coloured powder.   It abounds
in mucilaginous matter, which it readily imparts to water.
The mucilage is precipitated by acetate and subacetate of lead,
but not by alcohol.   Much of the bark brought into the
market is of inferior quality, imparting comparatively little
mucilage to water.   It has the characteristic odour of the
genuine article, but is much less fibrous and more brittle,
breaking abruptly when bent, instead of being capable, like
the better kind, of being folded lengthwise without breaking.
To what this inferiority is owing—whether to difference in
species, or the age, or to the circumstances of the growth of
trees producing it—we are unable to state."   Dr. C. W. Wright
Cincinnati, in communicating to the *Western Lancet* states that
slippery elm bark has the property of preserving fatty substances from rancidity, a fact derived from the Indians, who
prepared bears' fat by melting it with the bark, in the
proportion of a drachm of the latter to a pound of the former,
keeping them heated together for a few minutes, and then
straining off the fat.   The same process was tried with butter
and lard, and they were found to remain sweet for a long time.

MEDICINAL PROPERTIES AND USES.

Slippery elm is an excellent demulcent, applicable to all
cases in which this class of medicine is used.   It is especially
recommended in dysentery and diarrhœa, and diseases of the
urinary passages.   Like the bark of the common European
elm it has been employed in cutaneous eruptions, but neither
in these nor in any other cases does it probably exert any
greater power than demulcents generally.   Its mucilage is
nutritious, and we are told that it has proved sufficient to support

life in the absence of other foods. (Philadelphia Med. Times, Feb. 1874). Dr. J. Dowler of Beardstown, Ill., reports two cases of tapeworm—one in a child, the other an adult—in which the worms were discharged in consequence of the chewing of the slippery elm bark. Dr. Chase mentions a similar case, that of a child, to whom he gave the slippery elm for another purpose, but to his surprise it brought away several lengths of tapeworm. We know of its value as a food for invalids and children. For some years we have sold a digestive food, composed of one part of the powdered elm and three of sugar, with cinnamon to flavour. There are now in Dunedin and other parts children who have been brought up on it. For sucking babes it is also good when they are troubled with coughs. As a poultice we have seen it work wonders. We had two cases of poisoned fingers, so very bad that the attending doctors wanted to amputate, but with the elm and other help, such as our healing ointment, a cure was effected. We are conscious that all the foregoing is no more than can and ought to be said in praise of the slippery elm.

GUM ARABIC.

This is a well-known article, and a very useful demulcent, imported from Arabia, Egypt, and surrounding countries. Soluble in water and not in spirits. It is used for various purposes in medicine, such as making emulsions in which to suspend oils, in pills and cough mixtures, and as demulcent drinks in derangement of the bladder and scalding urine. One ounce of the gum dissolved in a pint of hot water, sweetened and strained, makes a good way to take it; about a wineglassful for a dose. On account of the disturbed state of Egypt this gum has risen to four times is former value, so that for the sake of economy many are now using gum tragacanth, which is three or four times stronger. We believe it has similar properties. The dose and uses will be found in the regular list.

COMFREY ROOT (SYMPHYTUM OFFICINALIS.)

This root is a native of Europe, but is now found in most civilized lands. It has long been held in high esteem as a demulcent. The early Britons called it Knit-Bone. The root was washed, scraped, and mashed, and applied in the form of a poultice over the broken limb, where it not only assisted the healing process, but hardening, it formed a splint. Dr Skelton strongly recommended it as a poultice in the rupture of young children, applied over the part. Of late years we have grown our own stock of this valuable root; it will be seen among our coloured lithographs. The Comfrey is cultivated by herbalists and used for making cough syrups and demulcent drinks. As a remedy for bleeding from the internal organs, it is affirmed that it will heal inward wounds better than any other agent yet discovered. It is a good ingredient in consumptive mixtures, also for leucorrhœa or whites. Dr. Fox recommends a syrup of it for this purpose, prepared thus :— Take two ounces of the fresh root, wash and slice it ; one ounce each of white pond lily root, stinking arrach, cudweed, and ginger root. Boil the whole gently in two quarts of water for half an hour, pour the whole hot upon two nutmegs powdered fine, half a teaspoonful of cayenne pepper, and half a pound of loaf sugar. A wineglassful of this four times a day, if persevered in, will cure this troublesome and weakening complaint. The decoction is two ounces of green or one ounce of dry to one pint. A wineglassful four times a day ; it may be sweetened.

COMMON MALLOW (MALVA SYLVESTRIS).

There are two varieties of the mallow, the garden and the marsh, the former growing in the form of a tree ; as most people are familiar with this kind we need not describe it. The leaves are good as a fomentation and poultice for inflammatory swellings, simply pour boiling water over them and lay them on the affected part, or bathe the part with the decoction, which is also recommended as a domestic remedy for coughs and colds. The root is the demulcent part. Infused or boiled, it gives out its mucilage. Take two to four ounces of the fresh dug root, wash and cut into small pieces, simmer in a quart of water for an hour, strain and sweeten, then you have a good demulcent drink, suitable for sore throats, soothing the stomach and bowels, and in bladder and urethra trouble.

MARSH MALLOW (ALTHŒA OFFICINALIS),

Is a smaller plant than the above, growing about a foot or eighteen inches high. Its leaves are smaller and harder, resembling the ivy. Its flowers, which are a bluish-purple, are followed by small button-like capsules containing the seeds. The root is white. The virtues of both are similar, and they can be used in the same way. The root powdered makes, with slippery elm, a fine poultice for swellings, also as a healing food for internal wounds. For colicky pains mixed with calamus it is excellent.

LINSEED (LINUM SEMINA).

The plant bearing the above seeds is one of the most useful we have, giving us food, medicine, and wearing apparel, and an oil which forms a most important article of commerce and manufacture. Medicinally, the seeds make a good demulcent drink. Simmer about one or two ounces in a quart of water, strain through a strainer, sweeten, and drink freely. If it is for coughs and colds, Spanish juice, or liquorice root, should be added, an ounce or two to the quart. The crushed seeds containing the oil make the regular poultice of the doctors. It is certainly good, but not equal to the slippery elm; the two combined sometimes make a desirable change for either. The oil is obtained by heating the crushed seed, and using hydraulic pressure. After the oil is extracted the remaining cake is used as a feed for cattle; it can also be eaten by man, but it is not so nutritious without the oil. Linseed tea is good in scalding urine, inflammation of the bladder, strangury, and as a soothing drink to the mucous membrane. The seeds taken whole in doses of teaspoonfuls, four times a day, will relieve chronic constipation. **This last** fact was discovered by an eclectic doctor in America, who was at his wits' end in treating a very bad case ; he affirms that the oil in the seeds seemed to lubricate the bowels in a better way than the usual remedy, castor oil.

DIURETICS.

The action of this class of remedies is upon the kidneys, stimulating and assisting them to secrete impurities from the blood. They alleviate and are useful in all dropsical affections, &c.

We desire, however, to inform our readers that diuretics are not to be given during an acute attack of inflammation of the kidneys or bladder, or if given it must be the mildest kind, as inflamed organs ought not to be stimulated. The reason of this must be apparent, as inflammation is the highest form of stimulation. The first essential is rest to the part inflamed till the acute condition has been overcome.

We will head this list of Diuretics with a medicine which we regard as not one of the best, but the very best medicinal gift which comes from the Father of Mercies We wish to impress this fact on the minds of our readers, as it must be admitted that we are all too ready to forget the source of all good gifts. As some doctors in writing their prescriptions put down the names of the makers of particular drugs, a Yankee M.D. takes such off in a prescription in one of the medical journals thus :—

Take Tincture delised iron	..	1 ounce, Werth's
,, fluid extract Sarsa Co.		2 ounces, P. D. and Co.'s
,, calamba ..	..	4 drachms, Squire's
,, syrup trifolium Co.	..	6 ounces, P. D. and Co.'s
,, water ad ..	..	12 ounces, God Almighty's.

That is it; water is the manufacture and gift of God. Some of our devout readers may say that all things come from God. That is true as far as the pure or crude material is concerned, but as Solomon says, man himself was first made pure, but he has found out many inventions, not only to debase himself, but also the gift of his Creator. Without further moralizing we affirm that water is the best diuretic, not only as the medium in which nearly all medicines are given, but in itself. It has been termed the water of life by some sufferers who took it hot as directed for the cure of foul stomach, chronic dyspepsia, &c. The faculty are now prescribing it in bladder complaints, which organ it washes out thoroughly; passing first through the kidneys, it cleanses them also, and in some forms of blood disease it must act beneficently in thinning it, and dissolving out the waste products of the body. While it thus cleanses the kidneys and bladder, there are other diuretics which stimulate the urinary organs, causing an increased secretion from the blood and drainage of dropsical accumulations in the cavities and cellurary tissue. Some of these we will now deal with. First beginning at home, we find our native

MANUKA SCRUB (Leptospermum),

Or tea tree, is a well-tried and approved diuretic. There is no need to describe it, at least to our New Zealand readers, as it grows in various parts of the colony. Still there may be many who have not had it made known to them, and who would like a description, which would enable them to identify it, for this purpose we will give a picture of it. (See illustration index.)

It is no use denying the existence of the form of folly which despises things because they are cheap and easily got. This is one reason why this valuable native plant is not more used. We know of a very estimable M.D. in Dunedin, who told a patient that had dropsy to go out to the bush and get this scrub, directing her to infuse a handful of it in a quart jug of water and drink it freely. She did so and was cured. This simple prescription, for which nothing was charged, reminds us of a contrast, a hypochondriac patient who took our medicine, as well as bucketfuls of others. He had visited the surgery of perhaps the most reputed doctor in the province, who, at last got tired of him, as his conscience might be accusing him for taking so many half sovereigns from a poor man. At the last visit the doctor addressed him thus : "Go home, my man, and don't take any more medicine ; go to work and try and forget your trouble, for it is only imaginary." His conscience, however, did not prevent him taking another fee. His advice did not suit, for he came to us and took about an hour to tell of his aches and pains. We gave him medicine, which we can only hope did him good. Returning to our subject, we do not know of a better way of taking this native medicine than that recommended by the liberal doctor just mentioned : a handful of the blossoms and twigs of the tree infused in a pint of boiling water, and half a cupful about two to six times a day. It may be made into a tincture, two ounces to the pint of proof spirit ; steep for a week, strain, press, bottle, and take from a tea- to a table-spoonful for a dose. This may be used in all cases when a diuretic is needed.

BEARBERRY (Uva Ursi).

This hardy shrub inhabits the northern latitudes and high mountains of Europe, Asia, and America. It prefers barren wastes and dry sandy tablelands. The leaves are the part used in medicine. They are small, pale green, not unlike senna, but smaller, thicker, and smooth, with slight shade of brown ; when powdered this brown shade is apparent. The best way we have found to get the whole of the virtues is to infuse the powder, two teaspoonfuls to the pint ; drink one or two wineglassfuls three or four times a day. It is usually combined in diuretic mixtures.

QUEEN OF THE MEADOW (Eupatorium Purpureum),
(Gravel Root or Meadow Sweet),

Is described as a perennial herbaceous plant, with a purple stem, five or six feet high. Its leaves are lance-shaped and toothed ;

it flowers are purple. It grows in swamps and low-lying grounds. The root is the strongest part, and may be prescribed as a diuretic. Where gravel is known or suspected, one ounce of the dry crushed root, simmered in a pint of soft or rain water makes the decoction, of which one or two wine-glassfuls may be given two or more times a day as the case may require; of the powdered root a teaspoonful in a cup of boiling water, drinking the clear, is perhaps the best way to take it. A tincture is made of two ounces to the pint of proof spirit. Dose, one to two teaspoonfuls.

BROOM TOPS (SCROPARIUS).

The broom is a cosmopolitan, and almost universally known. The common yellow variety is the medicinal kind; although the white, no doubt, has similar properties. It is put down in most books as diuretic, antiscorbutic, and cathartic. The decoction of the tops and flowers, one ounce to the pint, is good for dropsy, retention of urine, and water on the brain. The faculty use it in the expressed juice, which is made by chopping up the tops well and putting them through a powerful press. The juice is then fortified with 10 to 20 per cent. of alcohol. The dose is from a tea- to a table-spoonful three to six times a day. For preserving, when the plant is in bloom the tops are cut off about six inches long; should be carefully dried and put away in air-tight tins or strong brown paper bags till required.

BUCHU LEAVES (BAROSMA CRENULATA).

The name of this small shrub is from the Greek, signifying strong odour. It is found growing plentifully in South Africa and India. Its use was made known to us through the European doctors and English residents seeing the natives use it successfully in their practice. Recent trials have weakened faith in its power of increasing the flow of urine; but it is good in irritation and catarrh of the urinary organs and disease of the prostate gland (which is situated at the neck of the bladder). The leaves being hard, it is best to bruise or grind them before infusion. One ounce to the pint of hot water, cover up for ½ an hour, strain, and take one or two wineglassfuls three or four times a day. The tincture also is useful, made in the usual way, and dose one to two teaspoonfuls; or the fluid extract, dose half to one teaspoonful.

JUNIPER BERRIES (JUNIPERUS COMMUNIS).

This evergreen shrub is a native of Europe, but can be acclimatised as it is in America and the colonies. It grows in this city. Its height is usually from three to six feet, but it sometimes attains to 12 or 15 in the south of France and northern Italy. The leaves are small, sharp, deep green, shiny on the upper surface; the bark and wood have a characteristic aromatic smell, owing to the essential oil which pervades the whole plant. The berries are the best part for medicine. When ripe they resemble black currants; dried, they are nearly the same in appearance, only a little shrivelled. They have a sweetish warm taste, with a slight flavour of turpentine. As a diuretic the best and quickest way to extract their virtue is an infusion in hot water of the bruised berries, 1 oz. to the pint, the whole of which may be taken in the day; used in dropsy and similar troubles, when the kidneys need stimulating. A tincture may be prepared with two ounces to the pint of proof spirits. This will be found better than gin or schnapps, which have very little of juniper berries in them. The chief objection to families preparing the tinctures is the high price of the spirits of wine. However, by permission of our N. Z. Government, we manufacture in bond these tinctures at half the price of the spirits alone. The oil of juniper, made from the berries, is good in mucous discharges from the urethra and vagina, also pains in the back, and suppression of urine. Dose: 5 to 15 drops on sugar three times a day.

PARSLEY PERT (PERCICIER),

Is a well-proved herb for gravel. It is a good diuretic. Was formerly called parsley-break-stones; alluding to its power in gravel. It is said to have a small fibrous root, which continues in the ground for many years, from which many leaves rise along the surface. The stems are 9 to 12 inches high, but so thickly covered with small leaves that they can hardly be seen ; they are about the size of a finger nail and toothed at the edges. The flowers are small, so also are the seeds. The whole plant is used in infusion of an ounce of the dried herb or two ounces of the green. (This rule of two of the green for one of the dry holds good in nearly all cases). The dose, one or two wineglassfuls three or four times a day. Dr. J. Skelton says it is excellent in obstructions of the urine, liver, and jaundice.

PARSLEY ROOT (Petroselineum Sativum).

The top, used as a vegetable, has some diuretic effect, but the root is well-known to possess it. The roots should be used if they are to be had fresh ; cut up and boil gently, strain, and drink the decoction freely. In obstruction of the kidneys, liver, &c., the leaves are held in high repute by some. Bruised and applied as a poultice to contusions, inflamed breasts, and swelling of glands, they have a beneficial effect. The powdered seeds sprinkled on children's heads kill vermin. A poultice of the bruised leaves is used to dry up the milk in women's breasts, when it is desirable to do so.

PELETORY OF THE WALL (Parietaria Officinalis).

It is so called on account of its affinity for old walls and ruins as growing places. Dr. Robertson thus describes it : " It rises with brownish, tender, weak, and almost transparent stalks two feet high, on which grow at the joints two leaves, rather broad and long, of a dark green colour, rough and hairy, as the stalks are also. At the joints from the middle of the stalk upwards, where it spreads into branches, stand many purplish flowers in hairy, rough heads, after which come small black seeds, which will stick to any garment that comes against them. The root is rather long, with small fibres of a dark reddish colour." This is one of the best diuretics that we know; for dropsy it is unrivalled. Many cases where it was thought the patient would have been drowned, so to speak, have been cured with this. We have given it to consumptive patients whose legs were swollen, with the satisfaction of seeing the water disappear. We do not say it will cure in all cases, but where the disease is not the result of serious organic derangement it is seldom known to fail. It is also said to be good in shortness of breath and wheezing of the chest. The decoction made in the usual way and sweetened with honey makes an excellent gargle for sore throats. The juice of the herb injected into fistulas is also mentioned as a cure for them. A poultice of the leaves, mixed with bran and linseed meal, applied warm will mitigate the pain and cure bruises. This valuable herb will be found in our list of pictures. (See illustration index.)

HYDRANGEA ROOT.

This root is a very good diuretic in gravelly complaints: two ounces of the root simmered in a pint of water; the dose is from a tablespoonful to a wineglassful three or four times a day. In the *Chicago Medical Times*, for December 1888, is an article upon a common trouble that has grown out of the fast life of the people of America, nervous prostration, accompanied by symptoms of diabetes. The patients lose flesh and are unfit for business. When the urine is examined it is found loaded with phosphates, showing a great waste of nerve material. For this condition, the writer, an M.D. in good standing, recommended rest, change of habit, and a decoction of Hydrangea, one tablespoonful, and five grains of citrate of lithia. We have tried it, and can recommend it to anyone suffering with the above symptoms.

HAIR CUP MOSS

Is another mild and good diuretic; dose and directions are one ounce to pint infusion, of which a wineglassful three times a day may be taken.

DANDELION (Taraxacum.)

This is the celebrated plant in which the common people of every land have faith. We have adopted it as our trade mark. As we give it in illustration there is no need to describe it, seeing also it is so well known; but there are many who confuse it with a plant not unlike it, namely, the Cape weed. The one point of difference that will alone prevent mistake is that the true dandelion has a hollow stem; the Cape weed has not, but its stem is jointed, while the dandelion is straight, and when ripe has a brownish shade. The dandelion root is brownish white, the Cape nearly white and not so large. It is more bitter than the other. On this account it is a tonic and can be taken by experimentalists without fear in reasonable doses. We would suggest 1½ ounces of the Cape weed root simmered in a pint and a half of water down to a pint, a wineglassful three times a day. Of the dandelion root, two ounces to the pint; dose, the same. There are other preparations of it; the expressed juice, dose, a tea- to a table-spoonful; the solid extract, a half to a teaspoonful. In this form it is made into pills with other ingredients to increase its laxative power. Then the roots are washed, cut up, dried, roasted and ground into coffee, or without roasting, the powdered roots make a very convenient and efficient way of taking the medicine. As the dandelion has been such a friend to us in our business, we may be excused if we are somewhat jubilant in its praise. Our feelings are akin to those of a young man in London who was thrown out of employment and reduced nearly to starvation point, when a good Samaritan started him in the baked potato business. He got along famously, some weeks making as much as three pounds. Being a devout man and so much in love with his potatoes, he was surprised that he could not find them mentioned in the Bible, which he dearly loved to read. It is not too much to say that we have made millions of the dandelion pills. With the aid of machinery an assistant and myself turned out forty thousand in one day; as for the coffee, tons of it have been manufactured by us.

As a change from our long prosy articles we will put a few thoughts into meter. A certain poet has said that poets are born and not made, if this be so, then as we were born and not made, we must be a poet, or at least a doggrelist, as the following verses will show :—

> There is a flower that decks the plain,
>   And fills our hearts with pleasure ;
> The dandelion is its name,
>   We hold it as a treasure.
>
> This useful plant with jagged leaves
>   And pretty yellow flower,
> Is famous as a medicine
>   That gives the liver power;
>
> To properly prepare the blood,
>   And regulate the bile,
> Assist digestion, and induce
>   The pleasant healthful smile.
>
> The doctors may be sceptical
>   Of any virtue in it,
> Yet many who have tried it well
>   Can praise it any minute.
>
> Not only, as a medicine,
>   But also as a food,
> The root made into coffee
>   Most certainly is good ;
>
> And if you're ill and want a pill
>   You surely can rely on ;
> Don't take the old imported ones,
>   But try the dandelion.

There are several others in this class that we would like to mention, but must close with the above, which we believe are the best.

DIAPHORETICS.

These medicines act through the blood on the sweat glands of the skin. The way in which this is effected is explained by some physologists: "The heart's action being quickened, the blood is sent with greater force to the surface of the body. The capillaries or hair-like terminations of the arteries are filled a little more quickly than the veins can carry it off; thus the blood is left in the cooling parts of the body, the sweat glands are stimulated, and the watery elements expelled from the system with morbid matter; the natural temperature is restored, and the healthy functions of the body go on in the even tenor of their way."

The importance of these sweating medicines in fevers, catarrh, inflammation, cholera, and similar diseases cannot be ever-estimated.

The leader in this class is

YARROW (Achillea Millefolium),

Is a good old remedy, and one which is held in high esteem by those who have tried it. In our early days of herbalism we only heard and read of its excellence, but we soon had occasion to try it; having caught (according to the common phraseology) a severe cold, we felt the half-dead feeling which the French call *malaise*, we had also feverish symptoms. A trial of yarrow was determined upon. One ounce of the dry herb was put into a pint of boiling water with a teaspoonful of composition powder, infused one hour, strained and sweetened. We drank it hot in bed, put a hot bottle to our feet, covered up and went to sleep, and in the morning not a vestige of the cold was left. Ours was not an unusual experience; in thouands of cases the same has happened; yes, and we might say that all things being equal the same will be the result in every instance. Dr. Coffin in his "Guide to Health" tells us of an old Quaker herbalist (whom we might term a yarrowmaneist) who, when asked what was good for a cold said: "Thou shalt make a strong tea of yarrow, drink one pint hot on going to thy bed, put a hot brick wrapped in a cloth wet with vinegar to thy feet, and thou shalt verily be well in the morning." He was asked what was good for rheumatism, and he repeated the same cure and directions. Several other diseases were named, with a request for a cure, and his remedy was still the same, Yarrow, yarrow. This story reminds us of an old sea captain who had one cure for constipation, diarrhœa, fever, rheumatism, broken noses, arms, &c.—that was salts. Such men act on the principle of knowing only one good thing and sticking to it. This herb grows abundantly almost everywhere. We preserve about a quarter of a ton of it every year. Our celebrated Balm of Gilead owes much of its popularity to this plant, which is the chief ingredient in its composition. The above-mentioned doses are rather large for weak stomachs, especially if taken at one drink, but this is not needful, as it can be sipped. About half the dose for women and quarter for children. Yarrow will be found amongst our pictures.

The juice is, according to Dr. Fox, a specific for bleeding from the bowels. Sniffed up, or put on cotton into the nostrils, will stop the flow of blood. A strong decoction taken inwardly and bathed on them is good for piles.

PLEURISY ROOT (Aselepias Tuberosa),
Or Butterfly Plant.

The root is the part used. It is fleshy and large, and much esteemed by Botanics, Eclectics, and Regulars in America. It is given to promote perspiration and expectoration. As its name indicates it is the best thing for pleurisy, inflammation of the lungs, &c. Rheumatic fever, indigestion, and bronchial affections are benefited by this remedy, especially given in warm infusion.

To prepare this take one ounce of the bruised root, simmer in a pint of water, strain, sweeten, keep warm, and give a wineglassful every one, two, or three hours. The infusion is a teaspoonful of powdered pleurisy to a cup of boiling water, half of which may be taken every hour or so. When

treating of inflammation of the lungs, for which this root is
excellent, we will give full particulars. It is represented in
our pictures.

ANGELICA (Angelica Atropurpurea).

This is a large and beautiful plant, cultivated in gardens,
but also growing wild in some parts. It attains the height
of eight feet. The stems are strong and branching. The
leaves are large, notched at the edges, and of a bright green
colour. The flowers small and white, growing in round tufts.
Two seeds follow each flower : they are flat on one side, on
the other convex, and marked with three grooves. It flowers
at the end of summer; the seeds are ripe in autumn.

The whole plant is medicinal; the root, however, is the
strongest. Infusion and decoction made in the usual way,
and similar doses. Good for colds, wind, and colicky pains,
and heartburn. A good cordial is made by adding 2 ozs. of
the tincture to 18 of simple syrup, and 1 oz. of cardamons.
A wineglassful in water three or four times a day.

BONE-SET (Eupatorium Perfolatum),
Or Thoroughwort.

This, with the foregoing may be called in point of sweating qualities twin brothers. The appearance of the plant
is similar to the Pleurisy or Butterfly plant, only Bone-set
flowers are white, Pleurisy bright orange. Their properties
are somewhat analogous. As the Pleurisy is one of our
pictures we need not lose space by describing the appearance
of either. Bone-set is a native of America; it is found
growing on the borders of swamps and streams. The
medicinal parts are the tops and leaves. An infusion in hot
water, one ounce to the pint is the usual strength. Being
somewhat stronger than yarrow, the same dose as recommended by the Quaker would probably act as an emetic and
cathartic, so that if this effect is not desired, only half
the dose should be taken, *i. e.* a quarter to half a pint of the
infusion. It is strongly recommended in fevers, also as a

tonic, cold, in wineglassful doses three times a day. Combined with other herbs a good fomentation mixture is made for pains in the abdomen, inflammation of the bowels and other parts. The powdered herb can be taken, a teaspoonful to a cup of boiling water, strained and sweetened, being the largest dose. It may be useful here to remind those giving or taking these sweating medicines to see that the pores are closed before going into the cold. To do this the body should be sponged with tepid water and vinegar; rub with a dry, warm cloth. Or here is a better mixture: A teaspoonful of cayenne, a handful of salt, a cupful of vinegar, and a pint of water. Apply as above.

BALM (MELISSA OFFICINALIS).

This well-known plant is found in most gardens, and is called balm-lemon on account of its lemon flavour. It is a mild diaphoretic, useful in colds, fevers, and where it is desirable to produce a sweat. The warm infusion, sweetened and drunk freely will do this nicely. Dr. Skelton, in his "Science and Practice of Medicine," strongly recommends it in inflammation of the chest in children. A strong infusion given freely, and linen, or we should prefer lint, wrung out and wound twice round the chest, covered with two folds of flannel, and oiled silk over all, or some cloth that will keep in the steam. Renew every two hours.

The Mint family of plants, some of which we noticed before, are also good as diaphoretics, especially

CAT MINT (NEPETA CATARIA).

This is a large plant. When full-grown it is 3 feet high, has broad, pale green leaves and white flowers like spearmint. The stems are whitish, hairy, and straight. The leaves come out two at a joint; they are broadest at the base, tapering to a point. They are a little indented at the edge; the upper side of the leaf is bright green, the under side almost white. The plant has a strong, but not unpleasant smell, which is almost loses on drying.

The medicinal virtues of this plant are undoubted. It is good for hysteria and fits; also for headaches caused through colds. A strong infusion sweetened with honey is good for coughs; a poultice of the bruised leaves is recommended for piles. Infusion, 2 ozs. of green or 1 oz. of dry to the pint. Drink freely if a perspiration is desired.

HYSSOP (Hyssopus Officinalis).

A garden herb cultivated by the country people in Britain and elsewhere. We have grown it in Dunedin. It is a small plant, at the highest about 18 inches. The leaves are small and dark green, sharp pointed, and opposite the flowers, which are of a blue purple colour. The leaves and tops are the medicinal parts. They should be gathered just as the flowers begin to come out.

Hyssop, in addition to its diaphoretic property, is a pectoral, that is, for the chest. It is good for sore throats. In combination with sage, which has similar properties, the bruised leaves applied to bruises relieve the pain and remove the discolouration. It is also a good expectorant and may be taken in infusion and decoction, usual doses.

THYME (Thymus Vulgaris.)

This pleasant smelling little plant is a favourite with cooks and sausage makers, on account of the agreeable flavour it gives to stuffing, &c.; it is also a diaphoretic of some value. The warm infusion will bring out a perspiration. If sweetened it is pleasant to take. In this respect it may be given to young people who would not take some of the stronger. The wild thyme is stronger and better for some ailments. Whooping cough, asthma, bronchitis, and gout are said to be benefited and sometimes cured by it. An infusion used as a foot and leg bath, with the same drank freely, is generally successful in removing obstructed menses. The essential oil of thyme is a reputed cure for toothache; a drop is put into the hollow tooth and repeated if necessary.

BLUE VERVAIN (Verbena Hastata.)

This is a very valuable herb. Professor P. O. Brown, in the "Complete Herbalist," speaks of this herb in the most flattering terms. With him it is an emmenagogue, expectorant, diaphoretic, antispasmodic, hepatic, splenetic, febrifuge, stimulant, antiscorbutic, lithontriptic, emetic, astringent, stomachic, and a super-excellent tonic. We think he is just a little too much given to exaggerating, especially when he says he was the first to bring vervain to the notice of physicians twelve years ago. His book is dated 1885, while Coffin, in his lectures delivered in 1850, fully describes it, and tells of its great virtues. Dr. Dale, in his book, "The Botanic System," published in 1855, does the same ; also Fox, Stevenson, Skelton and Robinson. We can hardly understand why a man could fall into such an error unless it is his desire to appear original. Honesty in all things.

Still vervain is a first class diaphoretic. Coffin says it is the most powerful in nature. In intermittent fevers it is about the best remedy, and for what is known as cold and difficult menstruation. To bring and keep out eruptions in fevers, small-pox, measles, and scarlet fever. The green leaves bruised and mixed with slippery elm is reckoned the finest thing for bruises and discolourations resulting therefrom, and as a remedy for epilepsy, Mr Brown declares it unequalled, used in infusion in the ordinary way, half a teacupful every hour to produce a sweat, which may also act as an emetic on weak stomachs If this is desired the dose may be doubled. The powdered herb may be used, a teaspoonful to a cup of boiling water, strained and sweetened. For a tonic the cold decoction of an ounce to the pint ; dose, a wineglass three times a day is the best way to take it. For fits it is compounded with other medicines which will be found in our treatment of epilepsy. For a picture of this herb see illustrations. We are happy to say it is now introduced into the colonies. We saw it in Christchurch last summer and intend to get some of the seeds. The latest discovery that we know of as a diaphoretic is the

JABORANDI LEAVES.

The plant is found in Brazil. The dried leaves are smooth, pale green, hard and tough, varying in size from one to four inches long and half to two broad; no smell and when chewed, a slight balsamic taste. The infusion of the powdered leaves is the best way to administer it. One teaspoonful in half a pint of boiling water, strained and sweetened if patient prefers, will in about ten minutes bring out a profuse perspiration, beginning at the face and neck and spreading all over the skin. It has been estimated that in a robust person the amount of sweat poured out is nine to fifteen ounces. The temperature is slightly raised at first, but after the pores are opened it falls. From two to three hours the sweating usually lasts, after which the patient is more or less exhausted. To keep up a milder perspiration smaller doses are recommended. The indications for jalorandi are a hot dry skin, watery effusions in any part of the body, Bright's disease, acute inflammation of the kidneys. The sweats may be repeated daily, every other day, or as often as required. A tablespoonful dose, frequently repeated, acts as a gentle diaphoretic. The active principle (pilocarpine) is used as a hypodermic injection, when it is desired to induce perspiration immediately. This should only be done by an experienced person.

EXPECTORANTS.

This class of remedies act on the mucous membrane of the respiratory organ. They are abundant, and useful in colds, coughs, asthma, bronchitis, consumption, and all chest affections. Lobelia, skunck cabbage, pleurisy root, which stand high as expectorants, we have already described.

ARUM ROOT (ARUM TRIPHYLLUM).

(Indian Turnip, Dragon Root, or Wake Robin),

As this plant is variously called, has a perennial root, which, early in spring, sends up a large oval-shaped variously-coloured blade, convoluted at the bottom and bent over at the top like a hood, and supported by an erect, round, green or purplish neck. Within it is a club-shaped part, green, purple, black, or variegated, rounded at the end and contracted near the base, where it is surrounded by the stamens or germs in the double, and by both in the single plants; the female organs being below the male. The upper portions gradually decay, while the germs are converted into a compact bunch of shining scarlet berries. The leaves, usually one or two in number, and upon long sheathing foot-stalks, are composed of three oval-shaped leaflets, paler on their under than their upper surface, and becoming glaucous as the plant advances. There are three varieties of this species, distinguished by the colour of the tops, which in one is green, in another dark purple, and in a third white. The plant is a native of North and South America, and is common to all parts of the United States, growing in damp woods, in swamps, along ditches, and in other moist, shady places. All parts of it are highly acrid, but only the root was formerly recognized. This is roundish, flattened, an inch or two in diameter, covered with a brown, loose epidermis, and internally white, fleshy, and solid. In the recent state it has a peculiar odour, and is violently acrid, producing, when chewed, an insupportable burning, biting sensation in the mouth and throat, which continues for a long time and leaves an unpleasant soreness behind. According to Dr. Bigelow its action does not readily extend through its skin, as the bruised root may lie upon the skin till it becomes dry without producing pain or redness. The acrid principle is extremely volatile, and is entirely driven off by heat. It is not imparted to water, alcohol, or olive oil, but it is probably soluble in ether. The root loses nearly all its acrimony by drying, and in a short time becomes quite inert. It is a powerful local irritant, possessing the properties of stimulating the secretions either from the skin or lungs. It has been advantageously given in asthma, hooping-cough, chronic catarrh, chronic rheumatism, and various affections connected with the cachectic state of the system. As immediately taken from the ground it is too acrid to use. The recently dried root, which retains a portion of the acrimony, but not sufficient to prevent its convenient administration, is usually preferred. It may be given in the dose of ten grains, mixed with gum arabic, sugar, and water, in the form of an emulsion, repeated two or three times a day, and gradually increased to half a drachm or more. The powder, made into a paste with honey or syrup, and placed in small quantities upon the tongue so as to be gradually diffused over the mouth and throat, is said to have proved useful in the aphthous sore mouths of children.

ELECAMPANE ROOT (INULA HELENIUM).

This is a very useful expectorant; grows wild in some parts, but it is generally cultivated in gardens for its medicinal value. It has a resemblance to the sunflower, about five feet high. The leaves are large, long, and pointed; the flowers grow on the end of the branches, are a beautiful yellow, in pairs about two inches wide; the stem is round, thick, and of a reddish tint. It is highly recommended in chest affections and other troubles, as the following description from Dr. Robinson's "Family Herbal" will show : "The fresh roots of elecampane, preserved with sugar or made into a syrup or conserve, are very effectual to warm a cold windy stomach, or the pricking therein, and stitches in the side caused by the spleen ; and to relieve cough, shortness of breath, and wheezing in the lungs.

The dried root, powdered and mixed with sugar, serves the same purpose. The root is esteemed a good pectoral, and like angelica root, is candied and sold as sweetmeat. Dr. Hill says he has found an infusion of the fresh root sweetened with honey to be very successful for the whooping-cough. It operates by urine powerfully, and by sweat. The juice will cure the itch, applied externally. The decoction of the root in wine, or the juice taken therein, expels urine; and gargled in the mouth, or the root chewed, fastens loose teeth and keeps them from putrefaction. The decoction or juice in honey is good for those who spit blood. The root boiled well in vinegar, beaten and made into an ointment with hog's lard is an excellent remedy for scabs. In the root of this herb lies the chief effect.

WILD CHERRY BARK (Prunus Virginiana).

Old botanical books recommend the gum as a good remedy in coughs and chest disorders, but recently the bark only is used. The tree grows throughout the United States, flourishing in those parts where the soil is fertile and the climate temperate. The leaves have been found by Prof. Proctor to yield volatile oil and hydrocyanic acid on distillation, and in such proportion that a water distilled from them might with propriety be substituted for the cherry-laurel water. The fruit has a sweetish, astringent, bitter taste, and is used to impart flavour to spirituous liquors. The bark is obtained indiscriminately from all parts of the tree, but that off the roots is thought to be the most active; uniting with a tonic power the property of calming irritation and diminishing nervous excitability. This bark is adapted to the treatment of diseases in which debility of the stomach or of the system is united with general or local irritation; and when largely taken it diminishes the action of the heart. It has been employed in the hectic fever of scrofula and consumption. It may be used in the form of powder, infusion, fluid extract, or syrup. The dose of powder is from thirty grains to a drachm; of the infusion, which is properly directed in the pharmacopœia to be prepared with cold water, two or three ounces ; of the fluid extract a drachm ; and of the syrup half a fluid ounce.

LIQUORICE ROOT (Glycyrrhiza Glabra).

The liquorice plant has a perennial root, which is round, succulent, tough, and pliable, furnished with sparse fibres ; rapid in its growth, and in a sandy soil penetrates deeply into the ground. The stems are herbacous, erect, and usually four or five feet from the ground. have few branches, and are garnished with alternate pinnate or feather-shaped leaves, consisting of several pairs of elliptic-shaped, blunt leaflets, with a single leaflet at the end, of a pale green colour, and clammy on their under surface. The flowers are violet or purple, formed like those of the pea, and arranged in auxiliary spikes supported on long peduncles. The fruit is a compressed one-celled pod, containing from one to six small kidney-shaped seeds. The plant is a native of the south of Europe, Barbary, Syria, and Persia, and is cultivated in England and the north of France and Germany. Liquorice root is an excellent demulcent, well adapted to catarrhal affections, and to irritations of the mucous membrane of the bowels and urinary passages. It is best given in the form of a decoction, either alone or combined with other demulcents. It is frequently employed as an addition to the decoctions of acrid, irritating, and bitter vegetable substances, such, for example as the seneka and mezereon, the acrimony of which it covers, while it renders them more acceptable to the stomach. Before being used it should be deprived of its outside skin, which is somewhat acrid, without possessing the peculiar virtues of the root. The decoction may be prepared by boiling an ounce of the bruised root for a few minutes in a pint of water. By long boiling the acrid resinous principle is extracted. Perhaps, however, to this principle may in part be ascribed its virtues in chronic bronchial diseases. The powder is used in the preparation of pills, either to give due consistence or to cover their surface and prevent them from cohering. Used in some of our compounds.

SENEKA (POLYGALA SENEGA).

This plant has a perennial branching root, from which several erect, simple, smooth, round, leafy stems annually rise from nine inches to a foot in height. The stems are occasionally tinged with red or purple below, but are green near the top. The leaves are alternate or scattered, lance-shaped, smooth, bright green on the upper surface, paler beneath, and supported on very short footstalks. The flowers are small and white, and form a close spike at the summit of the stem. The calyx is their most conspicuous part. It consists of five leaflets, two of which are wing-shaped, white, and larger than the others. It is grown in North America. Seneka is a stimulating expeectorant and diuretic, and in large doses emetic and cathartic. It appears, indeed, to excite, more or less, all the secretions. Its action is especially directed to the lungs, as its expectorant virtues are those for which it is chiefly employed. As an expectorant it is prescribed in cases not attended with acute inflammatory action, or in which the inflammation has been in great measure subdued. It is peculiarly useful in chronic catarrhal affections and the secondary states of croup, employed so as to purge and as an emetic. It has proved useful in rheumatism and some cases of dropsy are said to have been cured by it. The dose of powdered seneka is from ten to twenty grains, but the medicine is never used in substance. The dose of syrup is one or two fluid drachms; of the extract from one to three grains. The decoction of an ounceof the bruised root to the pint; dose: half to two tablespoonfuls is, we think, the best way to get all its virtues.

BLOOD-ROOT (SANGUINARIA CANADENSIS),

(Red Puccoon),

Is second only to lobelia as an expectorant. The plant grows plentifully in Canada and the United States. It is perennial. The root is about the thickness of a finger, fleshy, of a reddish brown colour outside and red within. When it is cut or broken a bright red juice is exuded. From the root arises a short sheath, encircling the stalks, which are long and slender, with a groove running lengthwise. The folded leaves envelope the flower-bud, and roll back as it expands. The leaf is foliated, usually seven in number, one only on a stalk. The flowers are white, with yellow-tinged petals. It is reckoned one of the most beautiful spring flowers in America. We think it merits a place in our illustrations. It is a good medicine to use where an expectorant is required. The decoction of the dried root broken small is half an ounce to the pint, sweetened. As it is very strong, a table-spoonful will be a sufficiently large dose for an expectorant. Dr. Beach gives the following,' as, the properties of this valuable medicine :—

"The root is efficacious in bleeding of the lungs, croup, scarlet fever, jaundice, &c. We also use it in the form of snuff for the cure of polypus in the nose, and with other articles in pulmonary diseases ; also in the form of extract; and the powdered root an escharotic in foul ulcers."

Dr. Woodruff, a Botanic physician in Orange County, N. Y., informs me that he has recently had considerable practice in malignant scarlet fever which has prevailed as an epidemic in that section, and that he has treated the disease with remarkable success by the administration of mild vegetable emetics, purgatives, and diaphoretics, but the most signal benefit was derived from the blood-root, used in the following manner : Blood-root, pulverised, twenty to thirty grains, or a level teaspoonful in half a pint of boiling water. Let it settle, strain off the clear, sweeten it with honey : dose a teaspoonful for a child from two to four years; repeat every hour if the child can bear it. If the surface gets broken wash the parts with the same infusion. The Doctor further states that the virtues of the root are too little known. He uses it in bilious, hepatic, and pulmonary affections, as an expectorant, deobstruent, tonic, and antiseptic, creating a healthy action of the biliary organs and stomach.

Dr. Wholcott says that the sanguinaria, 2 drachms of the root put to half a pint of boiling water, is highly beneficial in pneumonia, attended with the expectoration of mucus streaked with blood. It should be given after the action of a mild emetic and gentle laxative. Dose of the above infusion, a teaspoonful every two hours throughout the day. An emetic dose is 10 to 15 grains. It has lately been employed with success in cancer. Used in several of our compounds.

MOUSE-EAR (PILOSELLA).

Mouse-Ear is a low-lying herb, creeping upon the ground by small strings, like the strawberry-plant, by which it shoots forth small roots and many short leaves, set in a round form together, very hairy, which being broken give a whitish milk. From among these leaves spring up two or three small hoary stalks, about a span high, with a few smaller leaves thereon. At the tops only one flower appears, consisting of many pale yellow leaves, broad at the point and a little dented, in three or four rows, very like a dandelion flower, and reddish underneath the edges. The seeds are winged with down. Mouse-ear is a good expectorant, recommended by some herbalists in the treatment of coughs, colds, and consumption, as well as in other troubles. The juice taken in wine, or the decoction drunk, is good in jaundice, even of a chronic character, to be taken in the morning and evening, abstaining from other drink three hours after. It is a special remedy against stone and the tormenting pains thereof, and griping pains of the bowels. The decoction, with succory and centuary, is very effectual in dropsy and diseases of the spleen. It restrains fluxes of blood, either at mouth or nose, and inward bleeding also.

The green herb, bruised and bound on a cut or wound, quickly heals it. The distilled water is a good wash for wounds

HOARHOUND (MARRUBIUM VULGARE).

This well-known herb is a great favourite with herbalists. It has several well-recognised virtues, in addition to its expectorant, which is the chief. We need not describe it, as most people are familiar with it. As is said of other common mercies, "their abundance causes them to be despised." So with hoarhound. It is growing by the acre in some places in nearly every land under the heavens. There are some people who have it growing at their doors, and yet are so ignorant of its virtues that they will go about with a sore throat or cold, or they will give money for medicine that is not so good, when a judicious use of this useful herb would cure them soon.

For a sore throat get 2 ozs of the green or 1 oz. of the dry. Simmer 10 minutes in a pint of water; strain through a cloth; sweeten with honey, and take a wineglassful three to six times a day. Taken this way it is good for hoarseness, coughs, and colds. As a tonic (and it is a good one), omit the honey. In our business we gather in yearly about half a ton of this plant, and generally find it is gone before the following season. We make a saturated tincture of the green herb, which preserves its virtues and flavour even better than in the dried herb. Hoarhound is one of the ingredients in our Balm of Gilead, Herb Beer Ext., Stomach Tonic, &c.

EMMENAGOGUES

Are medicines that promote the menstrual flow when it is checked by colds, &c. In removing obstruction and subduing pain they prove a blessing to women. There is a family of plants in America commonly called cohosh. Black, blue, and white are the three varieties. They are all good for the above purposes. Our space will only allow us to describe the most important one.

BLUE COHOSH (Caulophyllum Thalictroides).

(Squaw Root).

This plant grows with a high, round stem, from one to three feet high. The leaves ore oval, two to three inches long; when young it is of a purplish colour. It is found in all parts of the United States. The root is the part used. The decoction of the dry root is one ounce to the pint; dose, a wineglassful three or four times a day. There is a controversy as to the power of this agent being an emmenagogue; but the eclectics of America who have used it for many years affirm that it has this virtue, besides others, rendering it worthy of a place in the pharmacopœia of the United States. In proof of this there is the testimony of the Indians, who call it squaw root, squaw being their name for woman. Professor P. O. Brown says it is a valuable remedy in all chronic uterine diseases, and in combination for rheumatism, epilepsy, cramps, colic, hiccough, hysteria, &c.

PENNYROYAL (Hedeoma Pelegioides.)

An old mother's remedy and a great favourite in domestic medicine. As it is generally well known we need not describe it, seeing it has also a place in the illustrations

The Pennyroyal belongs to the mint family, having their common properties, i. e., carminative, diaphoretic, stimulant, and aromatic, and besides its distinguishing one, emmenagogue. When the usual term passes (or if disposed to obstruction), a warm tea of the pennyroyal should be drunk freely, two ounces of the green a handful, or cut up the herb and fill a pint jug, cover it with boiling water, and let it stand by the fire, covered, one hour; strain and press through a cloth; drink a teacupful, sweetened, if perferred, warm up the remainder when it is taken.

A very good way is to take this mixture at bed-time, that is the whole pint, along with a foot-bath. (See baths, index). If the suppression has been the result of a recent cold, this will generally remove it, if not take a similar dose three times a day: it cannot harm you. Where it is obstinate, the corrective pills or the essence of pennyroyal should be taken. Pennyroyal is also a simple and sometimes an effective remedy for colds; sweetened well it will be found especially good for children. Combined with agrimony and marigolds it makes a good mixture for scarlatina.

TANSY (Tanacetum Vulgare).

Is another old favourite herb, which, like pennyroyal, grows in all parts of the colonies. It is not so well known as the former, therefore we will give a short description as well as a picture, which will enable our readers to identify it, seeing it is really a valuable medicine. Tansy has a perennial root, which spreads. The stem is herbaceous, green when young, but as it ripens it becomes of a brown purplish colour and somewhat woody; the leaves are feathery, and the flower small and yellow, in shape like an old china shirt button. The size of the plant is from one to two feet high. It grows wild by the sides of creeks, in paddocks, and in the bush. The top leaves and flowers are the parts used; an infusion extracts its virtues. Two ounces of the green leaves or one of the dry to the pint of boiling water, covered beside the fire one hour. Dose: One or two wineglassfuls, sweetened, three or four times a day. The cold infusion in wineglassful doses three times a day makes an excellent tonic, especially for those who are convalescent from fevers or exhausting troubles; useful also as a worm medicine. Mixed with syrup the powdered flowers destroy those parasites which infest the human system

MUGWORT (Artemisia Vulgaris).

It has various leaves lying upon the ground, much divided or cut deeply in about the brims, like wormwood, but larger, of a dark green colour on the upper side, and hoary white underneath. The stalk rises four or five feet high, having on it such leaves as those below, but smaller, and branching forth towards the top, on which small pale yellowish flowers, like buttons, appear in tufts. The root is long and hard, with

many small fibres. It grows plentifully by water-sides and
by small water courses.

MEDICINAL VIRTUES.

Mugwort removes obstructions of urine caused by stone.
A decoction is said to cure ague. The Chinese use it to cure
wounds, applying the fresh plant bruised. A drachm of the
leaves powdered was given four times a day, by Dr. Horne, to
a woman who had been affected with hysteric fits for many
years. The fits ceased in a few days. All other medicines
had failed. Being made up with lard into an ointment, it
takes away wens and kemmels that grow about the throat.
It is made more effectual by adding a few field daisies.
Three drachms of the powder or the dried leaves taken in
wine are a certain remedy for sciatica. A decoction of it
with camomile and agrimony, and the place bathed while it is
warm, takes away the pains of the sinews, and the cramps.
For fomentation, with wormwood and camomile, it is good to
soothe inflammations, and as an emmenagogue to remove
obstruction to the menses. Taken in the warm infusion it will
seldom disappoint.

RUE (Ruta Graveolens),

Being a common garden plant, requires little or no description
except to those who have been brought up in large cities, who
have not had the opportunity of seeing these domestic
medicinal plants. Rue is a herb growing from one to two
feet high. The stem rises from a continuous fibrous root, and
spreads into many branches, covered with small leaves like
mouse ears. On the tops of the stems and branches are the
small yellow flowers, very numerous. We have it growing at
Caversham, and get two crops a year off the same plants. The
herb is the medicinal part, taken in infusion, decoction, juice, or
tincture. The ancients valued it very highly for its healing
virtues. So highly was it esteemed that the Pharisee thought to
commend himself to God on account of offering it with other
herbs. (See Luke xi. 42). Some may say that the reason why it
is comparatively neglected now is because other and better have

taken its place. This we doubt, for experience has convinced us that the ancients as well as the mothers and grandmothers of the past and present generations were right in their good opinion of rue. Dr. Robinson speaks of it so highly, and gives other authors' testimony, that we think our readers may find it interesting and useful to read. "It acts as a stimulant and tonic, but in large doses it is narcotic. It is very useful in hysterics and flatulent colic. It has been found useful in infantile convulsions, and as a destroyer of worms, especially thread-worms, used as an injection. In accumulations of flatulence in the bowels (tympanitis), a strong infusion of rue given as an injection, is of great use. In suppression of menstruation, when stimulants are required, the rue clyster is of great use. Boerhaave says that mixed with wine and salt it stops gangrene, restores vitality to the part, prevents suppuration and heals the wound. Medical men sadly neglect rue as a medicinal agent. Why go to foreign lands when we have medicines at our door? A decoction of it relieves colic and all inward pains. The leaves bruised and well rubbed on the parts relieves pain, sciatica, and inflammation of the chest. Some of the ancients believed that it arrested generation. They regarded it too as anti-pestilential, and the judges had their noses regaled with this fetid plant. Mithridate, in which rue had a principal share, repelled all poison. Rue, honey, and the gall of a cock, they said, cured dimness of sight; and ointment made of the juice, lard, oil of roses, and a little vinegar, cures erysipelas, running sores on the head, and ulcers. A decoction of the herb in wine used as a gargle is good for scurvy of the gums." Yesterday we received an order for "maiden rue." It is sometimes called by this name, which suggests its use for the stoppage to which young women are sometimes subject. There are other herbs which can be used as emmenagogues; some of them we have already described under other headings, some we shall notice further on. What we have given will, if used discreetly, prove a blessing.

LITHONTRYPTICS

are a class of remedies that dissolve gravel and stone, which sometimes form in the gall-bladder, the kidneys, and the bladder. None but those who have experienced it can realise how intense is the pain caused by the passage or the attempted passage of these sometimes sharp, angular concretions. We shall point out the different kinds, and how to cure them, under the proper name in the treatment of diseases. We will now describe one or two not yet put before our readers. As prevention is better than cure a timely use of some of these will do this, as well as dissolve and expel the particles if already formed.

HEMP AGRIMONY ROOT (Eupatorium Canabinum).

This plant grows several feet high. The stems are of a dark purple colour, with many branches growing apart. The leaves are wing-shaped, and toothed at the edge. The flowers grow at the top of the branches, are of a brown-yellow colour with black spots, somewhat resembling a daisy, in the centre. The seeds are long, and stick to clothing. It grows plentifully in Europe by ditches and damp cold ground, even in water. It is late in maturing. The root has most virtue in gravelly affections. The decoction of the usual strength, a wineglassful two to six times a day. It will be needful to regulate the dose, as it sometimes causes purging. Dr. Robinson says it heals and cleanses cancers. It has cured dropsy. It makes a good poultice for inflammation of the spleen, (or as the Americans, with whom this trouble is common, call it, ague cake.) The spleen lies on the left side of the backbone, and when it is inflamed or indurated, can be felt there.

Hemp agrimony is also a vermifuge. The farmers used to give it to their cattle for cold on the lungs and broken-windedness.

THE QUEEN OF THE MEADOW

will be found described as a diuretic. It is very highly commended as a gravel remedy; so is also slippery elm (one of the demulcents.)   A case occurs to our mind of a gentleman living in Invercargill.   We had been sending him some medicine for another complaint.   He wrote asking our advice as to the best doctor we knew at operating for stone, as he said he had made up his mind to undergo an operation.   We gave him our opinion along with a quantity of slippery elm bark.   He took it for about a month.   We heard from him then, and were agreeably surprised when he told us that he did not require the operation, as his painful symptoms were gone.   Uva ursi, formerly described as diuretic, is also a lithontryptic.   In fact nearly all the diuretics are.   When the stone or gravel is of an acid nature, the carbonate of soda and potash have been used with much benefit and success.

Dr. Skelton, in his large work, from which we have already quoted, gives the first place in this class to peletory of the wall, and parsley pert, or, as the old Saxons called it, "break-stone."

NERVINES.

The doctrine of special affinities in the suitability of certain remedies to separate parts of the system is doubtless correct in the main, although some philosophers in medicine carry it too far.   One proof that may be adduced is the action of poisons. One is fatal by its action on the stomach, another on the brain, another through the blood, &c.   The class of remedies which we shall now introduce have their power over the nerves, thus they are called nervines.

VALERIAN, ENGLISH (Valeriana Officinalis)

The great wild valerian is a large, handsome plant, with a perennial, fibrous root, an erect stem, and grooved, two to four feet high. The leaves are opposite, of a feathery character, terminating in flowering branches. The flowers are rose-coloured, though sometimes almost white; they have an agreeable smell. Our picture will enable it to be identified. Is growing in most botanical gardens, and can be cultivated privately. It is worthy of a place for its looks alone. The roots are the part used in medicine. They should be collected in the spring, dried, and separated from adhering earth, then kept from the damp and air. The decoction is made in the usual way, and ordinary dose. The tincture is two ounces to the pint of proof spirit; dose, from a tea- to a table-spoonful three times a day. The powder is taken in an infusion of one teaspoonful three times a day. For all nervous troubles and sleeplessness, valerian is a good remedy. It is generally used in combination with other nervines and tonics, according to indications.

LADY'S SLIPPER (CYPRIPEDIUM PUBESCENS.)

(American Valerian).

It will be seen from our picture of this plant that its appearance has suggested its name. It grows throughout the States. Several varieties of it are found, but the one with the yellow flowers is reckoned the best. It is described as rising on a single stem, which has a horny covering. The leaves being similar, lance-shaped and bent, about four or five inches long. The flower is yellow, and in four divisions, which taper, and give the slipper-shape. The roots are the medicinal part. They come to us in the form of slender broken pieces, from the thickness of a pin to a quill; of a brown clayish colour. It has a slight aromatic smell and taste, yielding its virtues to water and spirits. It is a good nervine; some affirm that it is as strong in its sedative power as the English valerian. We sell them both and find our customers take either, finding little or no difference in them. The dose of the powdered root is a teaspoonful infused in a cup of boiling water; cover, cool, strain, sweeten if required, and drink the clear three or four times a day. There are some who take a cupful at bed-time every night to induce sleep. The eclectics make a concentrated powder by first making a saturated solution, eight ounces of the coarsely ground root to one pound of spirit infused one week. It is then subjected to strong pressure, and the liquor is shaken up with water when it becomes opaque. It is then allowed to settle, the clear is poured off, the remainder filtered and dried. It is called cypripedium. The dose is from one to five grains. As a sedative and nervine, a good substitute for opium, it is perfectly safe and can be taken in double doses.

SCULLCAP (Scutellaria Lateriflora).

This plant is a native of America. It is thus described : A small, fibrous, perennial root, an erect and very branching stem, one to three feet in height. The leaves are about an inch long, thin, sharp-pointed, and coarsely indented or toothed. The flowers are small and of a pale blue colour. It grows in damp places, by the side of ditches. The whole plant is medicinal. It ought to be gathered just as it begins to flower, dried in the shade, and kept in air-tight tins or thick brown paper. It is a valuable nervine, tonic, and anti-spasmodic, used in chorea (St. Vitus' dance), convulsive fits, delirium tremens, and all nervous affections. The infusion is one ounce to the pint, half of which is a dose. The fluid extract (which represents weight for weight of the article), is from one quarter to a teaspoonful as a dose. The powdered herb is also a good way to take it; a teaspoonful in a cup of boiling water, sweetened or otherwise. It is an ingredient in our Nerve Powder.

WOOD BETONY (Betonica Officinalis).

This is an old herb. Dr Robinson says it ought to be kept in every house. It is described thus : It has many leaves rising from the root, which are rather broad, with rounded ends and indented at the edge ; standing upon long footstalks, from which rise small horny ones with some leaves on them, and small spikes of flowers of purple colour, like lavender. The seeds are black, the roots are fibrous and white; the stalks die in winter, but the root is perennial. As we mentioned in our "History of Medicine," Antonius, physician to the Roman Emperor Augustus Cæsar, wrote a whole book on its virtues, some of which he very much exagerated. Later experience has justified some of his statements about it. We have found it good in headaches of a nervous origin. As a nervine it may be taken in infusion of one ounce to the pint, and half a teacupful may be taken three or four times a day.

The green herb cut fine and simmered in lard makes a good healing ointment for ulcers, good also for fits and bloody urine. The powdered leaves made into conserve with honey, and a teaspoonful taken is a reviver for extreme weariness and fainting spells. The steam of the decoction, received by a funnel into the ear eases pain and will assist in healing running sores. The leaves of the betony, coltsfoot, and stramonium make a good smoking mixture for difficulty of breathing.

LACTUCA (Lactuca Elongata).

The long-leaved lettuce was commonly grown in gardens as a culinary herb. There are several varieties, some of them having no medicinal virtue. The one with the long dark leaves is the kind used. When it is broken a milky juice exudes, which becomes brown. The expressed juice is evaporated at a low temperature, till it is the consistency of thick treacle. The dose of this is from one to ten grains. In reading the various writers on medicine it is found that they all agree that this extract is a good substitute for opium, without its injurious effects. The herb may be infused in boiling water and the infusion drunk freely as a mild sedative for nervous excitement. The dose of the juice would be a tablespoonful for an adult.

GENSANG ROOT (Panax Quinquefolium).

Gensang has a perennial root which sends up annually a smooth, round stem, about a foot high, and divided at the top

NERVINES. 103

into three leaf-stalks, each of which supports a compound leaf, consisting of from three to seven leaflets, oblong, sharp-pointed, and indented at the edge. The flowers are small and of a greenish colour. The root is a mild tonic, and nervine, and demulcent. The decoction, usual strength and dose. It makes a good substitute for chewing instead of tobacco.

BLACK OATS (AVENA SATIVA).

Attention has been lately called to this variety of oats as a nervine and anti-narcotic. A strong tincture has been given as a cure for the opium habit, and in some cases a cure was effected by it. Dr. Pollock, in answer to an inquiry as to his experience with this remedy, says he has used it for some time with full satisfaction. He then gives some cases which show its power.

Case 1. A lady, 30 years old, troubled with nervous prostration, inclining to paralysis. He gave her 10 drops three times a day in hot water, and 15 drops in cold water on retiring to bed. Result: In less than two weeks sleeps well and is all right.

Case 2. Woman, 56 years old, had painful ulcers two years, and took morphia to allay pain, till the habit was formed. She had also used a quart of whiskey a week. Shut off the morphia, ordered her avena. After three weeks' use she sleeps well, has no morphia or whiskey. The Doctor says he is satisfied that avena will break up the opium and whisky habit, and for a depraved condition of the nervous system he knows nothing superior. This article is good also as a food for patients who are troubled with nervousness. We recommend either a light supper of porridge or what is known in Scotland as oatmeal brose, a spoonful or two of the meal put into a basin, and half a pint of boiling water poured on, and stirred gently, so as to keep the meal in little knots. This, with a little milk and sugar added, furnishes a good light supper. (See tinctures).

FEVERFEW (PYRETHRUM PARTHENIUM.)

This herb is a very common one, found in most gardens
It has small divided leaves and flowers like daisies. It grows
about two feet high. The small flowers standing at the top of the
stem, in bunches; they are white round the edge and yellow in
the centre. It has a strong smell, rather unpleasant. Many
mistake this plant for the camomile, to which it bears some
resemblance; but the similarity is only in the flowers. The
points of difference are that the feverfew rises up in straight
stalks, with leaves attached, the size of which might average
three-quarters of an inch, very much indented. The
camomile has a moss-like leaf, spreads along the ground
without stems, and smells much pleasanter. Both are good,
but the feverfew is best as a nervine. It is especially good
for hysterical complaints. The infusion is good for profuse
menstruation and chronic inflammation of the womb. In
domestic practice a medicine for coughs may be made by
simmering an ounce in a pint of water for ten minutes, and
straining hot upon half a pound of honey. Give a tablespoonful every two hours. For delicate persons a good tonic
made of the cold infusion, a wineglassful three times a day.
The flowers alone may be dried and used instead of the
camomile, as we doubt not they are as good for fomentations.
Combine them with wormwood, southern wood, and poppies,
and you will have a good mixture for bathing sprains,
swellings, &c.

There are many other nervines, some of which we have
noticed in the foregoing classes and some we will treat in the
tonic list; there are also some in the regular medicine division,
still as in the other classes we have given the chief.

STIMULANTS.

The collection includes several well-known and highly valued spices closely related to carminatives, yet not included under that head. They may be called the whip and spur to jaded nature, very good when required, but hurtful if long continued or taken when the system needs the opposite treatment. They are useful in certain kinds of dyspepsia, sore throats, debility, low fevers, &c.

Leading in this class is

CAYENNE PEPPER (Capsicum).

There are several kinds in the market; the large and long pods are grown in temperate climates, and while hardly ripe are used in pickles, to which they give an improved value; the smaller kinds are grown in hot countries. Of all the varieties the African Bird pepper, as it is called, is the best, and the one used by herbalists. Being an important medicine we will give an illustration of it. Samuel Thompson was the first to use and make known cayenne pepper as a medicine. He gave it freely, along with other remedies, to equalise the circulation, and thus remove obstruction, which is the first thing that ought to be attended to in treating the generality of troubles. Thompson, like most men, was not perfect. In his theory of fevers he affirms that the superabundant heat is only on the outside of the body (the clinical thermometer, as far as we know, was not invented in his early days, if even in his latter), so he gave cayenne to raise up the internal heat and reduce the outer. Although he was somewhat in error in his theory, yet he was most successful in his practice. At his time the regulars acted on the absurd adage (common then), viz.: "feed a cold and starve a fever;" he nearly reversed the treatment of both, especially the latter. The usual time in fevers was then 21 days, till what is called the crisis came, then another month recovering. Thompson generally brought the patients out of bed in a couple of days, and had them well in a week. His treatment, the steaming feeding process, was soon adopted by other progressive men on both sides of the Atlantic. It is said of a very successful doctor in London who when dying was asked what he would have on his tombstone, he replied, "only these words, I have fed fevers." That was the secret of his success. Now that cayenne is found in nearly all the text books, doctors are beginning to use it. Although acting on the doctrine of contraries, some of them decry its use in inflammation of the brain or some of the organs. It seems to us that their objection is very unreasonable. If we take, for instance, apoplexy, which is caused by an overflow of blood to the head, and becomes fatal when the vessels of the brain are engorged and congested ; it is not theory but actual practice that a half-teaspooonful of cayenne given in a little warm water sweetened, causing a heat in and stimulating the stomach, has lessened the blood pressure in the head and restored the patient. It is often said that a little knowledge is a dangerous thing. This may be true in some respects, but we think that even a little medical knowledge is good if it keeps people from following old and injurious customs. The temperance cause has helped to abolish the custom, which was to fly to spirits in all kinds of emergencies, as accidents, sudden pains. Many a time schemers have got a drink on the cheap from the false idea that it was a panacea for all ills. We have known of men doubling themselves up, rolling on the floor for a glass of whiskey. A complete cure for all that sort of thing is to substitute cayenne pepper as the stimulant *par excellence* for all who really need one; especially in fits, cramps, spasms, &c. The general opinion found in standard works on Materia Medica is that it stands first as a pure stimulant. Taken into the stomach it imparts a glow of heat which ramifies through the system, or as some express it, even to the tips of the toes. We remember reading of a young married lady who was foolish enough to ask a young brother-in-law, who professed to have some knowledge of medicine, for a cure for her cold feet, especially in church. He

told her to sprinkle some cayenne in her stocking before going.
She did so, and that day the meeting was interrupted by the
hasty withdrawal of the lady, followed by her husband;
the young villain who caused this joke having a hard time of
it to suppress his risibility. The young lady must have felt it
rather hot to be comfortable. Speaking of cayenne again we
must confess that some herbalists are a little too much in love
with it. In reading over their treatment of disease you will
almost invariably find a half to a teaspoonful put into all
mixtures. We hardly think this is justified in all cases, as in
prescribing care should be taken with each individual one,
and stimulants given or withheld as indications justify. Dose
of cayenne by itself is from five to thirty grains; an ingredient
in many compounds.*

GINGER (ZINZIBER).

This well-known root is a general favourite. It is grown
abundantly in China, India, and warm countries. A description
of the plant may be interesting. It has a biennial or perennial
tuberous root, and an annual stem which rises two or three
feet in height, is solid, round, erect, and inclosed in an
imbricated membraneous sheathing. The leaves are lance-
shaped, smooth, five or six inches long by an inch in breadth,
and stand alternately on the sheath of the stem. The flower-
stalk rises by the side of the stem, from six inches to a foot,
and is clothed with oval acuminate sheaths, but without
leaves, and terminates in a spike. The flowers are of a
dingy yellow colour and appear two or three at a time. The
roots are exported green or dried and bleached. We prefer
the dried root, as it has not been impaired in the process of

* Some of our critical readers may think that we are a little
contradictory, seeing that under the head of diuretics we cautioned
against stimulating an inflamed organ. We do not recommend stimulating
the inflamed one, but equalising the circulation, which will so far take
the stimulation from the point of danger; still there is no rule but has its
exception. Here is one or two: an inflamed sore throat is benefited by
gargling with cayenne in infusion or tincture; chronic inflammation of
the stomach is another form of trouble often removed or relieved by it.

bleaching. Ginger ranks next to cayenne as a stimulant; it is also a carminative and aromatic, and may be taken with safety and advantage in almost any trouble. The chief indications for its use are flatulance, pain in the stomach and bowels, indigestion, enfebled circulation. It is an excellent addition to bitter medicines, imparting to them an agreeable flavour and a warming sensation, which is grateful to the stomach. When chewed it produces heat and a large amount of saliva from the glands; on this account it will be found beneficial in a relaxed condition of the organs in the mouth and throat. Dr. Coffin strongly recommends it in consumption and for those who are accustomed to speak or sing in public. His custom was to put a piece in his mouth after lecturing, which he did very often. The dose of the powder is 10 to 20 grains crude or in infusion. A good way is to steep a ¼ of an ounce in a pint of boiling water. After stirring let it stand covered for half an hour, strain, sweeten, and take from a quarter to the whole; children much less. We make a strong tincture, which will be found a very good and handy preparation; dose : ½ to a teaspoonful in water, sweetened when required. In our compounds ginger will be found in many mixtures.

CARYOPHYLLUS (Aromaticus).

This plant is one of the most elegant of those inhabiting the isles of India. It has a pyramidal form, is always green, and is adorned throughout the year with a succession of beautiful rosy flowers. The stem is of hard wood, and covered with smooth greyish bark. The leaves are about four inches in breadth, and two in length; oval, long, sharp at both ends, with many parallel veins on each side, supported on long foot stalks and opposite. They have a firm consistence, and a shining green colour, and when bruised are highly fragrant. The flowers are arranged in clusters, and exhale a strong penetrating odour. It appears that the ancients did not know of the cloves. The first that we can learn of them was their introduction into Europe by the Arabs. Now they are exported in immense quantities from India, east and west. We presume our readers are all acquainted with the shape and colour of them. They are the unexpanded flowers of the tree. The clove is amongst the most stimulating of aromatics, but its stimulant quality can hardly be reckoned as diffusive, as it will generally be noticed that the pungency imparted is felt most in the mouth. However, they are valuable in some forms of trouble,—sick stomach, flatulency, gout, dyspepsia. The infusion of the powder is probably the best way to take it. A teaspoonful to a pint of boiling water, pour off the clear, sweeten and drink about a wineglassful. For a dose from 5 to 10 grains of the powder may be taken in substance. The essential oil is much used as a cure for toothache; also in combination for perfumes. This is another ingredient of the Composition and Stomach Bitters.

CAMPHOR (CAMPHORA).

This gum is obtained from a tree which is a native of China, Japan, and Eastern Asia. It is described as an evergreen of considerable size, with straight trunk below, but divided above with many branches, which are covered with a smooth greenish bark. The leaves stand on long foot-stalks, which are lance-shaped, smooth, and shining, with well-marked veins. Their colour is a greenish yellow on their upper surface, pale on the under, and two to three inches long. The flowers are small and white, arranged in clusters, standing on spikes. The fruit is a red berry, resembling that of the cinnamon. The leaves and all parts smell strongly of the camphor. The gum is separated by the following process :— The roots and branches are cleaned, cut into chips, and placed in a little water in large iron vessels, which have large earthen lids of dome-shape. This is filled with rice straw. A moderate heat is applied. The camphor condenses on the straw. Then it is melted and strained out. The gum runs into moulds of various shapes. As it is found in chemists' shops, it has been subject to another process of refining. This is done in the wholesale laboratories of Europe and America. The crude camphor is mixed with lime, and distilled over into bell-shaped rings and square cakes from one ounce up. Camphor is a diffusive stimulant in small doses, and it is also a safe one, exciting the heart's action, producing perspiration, and an exalted feeling. In immoderate doses it causes nausea, vomiting, anxiety, faintness, dizziness, convulsions, and probably death, as one case of poisoning by it has been recorded. It is largely employed by the faculty as a stimulant and corrective of griping cathartics ; also for its sedative qualities, being the chief ingredient in a comp. tinc. (paregoric.) In this form it enters into mixtures for coughs and colds. The dose of the crude is five to fifteen grains, given in pills, mixtures, &c. It is reckoned useful in hysteria, epilepsy, cramp, melancholia, gout, and acute rheumatism. As a strong liniment, one ounce dissolved in two ounces spirits of wine, and rubbed in, has been found good. Good also in rheumatic tumours, numbness, paralysis, and gangrene. The camphor water is made by putting about an ounce, broken into small pieces, in a pint of water. Dose a tablespoonful. Used in several compounds.

PRICKLY ASH (XANTHOXYLUM FRAXINEUM).

This is a shrub growing plentifully in America. Its height is from ten to fifteen feet. The branches are covered with prickles. The outside is of a yellow tinge ; the inside white. When chewed it is warm and aromatic, stimulating the salivary glands. When swallowed it is felt to impart warmth to the stomach, which diffuses through the system, increasing the pulse, and promoting perspiration. It has been well tried as a remedy for rheumatism ; so that in some parts it is called the rheumatic bush. The bark is the medicinal part for this purpose. The berries, which follow the small greenish flowers, are of a greenish red colour, and have an aperient and tonic property, useful in indigestion. An infusion of the bark taken inwardly, and the powder dusted on venereal ulcers, is recommended by Dr. Coffin. Chewing the bark is said to cure toothache. It has also been found good for paralysis. To make the decoction, simmer one ounce of the bark in three pints of water down to two. Take one to two tablespoonfuls four times a day. Begin with the smallest dose. An external application for rheumatism is prepared by adding an ounce of the powdered bark to four ounces of hot olive oil, and the affected parts rubbed well for at least five minutes, or better, ten ; rub gently downward.

HORSE RADISH (Cochlearia Armorica.)

The root is well-known everywhere, as it is a very hardy plant. Once into a garden it looks after itself. Although it is principally used as a condiment, it has good stimulant qualities, but not so lasting as any of the foregoing, being very volatile. Dr. Robinson's account of it is very good and temperate. He recommends the root to be grated, and applied instead of mustard in cases of rheumatic pains, hardening of the liver, spleen, and sciatica. It is a very good thing for hoarseness. We have given it, and can assure our readers of its virtue in this complaint. Scrape about a tablespoonful, infuse it in a pint covered vessel for half an hour, strain, sweeten with honey, if you can get it, if not, sugar. Swallow a dessert spoonful slowly every one or two hours. It makes a good article of diet for people subject to asthma, flatulency, and dropsy.

MUSTARD SEEDS (Sinapis).

There are two varieties of the mustard, white and black. The black seeds ground make the common condiment present at nearly all tables when meat is taken. It aids digestion in this form, as it stimulates the stomach and salivary glands. Made into poultice we are nearly all familiar with its irritant qualities. While there are some that decry all such applications to the skin as simply so much useless torture, affirming that the same end could be obtained by an application of boiling water applied carefully, yet the experience of several generations is that pain is alleviated, and often completely removed, by a mustard plaster, not kept on too long; if this is done it may leave behind a worse pain than it takes away. There is an oil expressed from the crushed seeds which is seldom seen or used now, but the distilled oil is one of the most pungent in existence; the smell of it is sufficient to knock a man down, and rubbed on the skin it will blister quickly. As a liniment for rheumatism and neuralgia, one fourth of it to three fourths of olive oil is highly recommended. The white mustard seeds are milder than the other. A teaspoonful swallowed is, it is confidently affirmed by some of our customers, a cure for rheumatism. There is no question but that it will raise the inward heat, and act as a good stimulant.

BLACK PEPPER (Piper Nigrum).

Another good stimulant, can be used as a substitute for cayenne. Double the dose. This article, in combination with elecampane, liquorice, fennel seeds, and senna, all in powder, made into a paste with treacle, and a teaspoonful taken in the morning, is good for piles. At one time it was used for intermittent fevers, but it is not much in favour as a febrifuge now. The dose is five to thirty grains in warm water, sweetened. As a carminative it is also good.

We will close the division with the great, but we must say much misused, alcohol. The evil which this inflammable liquor has wrought is beyond the power of mortal man to describe. Some temperance orators have affirmed that war, pestilence, famine, fever, accidents, all combined, have not destroyed more of the human race than this agent of destruction. We think the man that first found out the process of abstracting alcohol from fermented liquor, had he even dreamed of the evil consequences of the discovery, would have destroyed his still, and kept the secret hid in his bosom for ever. It is not our purpose to speak of the sufferings of starving wives and children, and the myriads of souls that have found at last a drunkard's grave. This, we all admit, springs from the abuse of spirits. That there is a use for it few will deny, but one thing is certain, that there are fearful odds against its use on the side of its abuse. Taking the most hopeful view of the temperance cause, we do not think it will succeed in abolishing the liquor traffic. At the same time we wish it God-speed, and are certain that as in the past so in the future it will carry its conquests in every land, and thus become a helper in the salvation of our race. However much some men may discount the value of the doctors, it must be conceded that they have a power over popular sentiment for good and evil. Their folly in the past has had a good deal to do with the pernicious drinking customs of the people. Many and many a one has blamed the doctors for making them drunkards. A man or woman, not having attended to the laws of health, feels languid and out of sorts. The family doctor is consulted, who, not finding anything much the matter with them, prescribes a stimulant, and as he knows they have an aversion to bitters, he writes " spiritus vinum Gallic." brandy, or some such spurious stimulant. The languid one likes the false stimulation given, which, however, is only temporary, and has to be repeated and repeated till the habit is formed, which is not improperly termed the devil's chain. We read an account of a lady in our native land who fell, after the above example, and came to a terrible end through it Her husband, who was a business man in a well-to-do position, was nearly heart-broken. One day he took the children to the coast for holidays. That night an old nurse, who was also an old drinker, spent a convivial evening with her. Whisky was drunk with such relish that both became drunk, and it is supposed upset the lamp. This is conjecture, but the following morning a heap of ruins was found, in the midst of which were the charred bodies of the unfortunate women. We should not like to be the doctor that started that woman on the downward course. But enough of moralizing. Spirits of wine, pure, are poison, if taken in over doses and undiluted. However, custom has so hardened some human beings' throats that a wineglassful of methelated spirits (enough to poison a horse) can be swallowed. The sensation caused by this fiery liquid passing over the mucous membrane of the throat has been said to be like a saw going down. We might ask, why on earth do men

take it? Why, for the stimulation it gives to their diseased
stomach, and because taken in small doses it imparts a warm
glow to the mouth, throat, and stomach, but only for a very
short time. It flies to the head. This can be understood
from its nature. Being volatile, the heat of the stomach
sends it upwards to the brain, which becoming (if much is
taken) sur-charged, the cerebrum or large brain, the seat of
consciousness and ideas, is confused, and the cerebellum,
(smaller brain), which is the seat of motion, being stupefied, the
legs are unable to carry the body with their wonted steadiness;
thus furnishing one of the inspired prophets with an
illustration of the earth under the wrath of the Almighty.
Jeremiah says : " The earth shall reel to and fro and stagger
like a drunken man." The stomach is the part most injured by
spirit-drinking. It first becomes inflamed, then congested, and
ultimately ulcerated. The brain next is diseased, and loss of
moral character and self-control follow in the order of ruin.
These are the abuses. Now what is the use of spirits in
medicine? We were about to quote Solomon's advice, viz. :
" Give strong drink to him that is ready to perish ; " but we
remember that spirits, as such, had no existence for 1800 years
after his time, for the process of distillation was only discovered
about the 12th century, by an Arabian named Gebar, so the
wise man's advice only referred to the milder intoxicants. But we
may apply them and give spirits in extraordinary cases to tide
men over critical times of trouble. Given only when needed, as
medicine little harm would be done Spirits have a strong
solvent property in dissolving out the medicinal properties
of gum, seeds, and for making essences and perfumes.
On this account they are useful; also in the arts and
manufactures ; varnishes, polishes, &c., owe their existence
to them. Probably our readers think they have had enough
of spirits at this time. Our advice to all is to take them only
in the form of medicine, for it is not safe to do otherwise.
Cures for alcoholism will be found under that name in the index,
which see.

SIALAGOGUES.

This is another class of remedies, that act on the salivary glands, stimulating them to secrete and discharge the saliva. As we have already noticed the principal ones, we will only name them now in their order of merit. These are:—

Prickly Ash Bark
Calamas Root
Cayenne Pepper
Lobelia Herb
Ginger
Stillingia Root

The indications for their use are fevers, inflammation, a dry and parched condition of the tongue and throat, and in the very rare affection, paralysis of the tongue.

TONICS.

This is the most numerous class of remedies that we have, required in most complaints, and especially in convalescence from acute disease, or when the system needs building up. Dr. Coffin in one of his lectures objects to the term tonic as not indicating the way in which these medicines improve the system, He affirms that they correct the digestive organs, improve their assimilating powers, then the food tones and builds up the body: the butcher and the baker furnish the true tonics. As it is not worth while to fall out with the ordinary name, we will call them tonics nevertheless.

The first in this list is a beautiful little plant, found in several parts of New Zealand and Australia, that is the

CENTAURY (Eyrthraea Centaurim).

Our artist has given a very good picture of it. It has long
been esteemed a very good tonic by the regulars, as can be seen
by looking up the Edinburgh Pharmacopœia. It yields its bitter
principle to water and spirit. The infusion or decoction is an
ounce to the pint; a wineglassful three or four times a day. In
cases of debility, indigestion, biliousness, chronic liver complaint, want of appetite, the centaury will be found a
beneficial medicine. The plant is an annual, flowers late in
summer, and is found growing wild in grass paddocks.

AMERICAN CENTAURY (Sabbatia Angularis).

The American Centaury is like the European, an annual
or biennial herbaceous plant, with a fibrous root and an
erect, smooth, four-sided stem, winged at the angles, simple
below, sending off branches above. The leaves, which
vary considerably in length, are single, oval, and entire,
smooth, embracing half the circumference of the stem at the
base. The flowers are white, numerous, growing on the ends
of the branches, and forming together a large terminal spike.
The virtues of the American centuary are almost identical
with the other, both being simply tonics. The infusion is
the usual way of taking it, one ounce to the pint; dose, a
wineglassful. The tincture, two ozs. to the pint; dose, from
a tea- to a tablespoonful three or four times a day.

GILANGAL ROOT.

Two varieties are described by authors—large and small.
According to Dr. Hance the small gilangal is derived from a
closely allied plant, called Alpina officinalarum. Both forms
are brought from the West Indies. The larger variety is
cylindrical, three or four inches long, as thick or often thicker
than a man's thumb; often forked; reddish-brown externally;
marked with whitish rings or orange brown internally; rather
hard and fibrous; hard to powder; of an agreeable aromatic
odour, and a pungent, hot, spicy, permanent taste. The small

gilangal resembles the preceding in taste, but is smaller, not exceeding the little finger in thickness, of a darker colour and of a stronger taste and smell.

This root, as a tonic, is very valuable in dyspepsia, accompanied with an engorgement of the veins and sluggish circulation. It is highly recommended for piles by those who have well tested it for that ailment. Many of our readers will remember the lady' doctor, Madame Duflôt, and her husband. When they came to Dunedin, before they opened their show in the golden chariot, they came into our shop and asked for some gilangal root in powder. This being the first time we were asked for it in that form, we did not have any in stock, but ground it for them. They said they could take fifty pounds of it. Soon afterwards we got some of their celebrated Dyspeptic Powder, and examining it carefully we found the gilangal was its chief ingredient, the other leading article in it being powdered aloes. No doubt it was a good mixture, but while it cost them about a penny a box, they sold it for 1s. 6d. We have often been asked what we thought of them, especially the woman. We replied that the wonderful cures she seemed to make were greatly due to her magnetic power, imparted to her patients by long rubbing, assisted by the liniment, which was a very good mixture of cloves, peppermint, glycerine, and spirits; but alas like most human cures they were not permanent. We scarcely know of one who was permanently benefited by the lady doctor. But returning to gilangal root, we must rank it as one of the best tonics. For the decoction one ounce bruised root to the pint ; powdered, one teaspoonful to the cup; a wineglassful of the former, and a half cup of the latter three times a day.

GOLD THREAD (Coptis Trifolia).

The root of the creeping plant, gold thread, is slender, and of a bright yellow colour. The leaves, which stand on slender footstalks, have a sharp-toothed margin, and a smooth-veined surface The flower stem is slender, round, rather longer than the leaves, and surmounted by one small white flower. The gold thread inhabits the northern regions of America and Asia, and is found in Greenland and Iceland. This is a valuable medicine for a stomach tonic. Professor Brown strongly recommends a mixture of one ounce of it with one ounce of golden seal, mixed into a decoction, with a quart of boiling water. Add one ounce to two ounces of elixir vitrol, and you have a medicine that if persevered with will take away the craving for alcoholic drinks. We might say the same of any other tonics. Add sufficient cayenne to give them pungency, and with a desire on the part of the drinker for a cure, the stomach will be brought back to a natural condition, and the craving allayed The gold thread cannot be excelled as a tonic to restore patients who, having passed through the acute stage, are suffering a recovery (as it is sometimes put.) To make it as palatable as possible, while conserving its tonic property, we would recommend the following :—

Gold thread	1 oz.
Ginger	¼ oz.
Cinnamon	¼ oz.
Sugar	2 ozs.
Boiling Water	1 pint.

Infuse one hour.

Strain, press through a cloth, and take from a half to a wineglassful three times a day. But if the weather is warm, it will be needful to fortify the mixture. This can be done by using one oz. each of the tinctures of ginger and cinnamon instead of the ¼-ounce crude.

SNAKE ROOT (SERPENTARIA ARISTOLCHIA).

This species of aristolchia is an herbaceous plant, with a perennial root, which consists of numerous slender fibres proceeding from a short horizontal head. Several stems often rise from the same root. They are about eight or ten inches in height, slender, round, jointed at irregular distances, and frequently reddish or purple at the base. The leaves are oblong, heart-shaped, pointed, of a pale yellowish green colour, and supported on long slender round peduncles, which are sometimes furnished with one or two small scales, and bend downwards so as to nearly bury the flowers in the earth or decayed leaves. The plant grows in rich shady woods in the United States of America. It is a very strong bitter. The Indians used it before the time of Columbus, and was given by them as a remedy for the bite of the rattlesnake. Formerly it had a reputation for curing pleurisy and other inflammatory conditions when the blood is loaded with fibrine ; being a grand tonic it is indicated in low vitality of the system, scurvy, indigestion, fevers, &c. The decoction is pre pared by boiling a ½ ounce of the bruised root in a pint of water for 10 to 20 minutes. Dose : from half to a wineglass three times a day. Smaller doses may be given with advantage to weak children troubled with worms.

CASCARILLA.

Cascarilla is the bark of a shrub from three to five feet high. The stem is white, and marked at intervals with white or grayish stains. The leaves are toothed, from two to three inches in length, and by an inch or more in breadth, often somewhat heart-shaped at the base, pale or grayish-green above, and densely covered beneath with shining silvery scales, appearing white a a distance. The shrub is a native of the Bahamas, and grows in abundance in Andios, Long, and Eleutheria Islands. The bark is intensely bitter, a strong tonic. Half an ounce in a pint of boiling water will make a useful medicine for impaired appetite in doses of a wineglassful three or four times a day. There is one peculiarity about this bark, it gives off a pleasant odour when it is burned. We sell it to smokers to perfume their pipes. One of its chief uses is that of making incense. If you want to fill a room with its sweet smell, burn about a teaspoonful of the powder slowly, and keep in the smoke. In the course of a year we import about 300 lbs. of the bark. See index for price list of all goods.

QUASSIA WOOD (QUASSIA AMARA).

The wood of this tree is another intensely bitter tonic, much used in regular practice. It was discovered by a negro, named Quassia, whose name it bears. So strong is the bitter principle in it that cups turned out of its wood, if filled with water and left standing a short time, give a very decided bitter drink. As they get used they have to stand the longer. The decoction is a half ounce to the pint; dose: a wineglassful three times a day. Tincture, two ounces to the pint; dose: one or two teaspoonfuls in water. The tincture is about the only one that will unite with the tincture of iron without becoming black.

BARBARY BARK (BARBARY VULGARIS).

This bush is not unlike the gooseberry. It has the same kind of thorny branches and small notched leaves; however it has flowers which are yellow, followed by red berries. The berries are pleasant acidulous, slightly astringent, used on the Continent as a drink in fevers and diarrhœa, and preserved as jam for table use. The shrub is growing in our city. It attains a height sometimes of 12 feet. In those places where it is cultivated for commerce, long hedges are planted like our hawthorn. The bark is cut off in long or short strips, which are again cut in pieces of an inch or two. Its colour is grey outside, yellow inside. Dr. Coffin, with whom this was a great favourite, says that he made a tincture of it, and compared it with one of bullock's gall. He found them in taste, smell, and colour, almost identical. Reasoning from this fact that the barbary must be a good liver medicine, he prescribed it freely, and was well satisfied with the results. Some of our customers have told us that they were cured of the jaundice by an infusion of the bark and twigs. There can be no doubt but that it is a valuable liver as well as tonic medicine. The usual decoction, infusion, and tincture, the active principle called Berberine is used, in doses of from three to ten grains for the above purpose. The bark was formerly used as a dye; it made a beautiful yellow.

CHAMOMILE FLOWERS (Anthemis Nobilis)

Are a universal favourite as a stomachic and tonic, useful in indigestion and debility, and as a tonic in fevers, &c. A fomentation and poultice, made by boiling an ounce in a pint of water, is very good in painful swellings, and to hasten the maturing of abscesses. The infusion may be made with an ounce to the pint or quart. Dose : a wineglass of the first, and two of the last; of the powdered flower, 10 to 20 grains ; of the essential oil, one to four drops ; solid extract, five to ten grains.

WHITE POPLAR BARK (Populus Tremuloides).

The bark of the white poplar tree has long been used by herbalists as a tonic. The ancients, as far back as the beginning of our era were well acquainted with it. Galen affirmed that it had a cleansing property, while Dioscorides, another old medico, says it will cure sciatica and strangury. The buds, which later on become the leaves, mashed with honey, are good for coughs, sore throats, hoarseness. &c. ; and according to Dr. Robinson this conserve is good for dull sight. The leaves bruised and pressed give out the juice, which, when warmed and a few drops put into the ear, eases earache. The white poplar bark makes as good a tonic as the celebrated quinine, one ounce to the pint. Dose : a wineglassful three or four times a day. The black poplar tree may be distinguished from the white by its being straighter in the stem and higher. Its leaves are broad and smooth at the edge, while those of the white are toothed and paler on the under side. The unexpanded buds, when simmered in lard or fresh butter, or better still, vaseline, make a very good healing ointment for fresh wounds, inflamed sores, and as a plaster to prevent the secretion of milk in the breasts. The seeds in decoction are recommended in epilepsy. The bark of the black is recommended by Dr. Coffin in the cure of dropsy ; usual decoction. The powder of the white enters into the Stomach Bitters, and various compounds.

PERUVIAN BARK (CINCHONA).

There are several varieties of this popular tonic and febrifuge, all of which may be passed over except the three principal kinds. The red comes to us in quills and flat pieces. Both are derived from different parts of the same tree—the one from the bark and larger branches, the other from the small branches. It is of a red colour internally, grayish outside. It has a bitter taste and the familiar smell of good bark. When boiled it yields a salmon-coloured, turbid decoction. The history of the discovery of its medicinal qualities is interesting. The wife of one of the Spanish governors lay dying of a fever; the doctors were powerless to save her; all their known remedies had failed. One of her husband's retainers had heard of a man who was cured by drinking the water out of a pool into which some of the branches of this medicinal tree had fallen. The decoction or infusion was given, with the result of a speedy cure. Her name (Cinchona) was given to the bark. Soon after, as she gave great quantities to the Jesuits, who administered it to the sick with success, it was also called Jesuit bark. It was introduced into Europe about the end of the sixteenth century. Since then it has gained a world-wide fame. Dr. Coffin, who was no friend to the faculty, seems to crow over the fact that the doctors did not discover this medicine. (We do not think the modern doctors has found out any of the herbal medicines, for the simple reason that they do not look for them.) However, our thanks for this and every other valuable medicine are due not to the discoverer but to the Creator, who gives us all good things.

The red Peruvian bark is the kind from which the most and probably the best quinine is made. The simplest way it is prepared is by adding acid to the infusion or decoction, then an alkali, so as to neutralise both. The salts are purified and dried, then we have the white powder, quinine, which at one time was sold weight for weight of gold. It may have been that its preparation being a secret made it so valuable. What a wonderful reduction has taken place in it since then, as the present wholesale price in London is about 2/- per ounce. Another reason for its famous price at one time was its fashionableness. Doctors prescribed it for everything. We heard an account of how the United States' Army doctors, during the Civil War, carried out this routine treatment. One soldier, who was ill, said it was no use going to the doctor, who simply gave one prescription. It was arranged among 20 men, who were on the sick list, to compare their prescriptions before getting them dispensed. They did so, and on each was written " Spiritus fermenti cum quinnun mixturia," which in plain English is whisky and quinine mixture. Some years ago it was found out that this good drug was being abused, especially in prescribing it for indigestion and stomach troubles, for which it is given too often now. Bitters are very good for the stomach, but it rebels against too much of a good thing, especially when it is not a natural product. In short, quinine is far too concentrated a bitter for the stomach. The decoction of the bark is quite strong enough for ordinary mortals, and like Dr. Coffin we question whether the discovery of quinine has been any benefit to the human race. In the southern States it seems to be next door to a failure in that dreadful scourge—yellow fever. One night's frost will do more good than a ton of it, has been the usual experience during epidemics. While in New York we came in contact with some old doctors who would swear by quinine in malarial fevers, which are sometimes, or always more or less difficult to diagnose. They said, if you don't know that the trouble is malarial fever give quinine, and if it is it will cure, if not it is some other disease. Quinine will be noticed in the regular medicine list.

THE YELLOW CALISAYA BARK,

which is a good tonic medicine, is used as a substitute for the red. Some affirm that it is better. The general opinion, in which we agree, is that both are alike good, and can be used for the same purpose. The decoction is an ounce to the pint, infusion the same. The powder can be taken crude or infused, and the clear only drunk. It is much used to put into wine, an ounce to a quart bottle, the dose being a wineglassful three times a day. The tincture is made simple and compound. The simple is four ounces to a pint of proof spirit, macerate a week, press, strain, and make up to a pint. The dose is one to two teaspoonfuls, three times a day. The compound is made up of the following :—

Red Peruvian Bark .... 2 ounces.
Bitter Orange Peel, cut .... 1 ounce.
Snake Root .... ½ ounce.
Saffron .... 55 grains.
Cochineal .... 28 grains.
Proof Spirit .... 1 pint.

Prepared same as former. Dose same also.

UNICORN ROOT (Helonias Dioica).
(Common names : Starwort, False Unicorn, Devil's Bit, &c.)

This plant has acquired a good reputation as an internal tonic, especially valuable in female debility. It exerts a power over kidneys, bladder, and generative organs. In all chronic diseases of these parts, where there is a tendency to miscarriage, the unicorn root will be found beneficial ; also in chronic inflammation of the stomach, known by the rejection of food and medicine. It will often be tolerated when other tonics are thrown off. The decoction of the bruised root is one ounce to the pint. The powder in infusion may be taken a teaspoonful to the cup of boiling water. It has been found that spirits extract its properties best. A tincture of two ounces to the pint. Dose: one to two teaspoonfuls three times a day.

BARBERIES AQUIFOLIUM.
This is another good tonic, of American origin. It has also an alterative quality, and is used by the eclectics as a blood purifier in cases where a tonic is also needed. The directions and dose same as last.

COLOMBO ROOT
is a well-known tonic used by all schools of medicine in weak conditions of the stomach and digestive organs. Used in the ordinary way and ordinary doses.

BALMONY (Chelonin Glabra).

The plant bearing this name is sometimes called snake head, thistle bloom, and salt rheum weed. It grows plentifully in America, where it is highly esteemed as a tonic, stomachic and vermifuge. As we deem it a very valuable herb, we intend to try and acclimatise it. We give a picture of it, so there is no need to supply a verbal description. The leaves are the part used. Decoction : one ounce to the pint. In powder they form the chief ingredient in the Stomach Bitters Powder. For worms in children, about a fourth of a teaspoonful in treacle, jam, or water, three or four mornings, followed with a purge, will be found generally effective. The decoction in wineglassfuls three or four times a day, with a dose of the worm pills at bedtime, is a good vermifuge treatment for adults.

BOGBEAN (Meganthus Trifoliata).

(Or Buckbean.)

This is a perennial plant growing in damp and marshy places. While in bloom it is one of those beautiful wild flowers that abound in Europe and America. It grows about a foot high. There are three leaves on each stalk, which are strong, round, and smooth. The leaves are oblong; the flowers small, white, and tinged with purple; the plant bearing a strong resemblance to our garden bean. The leaves are generally the only part used in Britain, but the Americans use also the root, which has the same properties, the chief of which is tonic, then antiscorbutic, astringent, and antiseptic, and in large doses purgative. Some of the German doctors affirm that it cures the worst forms of the ague. Haller says that intermittent fevers yield to it. In one of the German wars it was used with success instead of Peruvian bark. In malarial districts it is most providential that such a good medicine grows abundantly. We commend an infusion of the leaves for any one whose health is bad from want of appetite, and whose food does not seem to do them any good. It is a good and efficient blood medicine In skin

complaints, perseverance with it will prove its true value.
Preparation and dose as usual.

We will close our list of tonics as well as the other classes
with a recent introduction into the Materia Medica,

COCA LEAVES (Erythoxylon Coca)

Used by West Indians as a kind of stimulant, which enables
them to do long journeys without food, and to bear severe
fatigue by simply chewing the leaves. The plant is cultivated
in large plantations in Bolivia, South America. It grows in
the form of a bush from four to six feet high, and about
three feet in diameter. Its foliage is a bright green; its
flowers white; its fruit small and red. The young plants are
raised from seed sown in beds and transplanted. When about
18 months old, they commence plucking the leaves, which
are very carefully dried in the sun, packed in bales, and
exported. Dr. Albert Hamann of Goslar was the first to
separate the active principle, called Cocoaine, which is a most
remarkable and powerful local anæsthetic, (that is, when
applied to the mucous membrane or injected into the skin it
takes away all feeling). We have seen a few drops put into
the eye, and in five moments' time the oculist was able to
cut open the ball, take out the dim lens, close up the wound,
and the patient not feel it, thus doing away with the previously existing necessity of chloforming the patient, which
usually took an hour to recover from, and sometimes causing
death.

The leaves may be chewed as a stimulant, but the
decoction is preferable where the tonic effect is desired. The
fluid extract is also a convenient form to take it in. As a
substitute for the common tea it could be used in the infusion
of half an ounce to the pint, sweetened and with milk. In
this form it will act as a nerve tonic, but we would not
recommend it to be used continually, as it might in that case
undo all the good which an occasional use might do. When
the end is accomplished for which any medicine is taken,

reason teaches us to leave it off, or if not, it becomes an article of food instead of a medicine. In combination with other tonics and astringents it is highly beneficial in nervous debility, seminal weakness, &c.

In the foregoing pages we have briefly pointed out the prominent medicinal plants. There are many others, which time and space prevent us from describing at any length, but in order to bring a comparatively complete list under the eye of the reader, we will adopt the alphabetical catalogue, with abbreviated properties and doses, given by Dr. Dale of Glasgow, adding to it a few recent additions since his time.

AN ALPHABETICAL LIST OF SIMPLES USED IN THE BOTANIC PRACTICE.

In the following list of Simples, we have endeavoured to give at a glance the most common English and Botanical name of each plant, together with its chief properties indicated by abbreviations (*which see*), and as brief and clear an account of its general uses as possible to be given in so much space.

In order to save space we will add our price list for ounce lots. Discount on ¼lb., 10 to 25 per cent.; 25 to 50 on 1lb.; trade parcels, special quotations.

Inf., Infusion, is a simple preparation of an Herb or Bark, either in its *cr.*, crude, or *pulv.*, powdered state. Pulverizing, or powdering, is effected by simple grinding in a mill. To infuse, put one ounce of Herb, if crude, in a pint imperial of boiling water, cover it over, and let it stand to keep hot from fifteen minutes to two hours, and strain.

Dose—a wineglassful from two to six times a day.

If the Herb is pulverized, a teaspoonful of the powder to a teacupful of boiling water is a proper quantity, the half or whole of which, except the sediment, is taken at a dose; drank warm or cold; if to produce perspiration, *warm*. Infusion may be sweetened with sugar or not.

Dec., Decoction, is a stronger preparation of a vegetable medicine; it consists in boiling one to two ounces of Herb or Bark in a pint and a half, or two pints of water, down to one pint; strain, sweeten, or not. *Dose*—from half a wineglassful three times a day to a wineglassful two or three times a day; drank warm or cold; if to produce perspiration, as a decoction of Yarrow, &c., warm, and three wineglassfuls of such may be drank within an hour before going to bed. As a general rule, Relaxants, Alteratives, Anti-Scorbutics and Diuretics, &c., should be taken on an empty stomach. Tonics or Bitters, to promote digestion, may be taken about an hour after meals, or a little while before. Only violent cases of disease require medicine more than three times a day.

The above proportions and rules refer to all the following Medicines, except where specially mentioned otherwise.

Amer. indicates that the plant is usually obtained from America, or that it is indigenous to that country. *Brit.*, that the plant is either found wild in Great Britain, or cultivated in our gardens.

Ext. implies that the medicine is occasionally used in the form of Extract, or inspissated juice, prepared by macerating the fresh plant in hot water, or water and spirit, or spirit alone, for a length of time, and then evaporating the juice obtained at a low temperature till it becomes the consistence of treacle, or thicker. The best extracts are now prepared by a very superior method, termed, *in vacuo*, by approved machinery.

Inhal., Inhaling the smoke or steam in Asthma, Catarrh, &c.

Oint., Ointment.

Syr., Syrup, is a strong decoction, or infusion, or the juice of the plant simmered with an equal weight of sugar, or mixed with sufficient honey.

Sub signifies that the substance of the powder should be taken in water; the dose, half to a teaspoonful.

Tinc., Tincture, is a spirituous infusion of the medicine; two ozs. of the powdered herb to one pint of spirit is the usual proportion, macerated from one to fourteen days, according to the nature of the plant.

ABBREVIATIONS AND PROPERTIES EXPLAINED.

ALT   .. Alterative—changing the morbid actions of the secretions.

ANO   .. Anodyne—quieting, easing pain.

ANTH   .. Anthelmintic—expelling or destroying worms.

A-BIL .. Anti-bilious—correcting the bile or bilious secretions.

A-SCOR.. Anti-scorbutic—useful in scurvy.

A-SEP .. Anti-septic—preventing mortification.

A-SPAS.. Anti-spasmodic—relieving spasms.

APE   .. Aperient—opening.

AROM   .. Aromatic—agreeable, spicy.

AST   .. Astringent—contracting the fibres or solids.

BAL   .. Balsamic—mild, healing, stimulant.

CAR   .. Carminative—expelling wind.

CATH   .. Cathartic—purgative, cleansing the bowels.

CEPH   .. Cephalic—remedy for diseases of the head.

DEM   .. Demulcent—softening, and sheathing from the action of acrid substances.

DEO   .. Deobstruent—correcting the secretions, or removing obstructions.

DIA   .. Diaphoretic—producing insensible perspiration.

DIU   .. Diuretic—increasing the discharge of urine.

DIS   .. Discutient—dissolving, discussing.

EME   .. Emetic—causing vomiting.

EMOL   .. Emollient—softening, causing warmth and moisture.

EMM   .. Emmenagogue—promoting menstruation.

EXP   .. Expectorant—producing discharge from the lungs.

FEB   .. Febrifuge—dispelling fever, allaying fever heat.

HER   .. Herpetic—curing diseases of the skin.

INHAL .. Inhalant—drawing the steam or smoke into the lungs.

LAX   .. Laxative—mild purgative.

MUC   .. Mucilaginous—glutinous, lubricating.

NER   .. Nervine—strengthening the nerves.

PEC .. Pectoral—useful in diseases of lungs and chest.

REF .. Refrigerent—cooling, mitigating heat.

RELAX.. Relaxant—relaxing constriction, reducing inflammation, allaying action, &c.

RUB .. Rubefacient—producing heat and redness of the skin.

SED .. Sedative—depressing the vital powers.

SIAL .. Sialogogue—promoting a flow of saliva.

STIM .. Stimulating—exciting action, giving strength.

STOM .. Stomachic—to excite the action of and strengthen the stomach.

STYP .. Styptic—stopping bleeding.

SUD .. Sudorific—causing sweat.

TON .. Tonic—permanently strengthening.

VER .. Vermifuge—destroying worms.

VUL .. Vulnerary—medicines which heal wounds.

AGRIMONY, Herb *Agrimonia eupatoria.* Ast. Ton. Diu. Alt.

Used in Fevers, Coughs, Bowel Complaints, Asthma, Diseases of the Kidneys and Liver, and by some persons instead of China Tea. Cr.-Dec. Pulv.-Inf. Brit. Wild. 4d per oz.

ALMONDS, Bitter *Amygdalus communis.* Ton.

Useful with other articles in a debilitated state of Stomach and Bowels. Given in emulsion (bruised and beat up with liquid), half an ounce to a pint of Dec. or Inf. of Herbs. 3d per oz.

ANGELICA, Leaves *Archangelica.* Stim. Arom. Ton.

For Colics, Colds, and for producing perspiration. Inf. or Dec. Brit. 3d per oz.

ANGELICA, Root and Seeds *Archangelica.* Stim. Arom. Ton.

For same purposes as Leaves, but more powerful in effect. Inf. or Dec. 3d per oz.

ASSAFŒTIDA, Gum *Ferula asafœtida.* Ton. A-spas. Exp.

To quiet Nervous Irritability, relieve Spasms, Cramps, &c. Given in Pills ordinary size. Dose—two, two or three times a day. 6d per oz. Pills, 4d per dozen; 4 dozen 1s.

AVENS ROOT   *Geum rivale.*   Ton. Ast. Stom.

Valuable in Debility, Dyspepsia, Internal Bleedings, Relax, &c.   Cr.-Dec. Pulv.-Inf. Brit. Wild.   3d per oz.

BALM, Lemon, Herb   *Melissa officinalis.*   Relax. Diu. Ner.

Infusion, excellent as a drink in Fevers, and for allaying headache.   Used in country places in England instead of Tea. Cr. or Pulv.-Inf.   3d per oz.

BALMONY, Herb   *Chelone glabra.*   A-bil. Ton. Ver. Ape.

For Indigestion, Affections of the Liver, and expelling Worms.   And to restore the Tone of the Stomach after Fevers, Dysentery, &c.   Cr. or Pulv.-Inf. Amer. Wild and Gardens.   Thomsom's No. 4.   4d per oz.

BARBERRY BARK   *Berberis vulgare.*   A-scor. Ref. Ton. A-Bil.

For correcting the secretions of the Liver, Jaundice, Indigestion, &c.   Cr. or Pulv.-Inf. or Dec.   Brit. Shrub. Amer. Wild.   3d per oz.

BAYBERRY, Bark of Root   *Myrica cerefera.*   Ast. Stim. Deo.

Most effectual in removing Canker from the Stomach and Bowels, and unequalled in Scurvy, Scrofula, and Ulcers.   Internal, and external as a wash, and in poultices.   Cr.-Dec. Pulv.-Inf. Amer.   Thomson's No 3.   3d per oz.

BETH ROOT   *Trillium latifolium.*   Ast. Ton. A-sep.

Beneficial for Bloody Urine, excessive Female Evacuations and uterine Debility.   Pulv.-Inf., or Sub. Amer. and Brit. Wild.   3d per oz.

BLUE GUM, Leaves   *Eucalyptus globulus.*   Ast. A-sep Feb. Inhal.

A valuable remedy for Diarrhœa, Fevers, Rheumatism, colds and gangrene.   Inf., Dec., Ext. Oil.

BISTORT ROOT   *Polygonum bistorta.*   Ast.

Useful in Hemorrhages or Fluxes, externally or internally, Diarrhœa, and Cholera, a powerful astringent.   Cr. Bruised, Dec. Pulv.-Inf.   3d per oz.

BITTER ROOT   *Apocynum androsæmifolium.*   Ton. Cath.

For Liver Complaints and Dropsy, to remove Costiveness, and correct Digestion. Pulv.-Inf. Amer. Wild. 4d per oz.

BLACKBERRY, Bark of Root   *Rubus occidentalis.*   Ast. Ton.

Effectual in Diarrhœa, useful in Consumption and Wastings. Cr.-Dec., or Syrup. Pulv.-Inf. Brit. and Amer. Wild. 4d per oz.

BLACK SNAKE ROOT—(See COHOSH, Black). 4d per oz.

BLOOD ROOT   *Sanguinaria canadensis.*   Eme. Emm. Exp. Ast.

Used in Pulmonary Affections, Scarlet Fever, Jaundice, and for bleeding at the Lungs—powerful. Pulv.-Inf., or Syrup, Tincture, or in Pills. One-sixth of the usual dose. 4d per oz.

BOGBEAN, Herb, *Menyanthes trifoliata.* Ton. Deo. A-scor. A-bil.

Used in Scurvy and Cutaneous Eruptions, and all diseases arising from Obstructions in the Liver. Cr. or Pulv.-Inf. Brit. and Amer. Wild, in Bogs and Lochs. 3d per oz.

BONESET, Herb *Eupatorium perfoliatum.* Sud. Ton. Eme. Cath.

Unequalled in Fevers of every description—good in asthma, &c. Cr.-Dec. or Syrup. Pulv.-Inf. Amer. Wild. 4d. per oz.

BOXWOOD BARK   *Cornus florida.*   Ast. Ton. Emm.

To correct morbid state of Stomach, and remove Female Weaknesses. Excellent for Whites and Gleet. Cr.-Dec. or Syrup. Pulv.-Inf. 4d per oz.

BOXWOOD FLOWERS   *Cornus florida.*   Ast. Ton. Stim.

Highly serviceable in removing Fluor Albus, or Whites. Shrub. Prep. as the Bark. 6d per oz.

BUCKHORN BRAKE   *Osmunda regalis.*   Ast. Ton. Muc.

Good in Soreness of the Stomach and Bowels, Female Weakness, Dysentery, &c. Pulv.-Inf. or Syrup. Brit. and Amer. Wild. 4d per oz.

BUGLE, Sweet Herb   *Lycopus virginicus.*   Ast. Ton. Deo.

Unequalled in spitting of Blood, Coughs, and Diseases of the Lungs. Cr.-Dec. or Syrup. Pulv.-Inf. Brit. Wild. Amer. Wild and Gardens. 6d per oz.

BURDOCK ROOT   *Arctium lappa.*   Diu. Ton. A-scor.

In strong decoction for Scurvy and Eruptions, Diseases of the Kidneys, &c. A general purifier of the Blood. Cr. Bruised, Dec. Pulv.-Inf. 3d per oz.

BURDOCK SEEDS   *Arctium lappa.*   Diu. Ner. Ton.

Good for Inflammation of the Kidneys, Epilepsy, Spasmodic Convulsions, &c. The fresh leaves of this plant are used bruised, applied as cataplasms or poultices to the feet in Rheumatism, &c. Pulv.-Inf. 6d per oz.

BUTTERNUT, Extract of   *Juglans cineria.*   Cath Ton. Emm.

A good aperient, and a gentle cathartic for Worms. Dose —for a child of three and four years ¼ to ½ drachm once or twice a day. Amer. Wild. 1s per oz.

CALAMUS, Sweet Flag (Root)   *Acorus calamus.*   Arom. Stom.

Excellent in Flatulence, Colic, and Wind in the Stomach. Cr. or Pulv.-Inf. 3d per oz.; peeled 4d per oz.

CHAMOMILE FLOWERS   *Anthemis nobilis.*   Ton. Feb Stom.

Good in Dyspepsia, Loss of Appetite, Colics, and General Debility. Cr. or Pulv.-Inf. Brit. Gardens.

CARAWAY SEED   *Carum carui.*   Car. Arom.

A good ingredient in Stomachic compounds. Cr. or Pulv.-Inf. 3d per oz.

CARDAMON SEED   *Alpinia cardamomum.*   Arom. Stim.

Used as a corrector of Purgative and Tonic Medicines. Inf. or Tinct. 1s per oz.

CARROT SEED, Wild   *Daucus carota.*   Diu. Emm.

Given in Stranguary, Calculus, or Stone, and other Affections of the Kidneys, Bladder, and Urethra, and for Dropsy. Cr.-Dec. Pul.-Inf. 6d per oz.

CASCARA SEGRADA, Bark   A-bil. Cath. Ton.

About the finest anti-constipation Medicine yet discovered, or for Rheumatism and Dyspepsia. Amer. Dec. fluid Ext. 6d per oz.

CATNIP, Herb   *Nepeta cataria.*   Stim. Car. Sud.

For Colds, Suppressions, Fevers, and to induce Perspiration; excellent for Headache. Inf. Brit. and Amer. Wild and in Gardens. 4d per oz.

CAYENNE PEPPER, African   *Capsicum anuum.*   Stim. Car. Ton.

The strongest and purest stimulant known, and universal in its application where stimulants are required, being free from inflammatory action. This, of course, only applies to the unadulterated article—that sold as Cayenne in some grocers' shops generally consists of pepper, salt, logwood, red lead, and other ingredients. Used for Flatulence, Indigestion, Colic, Dysentery, Diarrhœa, and Cholera. Dose: ¼ to ½ teaspoonful. Pulv.-Inf. or tincture, or in Golden Syrup in substance. 6d per oz.

CELEDINE, Herb   *Cheledonium majus*   Acr. Ton. Her.

Excellent for Tetters, Ringworms, Warts, and the Itch; for sore eyes and blindness as a wash; also in ointment. Cr. or Pulv.-Inf. or Tinct. 6d. per oz.

CENTAURY, Herb   *Chironia centaurium.*   A-bil. Ton.

Good in Dyspepsia, Jaundice, Liver Complaints, Scurvy, and Scrofula, especially in children. Cr.-Dec. Pulv.-Inf. Brit. and Amer. Wild. 4d per oz.

CHERRY-TREE BARK   *Prunus virginiani.*   Feb. A-scor. Ton.

Excellent in compounds for purifying the Blood, and affections of the Bladder. Cr.-Dec. Pulv.-Inf. Brit. and Amer. Wild. 4d per oz.

CLIVERS, Herb   *Galium aparine.*   Relax. Diu. Sud.

Good in Gravel, Dropsy, Fevers, Obstructions, Eruptions, and Scurvy. Cr. or Pulv.-Inf. in cold or hot water—if in cold, for twelve hours. Brit. and Amer., wild, by every hedge-side. 3d per oz.

CLOVER FLOWERS, Red   *Trifolium pratense.*   Acr. Deo.

The extract good for Cancers and Ulcers and to purify the blood. Thomson's Cancer Plaster. Extract and crude infusion. 4d per oz.

CLOVES,   *Eugenia caryophyllata.*   Stim. Arom. Car-

For Flatulency, Dyspepsia, and to correct the action of Purgatives, &c. Inf. Half the usual dose. 4d per oz.

COCA LEAVES,   *Erythroxalon coca.*   Stim. Ton. Nerv.

Good for Debility, Exhaustion, Nervousness, Seminal Weakness, &c. S. Amer. Inf. Dec. Ext. 9d per oz.

COHOSH, Black   *Macrotis racemosa.*   Dea Emm. Stim.

Serviceable in Rheumatism, Female Obstructions, Glandular Swellings, Whooping-cough, Fevers, and Scrofula   Cr.-Dec. Pulv.-Inf. Amer. 4d.

COLOMBO ROOT   *Coculus palmatus.*   A-Bil. Ton.

Excellent for Weak Stomachs, for Jaundice, and Disordered Liver. Pulv.-Inf. Cr.-Dec. 3d per oz.

COLTSFOOT FLOWERS   *Tussilago farfara.*   Exp. Pec. Relax.

Esteemed in Coughs, Asthma, and Consumption. Cr.-Dec. Common. 6d per oz. Leaves, similar properties. 3d per oz.

COMFREY ROOT   *Symphitum officinalis.*   Pec. Dem. Ton.

Valuable in Dysentery, Gleets, Diseases of the Bladder, Kidneys, and Bowels. Cr-Dec. and Syr.; or Pulv. in substance, in milk. 3d per oz.

CORIANDER SEED   *Coriandrum sativum.*   Stim. Car. Stom.

An excellent Carminative in Stomachic compounds. Inf. and Tinc. 3d per oz.

CRANESBILL   *Geranium maculatum.*   Styp. Ast. Stom.
A well established remedy for Diarrhœa, Hemorrhage, and
Fluor Albus.   Cr.-Dec. Pulv.-Inf.   Brit. and Amer. Common.
3d per oz.

CUBEBS   *Piper Cubeba.*   Arom. Car. Diu. Ton.
Good in compounds for Gonorrhœa, Gleet, Seminal
Weakness, &c.   Pulv. in substance, in water.   1s per oz.

CURCUMA   *Curcuma longa.*   Feb. Diu. Ton.
Good for Debilitated Stomach and Liver, Fevers, &c.
Pulv.-Inf.   3d per oz.

DANDELION ROOT   *Leontodon taraxacum.*   Deo. Diu. Ton.
A favourite remedy in Diseases of the Liver, Gravel, and
Constipation.   Cr.-Dec. Pulv.-Inf. Ext.   Brit. Common.
Double ordinary dose.   3d per oz.

DEVIL'S BIT   *Scabious, Scabiosa.*   Stim. Dem. Feb.
Useful in Coughs, Fevers, and Inflammations.   Cr.-Dec.
Brit.   4d per oz.

DOCK ROOT. Yellow   *Rumex Crispus.*   Ton. Deo. Her.
Highly serviceable in Diseases of the Skin, and Scrofulous
Disorders.   Cr.-Dec. Pulv.-Inf.   Brit. Common.   3d per oz.

DOCK ROOT, Water   *Rumex Aquaticus.*   Ast. Dia. Deo. Her.
Good in Scurvy, Cutaneous Eruptions, and Cancerous
Tumours.   Cr.-Dec. Pulv.-Inf.   Brit.   3d per oz.

ELDER BARK   *Sambucus niger.*   Diu. Deo. Sud. Stim.
Used in Obstinate Glandular Obstructions, and Dropsy.
Cr.-Dec. Pulv.-Inf.   3d per oz.

ELDER FLOWERS   *Sambucus niger.*   Alt. Sud. Stim.
Infusion popular for Erysipelas, Fevers, Rheumatism,
Colds, &c.

ELECAMPANE ROOT   *Inula helenium.*   Exp. Ast. Stom.
Useful in Coughs, Colds, and Pulmonary Affections.   Cr.-
Dec. in water or tea.   Pulv.-Inf.   Brit. Gardens.   4d per oz.

ELM BARK, Slippery   *Ulmus fulva.*   Emol. Diu. Dem. Relax.

Used in Urinary and Bowel Complaints, Scurvy and Inveterate Eruptions, Inflammations, as a diet in Fevers, and externally in poultices. The best of all poultices for Inflamed Sores, Burns, &c. In substance, or mucilage by Dec. Amer. 3d per oz.

FEATHERFEW (FEVERFEW) *Chrysanth. parthenium.* Ner. Stom Stim.

Serviceable in Female Obstructions, and Hysteric Complaints. Cr.-Inf. or Dec.-Pulv.-Inf. Brit. Gardens. 3d per oz.

FERN, Female (Polypody) *Aspidium filix femina.* Pec. Dem. Relax.

Good in Lumbago, and in syrup for Coughs. Cr.-Dec. Pulv.-Inf. 4d per oz.

FERN, Male   *Aspidium filix mas.*   Ver. Ton. Ast.

Considered a good remedy for Tape Worm. Cr. Dec. Pulv. in Sub., or Inf. 4d per oz.

FROSTWORT   *Cistus canadensis.*   Deo Ast Ton.

Of great value in Scrofulous Affections, as a poultice, and a tea. 4d per oz.

GARLIC   *Allium sativum.*   Stim Exp Ton.

Beneficial in Feeble Digestion, Chronic Catarrh, Asthma, &c. Cr.-Inf. or Syr., or eaten. Brit. Gardens. 3d per oz.

GENTIAN ROOT   *Gentiana lutea.*   Ton. Stom. Ast.

Of great celebrity in Dyspepsia, Hysterics, &c. Inf., or Tinc. 3d per oz.

GINGER ROOT   *Amomum zingiber.*   Stim. Car. Stom.

Given in Dyspepsia, Flatulent Diseases, Tonic Compounds, &c. Cr.-Dec. or Syr., or chewed. Pulv.-Inf. Jamaica Best. 2d per oz.

GOLDEN SEAL   *Hydrastis canadensis.*   Ton. A-bil. Stom.

An excellent tonic and corrective of Bile and Bilious habits; a good wash for sores. Pulv.-Inf. or Sub. Amer. 6d per oz.

GOLD THREAD   *Coptis trifolia.*   Stom. Ton. Ast.
Excellent to restore the appetite and strength after Fevers.
Cr. or Pulv.-Inf.   Amer. Gardens.   6d per oz.

GOOSEFOOT (WORMSEED) *Chenopodium anthelminticum.* Ver. Ton.
Very successful in expelling Seat Worms.   Cr. or Pulv.-Inf.
Brit.   6d per oz.

GOOSEGRASS—(See Clivers).   Called also *Airiff and Stickaback.*
3d per oz.

GRINDILI ROBUSTA   Relax. Exp. Ner.
Remedy for Asthma, Colds in the Chest, &c.   Amer.
Inf. Dec., and fluid Ext.   Ordinary dose.   6d per oz.

GROUND IVY   *Glechoma hederacea.*   Ast. Diu. Ton.
Good for Coughs and Internal Ulcers, and for purifying
the Blood.   Cr. or Pulv.-Inf.   Brit. Common.   4d per oz.

GUAIACUM CHIPS   *Guaiacum officinalis.*   Stim. Dia. Det.
Strengthens the Stomach and cleanses the Blood.   Gum.
Tinc. and Dec.   3d per oz.

HEMLOCK SPRUCE FIR, Bark *Pinus canadensis.*   Ast. Ton. Diu.
Good for Diseases of the Bladder and Kidneys, and as a
wash for old Ulcers.   Cr.-Dec. Pulv.-Inf. and Sub., also Ess.
Oil.   Amer.   3d per oz.

HOLLYHOCK FLOWERS   *Althea rosea.*   Ast. Dem.

Useful in all cases where a Demulcent is requisite.   In
Conserve or Cr.-Dec.   Pulv.-Sub.   Brit. Gardens.   6d per oz.

HOARHOUND   *Marrubium vulgare.*   Exp. Stim. Ton.

A well-known remedy for Coughs, highly serviceable in
Asthma.   Cr-Dec. Pulv.-Inf. Tinc. or Syr.   Brit. Gardens.
3d per oz.

HYSSOP   *Hyssopus officinalis.*   Exp. Ceph. Relax.

Used in Humoral Asthma, Coughs, Headache, &c.   Dec.
or Inf.   Brit.   3d per oz.

ICELAND MOSS   *Lichen Icelandicus.*   Dem. Ton. Ast.
Used as medicine and diet in Consumption : Elm is better.
3d per oz.

JUNIPER BERRIES   *Juniperus communis.*   Diu. Car. Stim.
The infusion excellent for Dropsies. Cr. or Pulv. 3d
per oz

LIFE EVERLASTING *Gnaphaleum polycephalum.* Stom. Sud. Ast.
Excellent in Quinsy, Weak Lungs, Consumption, and
Fluor Albus. Cr-Dec. Amer. 6d per oz.

LILY, White Pond   *Nymphæ odorata.*   Pec. Emol. Ast. Ton.
Employed in Scrofulous Tumours, Gleet, Whites, &c.
Cr.-Dec Pulv.-Inf. 4d per oz.

LILY, Yellow Water   *Nuphar advena.*   Pec. Emol. Ast. Ton.
Use same as White Pond Lily. 4d per oz.

LIQUORICE ROOT   *Glycyrrhiza glabra.*   Dem. Exp. Relax.
Useful in compounds for Coughs, Hoarseness, Asthma,
&c. Cr.-Dec. 3d per oz.

LIVERWORT   *Hepatica triloba.*   Ast. Dem. Pec. Deo.
Celebrated in bleeding at the Lungs, Consumption, Coughs,
Liver and Kidney Complaints. Cr.-Dec. Pulv. Inf. Brit. Amer.
Wild. 4d per oz.

LOBELIA, Herb   *Lobelia inflata.*   Eme. Relax. Exp.
A most valuable emetic, and highly esteemed in Asthma
and other affections of the Lungs. Dr Thomson's No. 1. Cr.
or Pulv. in Tinc. or Acid. Pulv. in composition tea or warm
water, or in Sub. (See COMPOUNDS). 6d per oz.

LOBELIA SEED   *Lobelia inflata.*   Eme. Relax. Exp.
Propertices same as Herb, but much stronger. *Not used
alone.* 1s per oz.

LUNGWORT   *Variolaria faginea*   Pec. Ton. Dem.
Used with much benefit in Consumptions, Coughs, and,
Defluxion of the Lungs. Cr.-Dec. Pulv.-Inf. Brit. and Amer.,
on rocks by the shore. 4d per oz.

MAIDENHAIR   *Adianthum pedatum.*   Exp. Ast. Stom.
   Much esteemed in Coughs, Asthma, and Disorders of the
Chest. Cr.-Dec. and Syr. 6d per oz.

MANDRAKE ROOT   *Podophyllum peltatum.* Relax. Cath. A-bil
   Powerful in Dropsies, Liver Complaints, Venereal and
Scrofulous affections. N.B.—This is not the British Mandrake
—*Atrossa Mandragora.* Ext., Pulv.-Inf. or Sub.; one-fourth
of an ordinary dose with an arom. 3d per oz.

MARSH MALLOW, Herb *Althæa officinalis.* Emol. Dem. Relax.
   Serviceable in Asthma, Dysentery, and Affections of the
Kidneys; also as fomentation and poultice to allay Swellings,
&c. Cr.-Dec., or Syr. 3d per oz.

MARSH MALLOW, Root *Althæa officinalis.* Emol. Dem. Relax.
   Properties same as Herb; used the same. 3d per oz.

MARSH ROSEMARY ROOT   *Statice limonium.*   Ast. A-sep.
   Beneficial in Gleet, Whites, Canker, and Sore Throat.
Cr.-Dec. Pulv.-Inf. Amer. 4d per oz.

MILFOIL—(See YARROW).—Called also *Thousand Leaf.* 3d
   per oz.

MOUNTAIN FLAX   *Linum catharticum.*   Dem. Cath. Relax.
   An excellent purge for children and adults. Cr.-Inf. or
Dec. with Ginger. 6d per oz.

MUGWORT   *Artemesia vulgaris.*   Deo. A-bil. Ton. Emm.
   The infusion promotes Perspiration, Urine, and the
Menses. 3d per oz.

MULLEIN LEAVES AND FLOWERS *Verbascum thapos.* A-spas. Pec.
                                                    [Relax.
   Useful in Dysentery, Hemorrhage, Chest Affections,
Wasting, and the Piles. Cr.-Dec. 3d per oz.

MUSTARD SEED, White   *Sinapis alba.*   A-scor. Stim. Rub.
   Used in compounds for Dyspepsia, Obstinate Costiveness,
Dropsies, Rheumatism, &c. Cr.-Inf. 3d per oz.

NETTLE TOPS OR ROOT   *Urtica dioica.*   Ast. Ton.
   Useful in incipient stages of Consumption and Bloody
Urine. Cr.-Dec. 3d per oz.

NUTGALLS   *Quercus tinctoria.*   Ast.
   A good ingredient in Astringent Ointments and Gargles.
3d per oz.

NUTMEGS   *Myristica moschata.*   Arom. Ast. Stom. Stim.
   Powder good in violent Headaches, Diarrhœas, and
Dysenteries. 6d per oz. Use with care. (See Index).

OAK BARK, White   *Quercus Alba.*   Ast. Ton. A-sep.
   Beneficial as an astringent and antiseptic Gargle, and
wash for Putrid Sore Throat and Offensive Ulcers, &c. Cr.-
Dec. Pulv.-Inf. 3d per oz.

PARSLEY, Root   *Apium petroselinum.*   Ape. Relax. Diu.
   Highly esteemed in Kidney and Dropsical Affections.
Cr.-Dec. 3d per oz.

PARSLEY, Pert   *Percicier.*   Relax. Diu.
   Excellent in all obstructions of Urine, Jaundice, and
Affections of the Liver. Cr.-Inf. 4d per oz.

PEACH PITS, or KERNELS   *Amygdalis persica.*   Ton. Stom.
   In syrup or tincture, good for strengthening the Stomach
and Digestion. Half dose. 6d per oz.

PELLITORY OF THE WALL   *Parietaria officinalis.*   Relax. Diu.
   Excellent in Stone, Gravel, and Suppression of the Urine.
Inf. or Dec. 4d per oz.

PENNYROYAL   *Mentha pulegium.*   Car. Stim. Stom. Arom.
   A strong infusion, good for suppressions of Urine,
obstructed Menses, and the Gravel; also for Colics and
Eruptive Diseases in children. 3d per oz.

PEPPERMINT   *Mentha piperita.*   Stom. Stim. Sud.
   Good in Nervous Affections of the Stomach, Flatulence,
and to allay Vomiting. Inf. 3d per oz.

PERUVIAN BARK   *Cinchona officinalis.*   Ton. Ast.

Highly esteemed for want of Appetite, General Debility, &c. Pulv.-Sub., Dec., and Inf. 6d to 1s per oz.

PINUS CANADENSIS—(See HEMLOCK SPRUCE FIR). 3d per oz.

PIPSISSEWAY   *Chimaphila umbellata.*   A-Scor. Diu. Stim.

An excellent Purifier of the Blood, and for Rheumatism. Dec. Pulv.-Inf. 4d per oz.

PLEURISY ROOT   *Asclepias tuberosa.*   Dia. Sud. Relax.

Beneficial in Pleurisy, Inflammation of the Lungs, Colic, and all Flatulent Disorders. Pulv.-Inf. 4d per oz.

POKE ROOT   *Phytolacca decandria.*   Relax. Deo. Cath. Alt.

Valuable in Rheumatic Complaints, and for Indolent Tumours. Cr.-Dec. Pulv.- Inf. Amer. 4d per oz.

POLYPODY—(See FERN, Female).

POMEGRANATE BARK   *Punica granatum.*   Ver. Ast. Ton.

A specific for Tape Worm. Cr.-Dec., Pulv.-Inf., or Sub. 4d per oz.

POPLAR BARK, White   *Populus tremuloides.*   Ton. Diu. Ast.

Excellent in Diarrhœa, Debility, and Digestive Complaints. Cr.-Dec. Pulv.-Inf. 3d per oz.

POPLAR BARK, Black   *Populus Balsamifera.*   Ton. Arom. Ast.

One of the best articles in use for Debility of the Stomach and Bowels. Cr.-Dec. Pulv.-Inf. 3d per oz.

PRICKLY ASH BARK *Xanthoxylum fraxineum.* A-Scor. Stim. Diu.

Powerful in Rheumatism, Scurvy, Paralysis, &c. Cr.-Dec. Pulv.-Inf. 4d per oz.

PRICKLY ASH SEEDS *Xanthoxylum fraxineum.* A-scor. Stim. Dia.

Properties similar to Bark, but more powerful. Half dose. Pulv.-Inf. 1s per oz.

PRINCESS PINE—(See PIPSISSEWAY).

QUASSIA CHIPS   *Quassia excelsa.*   Ton. Feb.
Useful in Dyspeptic Cases and Debilitated Digestive
Organs. Inf. 3d per oz.

QUEEN OF THE MEADOW   *Eupartoreum purpureum.*   Diu. Ast.
Most valuable in all cases of Stranguary, Gravel, Stone,
Dropsy, and Impurities. Inf. of the leaves is a good
substitute for China Tea. 4d per oz.

QUEENSLAND, Herb, *Euphorbia pilulifera* Exp. Anti. Spas. Pect.
A new Asthma remedy. Dec. Inf. Exp., and inhale smoke.
6d per oz.

QUEEN'S DELIGHT, Root *Stillingia sylvatica.* Relax. Alt. Cath.
Valuable in Ulcers, Leprosy, and Syphilis. Dec., Pulv.-
Inf., or Tinc. 4d per oz.

RASPBERRY LEAVES   *Rubus strigosus.*   Ast. Ton.
Good for Bowel Complaints and Canker, Invaluable
during Childbirth. Crude Inf. 3d per oz.

RHUBARB ROOT, East India *Rheum undulatum.* Carm. Ast. Ape.
    „   „   Turkey   „   „   „   „   „
A well-known useful Tonic and Aperient. Half dose.
Inf.-Syr., or Sub. 1s 6d per oz.

ROSEMARY LEAVES   *Rosemarinus officinalis.*   Ast. Ton.
Good in Nervous and Hysterical Affections. Cr.-Inf. 3d
per oz.

RUE   *Ruta Graveolens.*   Ver. Ton. Diu. Stom.
Useful in Epilepsy, Hysterics, Female Obstructions, and
as a Stomachic. Cr. or Pulv. 3d per oz.

SAGE, Garden   *Salvia officinalis.*   Ast. Stim. Ner.
Excellent to allay griping pains in children, and to quiet
nervous excitement. Inf. 3d per oz.

SAGE, Wood and Mountain *Teucrium scorodonia.* Ton. Diu. Deo.
Excellent in removing obstructions from the Kidneys and
Liver. Cr.-Dec. Pulv.-Inf. 3d per oz.

SARSAPARILLA, Jamaica   *Smilax sarsaparilla.*   Alt. Ton. Deo.
Good for Scrofulous, Venereal, and Eruptive Diseases.
Ext. or Dec.   6d per oz.

SARSAPARILLA, American   *Aralia nudicaulis.*   Alt. Ton. Deo.
Properties same as Jamaica Sarsaparilla, and by some of
the American botanists considered equally as good.   Ext. or
Dec.   4d per oz.

SASSAFRAS CHIPS   *Laurus sassafras.*   Stim. Ape. Ton. Alt.
Very good in Rheumatic. Complaints and Eruptive
Diseases.   Dec.   2d per oz.

SASSAFRAS, Bark of Root *Laurus sassafras.* Stim. Ape. Ton. Alt.
Properties same as Chips, but much more powerful.   Cr.-
Dec. Pulv.-Inf.   4d per oz.

SELF HEAL   *Prunella vulgaris.*   Ast. Vul.
Good in Hemorrhage, Diarrhœa, and as a Gargle for sore
Throats.   Dec.   4d per oz.

SCULLCAP   *Scutellaria laterifolia.*   Ton. Sud. Ner.
Remarkably efficacious in St. Vitus' Dance, Convulsions,
Lockjaw.   It is also said to be a specific for Hydrophobia.
Pulv.-Inf.   Amer   6d per oz.

SENNA LEAVES   *Cassia acutifolia.*   Relax. Cath.
A valuable Cathartic, operating mildly.   Inf.   3d per oz.

SKUNK CABBAGE ROOT   *Ictodes fœtida.*   A-spas. Relax. Stim.
Good for bleeding at the Lungs, Coughs, Asthma, and
Obstructed Menses.   Pulv.-Inf.   4d per oz.

SNAKEHEAD—(See BALMONY).

SNAKE ROOT, Virginia *Aristolochia serpentaria.* Ton. Dia. Sud.
Promotes Perspiration, and strengthens the Stomach.
Half Dose.   Pulv.-Inf.   6d per oz.

SOLOMON'S SEAL ROOT   *Convallaria multiflora.*   Ast. Dem. Bal.
Good in Fluor Albus and Female Weakness, and as a
Poultice for Bruises and Rheumatism.   Cr.-Dec.   4d per oz.

SPEARMINT   *Mentha viridis.*   Feb. Diu. Stim.

Inf. allays Nausea, and an excellent remedy in Flatulence, Gravel, and Suppressions.   3d per oz.

SPIKENARD   *Aralia racemosa.*   Pec. Ton. Stom.

Good in Coughs, Colds and Gout in the Stomach.   Cr.-Dec. Pulv.-Inf.   4d per oz.

STRAMONIUM LEAVES   *Datura Stramonium.*   Exp. A-spas.
The smoke inhaled.   [Inhal.

An almost universal remedy in Asthma, internally in very small doses as a cure for the opium habit.   Tinc., 5 to 20 drops; also a valuable Ointment. (See Compound). 3d per oz.

SUMACH BERRIES   *Rhus glabra.*   Ast. Ref. Diu.

Good in Putrid Fevers, and as a Gargle in Sore Throat. Inf. or Dec.   6d per oz.

SUMACH LEAVES   *Rhus glabra.*   Ast. Ton. Diu.

An excellent addition to Astringent Compounds.   Cr.-Inf., or Dec.   4d per oz.

TANSY   *Tanacetum vulgare.*   Diu. Emm. Ton Stom

Good in Feminine Weaknesses, pains in the Back and Kidneys.   Inf.   3d per oz.

THOROUGHWORT—(See BONESET).

TORMENTIL ROOT   *Tormentilla erecta.*   Ast. Styp.

A favourite remedy in Looseness and Bowel Complaints. Cr.-Dec., Pulv.-Inf., or Sub. in boiled milk.   3d per oz.

TURNIP, Wild—(See WAKE ROBIN).   4d per oz.

UNICORN ROOT   *Helonias dioica.*   Ton. Exp. Stom.

Highly serviceable in weakness of the generative organs, pains in the back and chest.   Pulv. in Sub. in hot water. Amer.   4d per oz.

UVA URSI   *Arbutus uva ursi.*   Diu. Ast. Ton.
Efficacious in Ulcerations of the Kidneys and Bladder.   Dec. or Inf.   4d per oz.

VALERIAN ROOT, American *Cypripedium pubescens*. Relax. Ton.
[Ano. Nerv.

Applicable in all cases of Nervous, Hysteric, and
Spasmodic Affections; considered by some writers as being
much superior to the English Valerian. Pulv.-Inf.   4d per
oz.

VALERIAN ROOT, English *Valeriana officinalis*. Relax. Ton. Ano.
[Nerv.

Useful in all Nervous and Paralytic Diseases.   Pulv.-Inf.,
4d per oz.

VERVAIN   *Verbena hastata.*   Sud. Ton. Eme. Diu.

Good in Fevers, Colds, Scrofula, Gravel, &c., and as an
Emetic.   Inf.   4d per oz.

VIRGINIAN SNAKE ROOT *Aristolochia serpentaria*. Ton. Dia. Sud.

Promotes Perspiration and strengthens the Stomach.
Pulv.-Inf.   6d per oz.

WAKE ROBIN, Root   *Arum tryphillum.*   Stim. Exp.

Valuable in Coughs, Colds, Cramps, and Consumptive
Affections.   Sub.   4d per oz.

WILLOW BARK   *Salix alba.*   Ton. Ast.

Superior to Peruvian Bark in Intermittents, and as a
general Tonic.   3d per oz.

WITCH HAZEL LEAVES   *Hamamellis virginica.*   Ton. Ast. Her.

Useful in Bowel Complaints, Hemorrhage, and Painful
Tumours.   Inf.   4d per oz.

WORMWOOD   *Artemisia absynthium.*   Ton. Stim. Her.

Promotes the Appetite and Digestion ; good in Dyspepsia,
&c.   Inf.   3d per oz.

YARROW   *Achillea millefolium.*   Stim. Sud. Ton. Ast.

An herb of universal application in the first stages of
disease; it equalises the circulation, opens the pores, and
removes obstructions.   Cr.-Dec. Infus. Pulv.-Inf.   6d per oz.

YERBA SANTA   Exp. Pec. Sim.

Beneficial in Coughs, Asthma, and Bronchitis.   Dec.-Syr.
Inf. Tinct. Ext.   Amer.   6d per oz.

PRICE LIST.—In order to save the space that would be
occupied at the end of the book by the usual price lists, we
have added the retail price for the crude articles in ounce lots.
In ¼lb. we make a reduction of 10 to 25 per cent.   Those
marked 4d are generally 1s per ¼lb, 1s 4d to 1s 9d per ½lb, and
2s 6d to 3s per lb ; those at 6d per ounce, 1s 6d per ¼lb, 2s 6d
per ½lb, 4s to 5s per lb.   The powdered article is generally
from ½d to 2d per oz. higher.   This list is only intended for private
use.   Special quotations to the trade and those who sell again.

CULTIVATION OF HERBS, ROOTS, &c.

There are some plants that thrive best in the uncultivated
soil ; being of a hardy nature they can, so to speak, fight
for and maintain their existence against all competitors, even
the collecting raids of the herbalist and hunger of herbivorous
animals who have a keen appetite for some of our medicinal
herbs ; there are others that need protection and care in order
to keep them from being destroyed by weeds.   As a rule few
will seek to cultivate those that experience has taught us grow
best wild ; the more delicate kind will generally compensate
for the toil spent upon them by their outer adornment of
colour or fragrance.

As a foundation for successful gardening we need hardly
say the first thing is to prepare the ground well, weed, and
manure it thoroughly.   If the herbs grow from seeds (and
most that we import must be started in this way), it will be
needful or better to get a small hot-bed to start them.   Smooth

the surface, sprinkle the seeds, then simply cover them with a mixture of soil and dry horse manure. When grown sufficiently, from one to three inches, transplant them into beds of fine mould with sand. Let this be done after rain when the sun has gone down; if there has not been rain, water the ground in the evenings.

Herbs that grow well from cuttings, such as hoarhound and sage should be treated thus: At the beginning of summer cut off the strong branches; take off the top leaves for about six inches. Put in a well-prepared bed in rows about one to two feet apart, and about the same distance between the rows. If the weather is dry, water them well in the evening till they have got good hold of the soil and are showing signs of growth.

Rue, southern wood, hyssop, feverfew, wormwood, motherwort, and other hardy plants same time and directions as hoarhound and sage. The seeds of these should be sown two months earlier. Agrimony roots should be carefully shifted with the earth round them in the spring when the frost is over; in the winter it will be better to cover them well with earth to keep it from them. This is a delicate herb to rear.

Peletory of the wall is best raised from seeds, which should be sown at the beginning of summer. The soil must be fine; it is best to sift it. Lobelia, which we have several times tried to raise from the seeds and failed, probably on account of the seeds (which are very small) having perished. In order if possible to prevent this, the seeds should be mixed with earth in a hot-bed, and tended very carefully even after transplantation, which must be done by lifting the earth with the plants.

Elecampane roots should be planted in the spring with a part of the stem attached; one root may be divided up into several. Marsh mallows and rosemary may be treated the same way as hoarhound, or grown from the seed, sown in early spring. Vervain in a similar manner. When the whole plant is medicinal and an annual, it may be cut off above the root and hung over a line till it is dry, then cut up and kept air-tight and damp-proof. Great care must be taken to keep the plants dry, as dampness will spoil them.

Pressing Herbs, &c.—Gather them, as above in fine weather, and when dry, if you want to keep them a long time get a strong-made box, eight by four inches in the clear and six inches deep. Fill it with the herbs laid flat; put on top of this a wooden block which will just fit into the box; press and keep on the top a heavy weight or screw; let it remain thus all night, and you will have an oblong block, (8 x 4 x 4 in.), which wrap in thick brown paper, and it will keep good for a long time. The proper time for collecting herbs or leaves is when the flowers come out. If the leaves alone are wanted, pick them off with the footstalks, if they have any. Spread them in the sun, if sunlight does not take the colour out of them, (as it does to some very delicate plants); but if so, spread them upon paper on the floor, or on shelves, till they are dry; then put them in air-tight tins, boxes, or bags, labelled, and put in a dry place.

Roots ought to be dug up early in spring, before the sap has ascended into the tops. Clean, and brush the earth off them; if large, slice and run a string through them, making a knot between each to keep them apart. Let the string or twine needle be sufficiently strong to hold about a yard length of roots. These may be either hung at both ends or at one. When thoroughly dry, which may be determined by breaking the root, put them away, like the herbs, labelled, for future use.

Yarrow growing in beds must be thinned out every spring, or it will die out in time. Flowers ought to be gathered in full bloom, spread on cloths on a dry floor. They should be turned every day till dry, then put away as the others. Seeds must not be gathered till ripe, then dried and separated from the husks, spread on paper till bone dry; keep from the air in a dry place; look at them occasionally, as they are apt to draw the damp, get mouldy, and spoil. The one thing needful is care to get and keep good the herbs. We feel certain that if the above directions are attended to they will enable any one to cultivate many of our medicines.

In closing this division of our work we wish to inform our readers that we are now gathering all the information possible on our native medicinal plants. The result of our inquiries we will give in a separate chapter at the end of the book, along with those already described, so as to bring them together for the convenience of reference.

A LIST OF THE NAMES, PROPERTIES, AND DOSES OF MEDICINES, &c.,

USED IN THE REGULAR PRACTICE OF MEDICINE, WITH RETAIL PRICES

Although as a rule the prices of drugs vary little, still there are some slight changes, so this list is subject to any fluctuation in the market. Our object in giving our readers this list is not so much to recommend their use, but to give a knowledge of them, so that the thoughtful may be able to read prescriptions, and know what they are given in the shape of medicine. We do not wish to be understood as having no faith in any of the following, for we have both used them ourselves and known of many cases in which some of them have done good, and act in harmony with nature; but some of them are deadly poisons, and ought never in our judgment to have been made or given a place in any pharmacopœia.

Should our readers desire to try them, we will for their safety add a word or two as to their nature and use. The term safe after certain will signify, can be used without fear.

Use carefully : that over-doses would do injury. Dangerous : that the greatest care should be exercised in measuring. If in drops, a dropper should be used, or a minim or drop measure. Very dangerous : these, with the foregoing, ought not to be taken by any but the experienced, and their effects carefully watched ; being as it were sharp-edged tools, they require skill to use them safely. The signs and abbreviations used by medical men are as follows :—

Gr. stands for grain, which is the average weight of a grain of wheat. There are 480 of these to the ounce.

Ə represents scruple, one of which is equal to 20 grains, 24 to the ounce.

Ʒ stands for drachm, 8 of which make the ounce.

Ʒ represents ounce, 16 of which make one pound.

These signs do not represent any number unless the number is put down after them :—i. added to any of them signifies one scruple, one drachm, or one ounce, two is ii. ; three, iii. , four, iv. ; five, v., and so on, the Roman numerals being always used. Pounds are seldom written, the number being given in ounces. Fl. is fluid, and prefixed to show that liquid is meant. O represents pint imperial, 20 ounces. When a half is signified two ss. are used. Thus ss. behind the sign means only half of it. Behind any cypher following, they mean half of one only, immediately preceding. It is very important to know well these signs, as a mistake might cost some poor mortal his or her life. Doses are generally calculated from the smallest to the largest for adults. Delicate people should not take full doses, especially of the dangerous drugs. Abbreviations are generally the first part of the name, thus—sps. for spirits ; syr. for syrup , tr. for tincture ; pulv. for powder ; gtts for drops ; ung. for oint-ment ; emp. for plaster ; eth. for either ; nit. for nitre ; vin for wine ; ol. for oil ; treben. for. turpentine ; hydg. means mercury ; mag. for magnesia ; sulp. for sulphur, or sulphate. Now we do not think it is safe for prescriptions to be written

in this loose way, as many of these abbreviations are
similar, and mean very different articles, a substitution of
which would lead to very serious consequences.   For instance,
acid hydro. may mean hydrochloric acid (spirits of salts),
a poison or hydrocyanic acid (prussic acid), the very smell of
which is sufficient to poison; ammon. may mean ammonia or
ammoniac; aqua chlor. may mean chloroform water or
chlorine water; ext. col. either colchicum or colycynth; hyd.
chlor. may mean calomel or corrosive sublimate (a virulent
poison), or hydrate of chloral; sod. hypo. either hyposulphate
or hypophosphite; sulph. may mean sulphur, sulphate,
sulphide. These examples will show the danger of abbreviations
in naming such dangerous materials.   Our own opinion is
that men ought to be compelled by law to use the English
language in writing prescriptions.   This would not only
prevent imposition, but save accidents and lives, as many have
been poisoned by dog Latin.

ACETIC ACID.—An acid liquid obtained from wood by
distillation.   Dose of the diluted acid, 10 to 20 drops 2 or 3
times a day.   Given in alkaline conditions of the stomach and
urine.   Use carefully.   3d. per oz.

ACID ARSENIOUS.—Obtained by roasting arsenial ores and
purifying by sublimation.   Used in skin diseases.   Dose,
1-60th to 12th drop.   Very dangerous.   3d. per oz.

ACID BENZOIC.—Obtained from gum benzoin, and prepared by sublimation.   Combined with Buchu, and used in
urinary troubles.   Dose, 5 to 15 grains.   It is safe in small
doses.   1s. 6d. per oz.

ACID BORACIC.—Obtained by the action of sulphuric acid
on borax.   Dose, 5 to 10 grains.   Used as an antiseptic and
food preservative.   Safe.   6d per ounce.

ACID CARBOLIC.—Obtained from coal or oil.   Dose, ½ to
2 drops.   Disinfectant, one part in 20 parts of oil or water, as a
wash and liniment for wounds and sores.   Dangerous.   3d.
to 9d. per oz.

ACID CITRIC.—Prepared from lemon juice or the juice of the fruit of the citron. Used in acidulous drinks and making white wine vinegar. Dose, 5 to 20 grains. Safe. 6d. per oz.

ACID GALLIC.—Prepared by boiling nut-galls with diluted sulphuric acid. Properties astringent. Dose, 10 to 30 grains. Use carefully. 1s. per oz.

ACID HYDROCYANIC.—Commonly known as prussic acid. It is one of the deadliest poisons known; one or two drops of the pure acid will kill a large dog in a few seconds. Very dangerous. Diluted, 1s. 6d. per oz.

MURIATIC ACID.—Commonly known as spirit of salts, is obtained by the action of sulphuric acid on common salt. Properties, tonic, refrigerant, and antiseptic. Dose of the diluted acid, 10 to 30 drops, is in the proportion of six parts of the pure acid to thirteen parts of distilled water. Dangerous. 2d. per oz.

NITRIC ACID.—Is prepared from nitrate of potash or saltpetre, by distillation with sulphuric acid and water. Properties, tonic, antiseptic, and astringent. Should always be used in the diluted form, as it is a very fatal poison. Dilution, 1 of acid to 6 of water. Dose of the diluted acid, 5 to 20 drops. Dangerous. 3d. per oz.

ACID PHOSPHORIC.—Prepared by distillation from phosphorus and nitric acid. Generally used in the diluted form 1 of acid to 4 of water. Dose of the diluted acid, 10 to 30 drops. Dangerous. 3d. per oz.

SALICYLIC ACID.—Obtained from oil of wintergreen. Used as a preservative against fermentation, and also forms one of the principal ingredients in Cura Clava or corn cure. Given internally in the form of salicylate of sodium, for rheumatism, in doses of 5 to 15 grains four or five times in the twenty-four hours. Use very carefully. 1s. per oz.

SULPHURIC ACID, commonly known as vitriol, is obtained by burning sulphur and allowing the product of combustion to mix with nitrous fumes obtained from the decomposition of nitre. Used medicinally in the diluted form, and is sometimes given in typhoid fevers with advantage. It also makes a good gargle for sore throats. Dose of the diluted acid (1 part acid to 9 water) 5 to 30 drops. 3d. per oz.

SULPHUROUS ACID.—Made from sulphuic acid, charcoal, and water. Used externally for all parasitic affections of the skin. When locally used it should be diluted with 2 or 3 parts of water. Much advantage has been found by inhaling the acid in typhoid and typhus fevers, catarrh, hay fever, and rheumatism. Dose, ½ to a teaspoonful. Use carefully. 3d. per oz.

TANNIC ACID.—An acid obtained from galls. Is a very strong astringent, used internally and externally, for hemorrhages or bleedings, piles, chilblains, &c. Use carefully. 1s. per oz.

ACONITE, TINCTURE OF ROOT.—Is a powerful poison. Used in moderate doses it is very good in rheumatic neuralgia and fevers. Dose, 5 to 10 drops. Dangerous. 1s. per oz.

ALNUIN.—Active principle of the tag alder bark. Used for scrofula, eruptions of the skin, rheumatism. Dose, 2 to 10 grains. Use carefully. 4s. per oz.

ALOES.—Three chief varieties of aloes are known in commerce—the Cape, the Socotrine, and the Barbadoes, of which the last two are most used in this country. They are all cathartic, operating slowly but certainly. Owing to its excessively bitter and somewhat nauseous taste, it is most conveniently given in pills. Dose of the powder from 5 to 10 grains. Use with care. 6d. to 9d. per oz.

ALEOIN, the active principle of aloes. Dose 2 to 5 grains. Dangerous. 4s. per oz.

AMMONIA CARBONATE.—Manufactured by subliming a mixture of the chloride or sulphate with chalk. Chloride of ammonia and chalk are heated together in iron pots or retorts, and sublimed into large earthen or leaden receivers. There are a great many preparations of ammonia, of which the following are a few :—Bromide of ammonia, in conjunction with nervines, good for neuralgia; the chloride, sulphate, and several others. Dangerous in over-doses. Carb. 3d., bromide 9d per ounce.

NITRITE OF AMYL.—a liquid produced by the action of nitric acid on amylic alcohol. Care should be taken not to confound it with nitrate of amyl. The nitrate is not taken as a medicine. The nitrite is sometimes given in asthma with good effect. Dose 1 to four drops. Dangerous. 2s. 6d. per oz.

ANTIMONY.—All the different preparations of antimony are prepared from the native sulphide, of which the following are a few of the principal :—Oxide, dose 1 to 4 grains. Antimony and potassium (tartar emetic), dose diaphoretic and expectorant 1-16th to 1-6th grain; as an emetic ½ to 2 grains. Very dangerous. 1s. per ounce.

APIOL.—The active principle of parsley, Properties, diuretic; dose 3 to 8 drops. Use very carefully. 2s 6d per oz.

ARNICA (tincture of) is very seldom given internally, being principally used diluted with water for sprains and bruises. Dangerous. 9d per oz.

ATROPIA.—The active principle of belladonna. Atropia may be given internally for all the purposes for which belladonna is given, and it is largely used as a local remedy for application to the eye. Dose 1-120th to 1-50th part of a grain. Very dangerous. Poison. 1d. per gr.

AURUM CHLORIDE (chloride of gold). Dose 1-30th to 1-15th gr. Very dangerous. 3d. per grain.

BARIUM is a metal first obtained by Sir H. Davy. The compounds of barium are the chloride and the carbonate. The only pharmaceutical use of the carbonate is to prepare the chlorides. Very poisonous. 1s. per oz.

BELLADONNA (tincture of).—The leaves of atropa belladonna, commonly known as " deadly nightshade." Belladonna is mostly given in nervous diseases. Dose of the
tincture 20 to 30 drops. Dangerous. 9d. per oz.

BENZOIN GUM forms one of the principal ingredients in
that well-known preparation, Friar's Balsam.—Dose of the
compound tincture 1 to 2 drachms; used for fresh wounds
internally; for old coughs, dose 5 to 20 drops. Safe. 9d.
per oz.

BISMUTH.—A crude metal. Of the many preparations of
bismuth the subnitrate or white bismuth is mostly used.
Snuffed up the nose it will relieve cold in the head; taken
internally it will relieve indigestion. Dose: 5 to 30 grains.
Use carefully. 1s. 6d. per oz.

BROMIDE OF SODIUM.—Said to be a specific for sea-sickness.
Dose: from 5 grains to 1 drachm. Safe. 9s. 6d. per oz.

CAFFEIN, (an alkaloid).—Obtained from the seeds of
Arabian coffee. Said to be good for headaches. Dose: 1 to
5 grains. Care in using. 4s. per oz.

CAJEPUT, Oil of.—Employed in flatulent colic, hysteria,
and cholera. Dose: 1 to 4 drops. Care. 1s. 6d. per oz.

CANNABIS INDICUS (Indian Hemp).—Is a narcotic ; in its
anodyne and soporific action it resembles opium. It has been
given in the different forms of neuralgia, in spasmodic coughs,
asthma. Dose of the tincture, 5 to 30 drops. Dangerous in
over-doses. 1s. per oz.

CANELLA.—The bark of canella alba or laurel-leafed
canella, deprived of its corky layer and dried, mixed with
socratim aloes, forms the well-known Hiera Piera. Dose of
the powder 14 to 30 grains. Care. 6d. per oz.

CANTHARIDES.—The blister beetle or Spanish fly, collected
in Russia and Sicily, but chiefly in Hungary. Used externally as
a blister; internally it is given in chronic affections of the

nervous system. Dose of the tincture, 5 to 15 drops. Dangerous. 1s. 6d per oz.

CASTANEA VESCA (CHESNUT LEAVES).—Splendid remedy for whooping cough. Dose of fluid extract, ½ to 2 drachms. Safe. 9d. per oz.

CERIUM OXOLATE.—Appears to act as a local sedative and afterwards upon the system as a nervine tonic. Dose : 1 to 2 grains. Dangerous. 2s. per oz.

CHENOPODIUM, (Oil of Wormseed).—Used, as the name indicates, for worms. Dose : 5 to 10 drops. Careful use. 1s. 6d. per oz.

CIMICIFUGA EXTRACT (Black Cohosh).—The powder in conjunction with other herbs makes a good emmenagogue. It is also said to be good for rheumatism. Dose of extract 10 to 30 drops. Careful use. 4s. per oz.

CINCHONA (Peruvian Bark).—Is the bark from which quinine is extracted. It is a splendid tonic. It has also the reputation of being a cure for drunkenness. Dose of the tincture 1 to 4 teaspoonfuls. Safe. Crude best. 9d. per oz.; powder 1s.

COCA (Fluid Extract.)—Prepared from the leaves of Erythroxylon Coca. The leaves when chewed are said to exert a powerfully restorative and stimulant effect. The South American Indians can endure fatigue for days together without food if they can get coca. Coca contains an alkaloid called cocaine, which is being employed for its anæsthetic properties. Dose of the fluid extract, ½ to 2 teaspoonfuls. Safe. 1s. per oz.

CODEIA OR CODENIA.—An alkaloid contained in opium. Dose : ½ to 2 grains. Very dangerous. 10s. per oz.

CONIA.—The active principle of poison or spotted hemlock. Dose : 1-60th to 1-15th grain. Very poisonous. 4s. per oz.

CONDURANGO BARK.— This drug was introduced as a remedy for cancer. Dose of the powder, ½ to 1 teaspoonful. Safe 6d. per oz.

COTTON ROOT.—Used by the natives of Africa for its emmenagogue properties. Dose of fluid extract ½ to 1 teaspoonful. Use with care.

CROTON OIL.—A most powerful drastic purgative, used in obstinate constipation and apoplexy, also as a counter-irritant in very small doses; one part in ten of olive oil as an ordinary purgative. Dose: ½ to 1 drop. Very dangerous in over-doses. 1s. 6d. per oz.

DIGITALIS.—Better known as foxglove leaves. The dried leaves of digitalis purpurea (foxglove leaves) have a faint, agreeable, tea-like odour; their taste is somewhat bitter and acrid. At least five principles are said to be present in fox-glove leaves : digitoxin, digitalin, digitalein, digitonia, and digitin. The first three are cardiac poisons. Digitonia has an action like that of japonin, being a powerful irritant, a local anæsthetic, and a muscular poison. Digitin appears to be inert. Digitoxin and digitalin are insoluble in water, while digitalein is readily soluble. Digitalis is given as a cardiac sedative in almost all cases where there is excited action, whether it be of sympathic origin or due to organic disease of the heart or great vessels, as hypertrophy, valvular disease, aneurism, &c. Digitalis is also employed as a diuretic, more especially when the deficient flow of urine is due to heart disease and associated with dropsy. It should not be used in the dropsy of chronic Bright's disease. Dose of the powdered leaves, ½ to 1½ grains; of infusion 2 to 4 drachms; of tincture 5 to 30 drops; dose of digitalis, 1-60th to 1-30th grain We would not use any of these concentrations; the tincture or the infusion is strong enough, and must be used very carefully. Leaves, 6d per oz. Tincture, 9d per oz.

DONOVANS (solution).—Solution of iodide of arsenium and mercury. A very pale yellow liquid, having no odour, but a styptic taste. It has been used chiefly in obstinate skin diseases, and seems occasionally to be useful when other preparations of arsenium fail. It is peculiarly applicable to those depending on venereal taint. Externally, freely diluted, it has been used as a lotion in similar cases. Dose, 10 to 30 drops. Dangerous. 6d per oz.

DOVER'S POWDER.—Compound powder of ipecacuanha. A mixture of ipecacuanha, opium, and sulphate of potassium, generally given as a diaphoretic, and sometimes employed in catarrhal affections. Dose, from three to five grains. Use very carefully.

ELATERIUM.—The active principle of ecbalium elatorium or squirting cucumber. Elatrium is a powerful drastic, hydragogue purgative, used chiefly in dropsical affections. It sometimes causes nausea and great depression, hence should be carefully administered. Dose, 1-16th to ½ grain. Dangerous. 1s per drachm.

EPSOM SALTS.—Sulphate of Magnesia. Generally made from dolomite, a magnesian limestone, by treating it with sulphuric acid. Formerly made from the residual liquor of the crystallization of common salt, from sea water. The properties of Epsom salts are too well known to require mentioning. Dose, from ½ to 1 oz. Safe in these doses not too often repeated. 1d per ounce.

ERGOT.—Is a fungus which grows on ryegrass in the form of a spur, which is separated from the grain, dried and powdered. The oil, which has little or no medicinal properties, is separated by ether. In the preparation of the fluid extract, which is the form generally employed for administration, the dose is from 5 to 30 drops. Used to stop internal bleedings and cause contractions of the womb. Requires careful use. Fluid Extract and Powder, 1s per ounce.

ERIGIRON, Oil of.—Distilled from the French herb Canadian fleabane. Used in America in all forms of internal bleedings, dysentery, &c. Dose, 5 to 20 drops. Safe.

ÆTHER.—Sulphuric Æther. A volatile liquid prepared by the action of sulphuric acid on alcohol. Taken internally, ether is a powerful diffusible stimulant, more rapid in its action than alcohol. It is used for flatulency and to allay pain and cramp in the stomach, to diminish spasm in various other affections, as in spasmodic asthma, angina pectoris, and hysteria. When applied externally it produces cold by its rapid evaporation, and is occasionally made use of as a refrigerant in the reduction of hernia. Inhaled in the form of vapour, it acts as an anæsthetic. It is almost universally preferred to chloroform in America, and its use in this country has become very general during the last few years. Dose, 15 to 30 drops. Dangerous. 9d per ounce.

FEL BOVINUM.—Purified Ox Bile. Dried bile appears to act as a slight laxative on the alimentary canal when given in the ordinary medicinal doses. Its use is supposed to be indicated in cases attended with deficient excretion of biliary matter, as shown by the pale colour of the alvine evacuations. Dose, 5 to 10 grains. Safe. Fl. ext. 9d per ounce.

FELIX MAS (male fern).—Is used as an anthelmintic, and acts apparently by killing the worms, and thus aiding their expulsion from the intestinal canal. Its use has been attended with much success in cases of tape-worms. It should be given on an empty stomach, and followed after an interval by some mild purgative. Upon the whole the liquid extract of male fern is perhaps the most valuable and most extensively employed of any anthelmintic in this country for the removal of tape-worm. In emulsion and capsules (see treatment for tape-worm.) Dose of the liquid extract, ½ to 1 drachm. 6d per drachm.

FOWLER'S SOLUTION (arsenical solution).—A mixed solution of arsenite and carbonate of potassium. Employed in certain forms of skin diseases not of syphilitic origin. Dose, 2 to 5 drops. Dangerous. 1s per oz.

GAMBOGE.—The gum resin obtained from Garcinia Hanburii, imported from Siam. Gamboge acts as a drastic and hydragogue purgative, often causing vomiting and griping. It sometimes promotes the action of the kidneys. It is seldom given alone, but combined with cream of tartar or some vegetable purgative, usually in pills. Dose, 1 to 4 grains. Dangerous. 1s per oz.

GELSEMINUM (Yellow Jasmine Root).—The active properties of the root are due to an alkaloid, gelsemine. Gelseminum acts chiefly on the nervous system. It has been employed in various forms of neuralgia, rheumatism, and muscular spasm as a sedative. Serious results have occurred from an overdose. Dose of the tincture, 5 to 20 drops. Dose of the alkaloid, 1-16th to 1-30th grain. Use carefully. 1s 6d per drachm. Tincture of root, 9d per oz.

GENTIAN ROOT.—The dried root of Gentiana Lutea, growing chiefly in the European Alps and Pyrenees. Gentian is a simple bitter or stomachic tonic, improving the appetite and giving tone to the stomach, hence used in convalescence from acute disease, and in cases of dyspepsia. Dose of extract, 2 to 10 grains. Tincture, 1 to 2 drachms. Of the infusion, 1 to 2 ounces. Safe.

GINGER.—The dried root of the Zingiber Officinale, native of Hindostan and China, but cultivated in the West as well as in the East Indies. Ginger is an aromatic, stimulant, and carminative. When taken internally it produces an agreeable feeling of warmth, and appears to aid digestion by giving a healthy tone to the stomach ; hence it is used in atonic forms of dyspepsia, especially if attended with much flatulence, and as an adjunct to various purgative medicines, to correct their griping tendency. Dose in powder 10 to 20 grains ; of the syrup 1 to 4 drachm ; of the tincture 15 to 60 drops. Safe. Crude root, 2d per oz. Powder, 3d per oz. Strong tincture, 6d per oz.

GLYCERINE.—A sweet principle, obtained from fats and viscid oils. Glycerine is used on account of its physical properties as an adjunct to lotions in skin diseases to prevent the surface from becoming dry. It has been proposed as a substitute for sugar in the diet of diabetic patients. Taken internally it is slightly aperient. Dose : 1 to 2 drachms. Safe. 3d per oz.

GUARANA.—A dried paste prepared from the powdered seeds of Paullinia Soebilis, from Brazil. It has been recommended as a remedy for migraine or sick headache. One or two doses will frequently ward off a threatened attack in persons liable to recurrent paroxysms of the disorder, but its action is somewhat uncertain. Dose : 15 to 30 grains in powder or infusion, and repeated if necessary, in two hours ' Safe. 1s. 6d. per oz.

GUAIACUM WOOD (Lignum Vitæ).—The heart wood of guaiacum officinalis, native of St. Domingo and Jamaica. The chips of guaiacum are generally used in conjunction with sarsaparilla, sassafras, and other alteratives. The resin taken from the chips is employed in chronic forms of rheumatism, especially that form called cold rheumatism, in which the symptoms are relieved by warmth ; also in chronic gout, and many other affections, as skin diseases and dysmenorrhœa. Dose of the resin, 10 to 30 grains. Safe. Chips, 3d per oz. ; gum, 9d per oz.

HOFFFMAN'S ANODYNE.—(Compound spirit of æther) is a mixture of ether and spirits, two of the former and eight of the latter. Used in flatulency, colic, and as a diffusive stimulant. Half to two drachms. Use carefully. 9d. per oz.

HENBANE LEAVES.—The fresh leaves of Hyoscyamus Niger. Henbane appears to act as belladonna and stramonium, but is much milder, and is used chiefly as a sedative in certain excited conditions of the nervous system when opium is not advisable. It is also employed to diminish pain and allay irritation of the bladder, to prevent the griping of purgative medicines, ease cough, and diminish pain in many other diseases. Dose of the extract, one to two grains ; of the tincture, half to one drachm. Dangerous. Leaves 4d. per oz. ; extract 6d. per drachm ; tincture 6d. per oz.

IGNATIA BEAN.—The fruit of a tree growing in the Philippine Islands, having the same properties as nux vomica, yielding like it the powerful poison, strychnine. Dose of the extract, half to one grain. Used in paralysis and nerve diseases. Very dangerous. 9d. per drachm.

IODINE.—Is prepared from kelp, the vitrified ashes of sea wrack, found in the Western Islands. When applied externally, free iodine acts as an irritant, or vesicant, according to the mode of using it. Iodine is also used in chronic skin diseases, and over-enlarged and indurated parts, and diseased joints, to alter action or cause absorption, or as a parasiticide. For this purpose it may be used in the form of the liniment, solution, tincture, or ointment. Use carefully. 1s. per oz.

IODOFORM.—Iodoform results from the action of iodine in a mixture of alcohol and solution of carbonate of potassium. Iodoform is a powerful antiseptic and deodoriser. On account of its local anæsthetic and antiseptic properties, it is used in operations on the bladder or rectum ; in chancres and syphilitic sores; also to relieve the pain in cancers. Outward use safe. 1s. per oz.

IODIDE OF POTASSIUM.—The mode of preparing this salt consists in adding iodine to a solution of potash. It has been administered in large doses (20 to 30 grains three times a day) to patients suffering from aortic aneurism. Its depressent influence upon the circulation, aided by rest and low diet. probably explains the good results that have sometimes been obtained. It also has the power of causing the elimination of mercury from the system, and is administered with advantage after a mercurial course. It also removes lead. Ordinary dose, 5 to 20 grains. Use with care. 2s. per oz.

IPECACUANHA, (the dried roots of).—Cephælis ipecacuanha, growing chiefly in the Brazils, and sent from Rio Janeiro. Ipecacuanha, in large medicinal doses, is an emetic. It is well suited as an emetic in chest affections, accompanied with fever, as in bronchitis, consumption, phthisis, and croup, in which the after expectorant effect is of great service; also to unload the stomach in dyspepsia when of an inflammatory character. As an expectorant it is used in the various forms of bronchitic disease. Dose as an emetic, 15 to 30 grains ; as an expectorant, half to two grains. Safe in above doses. 1s. per oz. ; wine, 1s.

IRON.—Iron forms an essential part of the red corpuscles of the blood, as much as six and a half per cent. of the metal being contained in the pure colouring matter. This portion of the blood is apt from various causes to become deficient, and a state of system is then induced designated by anæmia. Iron preparations also produce a distinct and direct influence upon the nervous system, and hence their administration is indicated in debility of the system, as in many cases of chorea, neuralgia, hysteria, epilepsy, &c. Iron salts are often given in amenorrhœa as emmenagogues, but it is questionable if they act directly upon the uterus. They certainly do so indirectly by restoring the blood to its normal state, and hence causing the necessity of a catamenial discharge. There are about 20 different preparations of iron, but we have not space to describe them all, we will give the dose of a few of the most common preparations. Tincture of iron or steel drops, 5 to 30 drops, 6d. per oz., reduced, iron, 5 to 10 grains, 3d per oz.; carbonate, 3 to 20 grains, 3d. per oz. Used with care.

JABORANDI.—The dried leaflets of pilocarpus pennatifolius, imported from Brazil. Jaborandi is a powerful diaphoretic and sialagogue. In large doses it causes vomiting. It increases the rapidity of the heart's action, and diminishes arterial tension, causing flushing of the face, ears and neck, followed speedily by profuse perspiration and enormous secretion of saliva. Dose of the fluid extract, ½ to 1½ drachms; of the tincture, ½ to 2 drachms. Leaves, 6d per oz. Fluid extract, 9d per oz. Tincture, 6d per oz. Use carefully.

JALAP.—The dried root of Ipomœa Purga, True Jalap plant, imported from Mexico. It is named from the city

Xalapa. Jalap is a brisk purgative, causing watery discharge, much allied to but less irritant than scammony. Jalap is used as an ordinary purgative in costiveness and imflammatory affections, especially when combined with aromatics, which diminish the griping. It is also given as a hydragogue in dropsies. Dose of the powder, 10 to 30 grains. Of the tincture, ½ to 2 teaspoonfuls. 6d per ounce. Safe in above doses.

KAMALA.—The powder, consisting of minute glands and hairs obtained from the surface of the fruits of Mallotus Philippinensis (rottlera tinctoria), imported from India. A powerful anthelmintic found very efficacious in India in the treatment of tape-worms. It usually purges freely. Dose, 30 grains to ¼ ounce in honey or thick gruel. Safe. 6d per ounce.

KINO.—The juice hardened in the sun, flowing from the incised bark of pterocarpus marsupium or Indian kino tree, growing near the Malabar coast. A powerful astringent. May be given when tannin is indicated. Often employed in pyrosis and diarrhœa, and as a gargle in relaxed throat. Dose of powdered kino, 10 to 30 grains. Of tincture, ½ to two teaspoonfuls. Use carefully.

KOUSSO.—The dried panicles, chiefly of the female flowers of Hagenia Abyssinica, native of Abyssinia. Kousso acts as an efficient anthelmintic; whether it is superior to other remedies of the same class is as yet doubtful. It has little or no cathartic power, and the subsequent administration of a purgative is generally required to bring away the entozoa which the kousso seems to destroy. Dose of the infusion, 4 to 8 fluid ounces. Safe. 1s per oz.

KRAMERIA RADIX (Rhatany Root)—The dried root of Peruvian rhatany, growing in New Granada and Brazil. A powerful astringent. It is used in chronic forms of diarrhœa and dysentery, and may be given in the various forms of hemorrhage. The powder has much repute as a dentifrice where the gums are bleeding or spongy.   Dose of the powder, 20 to 60 grains.   4d per ounce.

LACTUCARIUM.—Is the name given to a substance which is prepared by pressing out the milky juice of the flowering tops of the wild lettuce.   The lettuce has been asserted to possess some narcotic power, and has been occasionally eaten at bedtime as a narcotic.   Extract of the fresh juice and lactucarium are employed, and have been prescribed in cases in which opium disagrees, to procure sleep, allay cough, &c. Dose, 5 to 15 grains.   1s per ounce.   Use with care.

LAVENDER, Oil of.—The oil distilled in Britain from the flowers of common lavender, a native of southern Europe. Oil of lavender is stimulant and carminative.   It is used in hysteria, flatulence, and colic.   Dose, 1 to 4 drops.   Safe. 1s to 2s. per oz.

LEAD, Acetate of.—Sugar of lead, prepared by dissolving oxide of lead in dilute acetic acid, and subsequent evaporation and crystallisation.   In small doses sugar of lead acts as a sedative and astringent, but it is more used as an external than an internal remedy.   Externally it is used in skin affections and to reduce inflammation.   Dose, 1 to 3 grs. Dangerous in internal use ; outward use with care.   3d. per oz.

LITHIUM, (Carbonate of).—A powerful diuretic, and in the same dose has more influence in rendering the urine alkaline than the corresponding salt of sodium or potassium.   Accordingly it may be given with great advantage in acute and chronic gout, in uric acid gravel, and renal calculus ; owing partly to its solvent, partly to its diuretic properties.   Externally it may be used as a lotion (4 grains to the oz.) to parts affected with gouty inflammations of joints or stiffened by chronic gout ; to gouty ulcers and to chalk stones covered with unbroken skin.   Dose of the carbonate, 3 to 6 grs.   Use carefully.   2s. 6d. per oz.

LITHIUM, (Citrate of).—The citrate of lithium resembles the carbonate as far as its remote antacid properties are concerned, but it has no direct antacid property; that is, it has no influence upon any acid it meets with in the alimentary canal. Dose, 5 to 10 grs. 3s. per oz.

LOGWOOD. — The sliced heart-wood of Hæmatoxylon Campechianum, a native of Campeachy. Logwood is chiefly employed as an astringent in affections of the alimentary canal, as diarrhœa, chronic dysentery, and some forms of atonic dyspepsia. It is often given to children. Dose of decoction of logwood, 1 to 2 fl. ozs.; of extract, 10 to 30 grs. Safe.

MANGANESE, (Oxide of, called also black oxide of manganese).—Is found native, sometimes crystallized, sometimes amorphous. As met with in commerce it is a black, heavy powder, devoid of odour and taste, and when heated to redness evolves oxygen. The black oxide is not used in medicine. 2d. per oz.

MANNA.—A concrete saccharine exudation from the incised bark of Fraxinus Ornus, obtained by making incisions in the stems of the trees, which are cultivated for the purpose chiefly in Sicily and Calabria.—A very mild laxative, adapted for children, also a pleasant adjunct to some purgative draughts, though it sometimes causes flatulence and griping. Dose, 1 drachm to 1 oz. 6d. to 1s. per oz.

MORPHIA, Muriate of.—The hydrochlorate of an alkaloid prepared from opium. Morphia has both a soporific and a convulsant action. Clinical experience has shown that morphia possesses the anodyne and soporific powers of opium, and gives to the drug most of its valuable properties. At the same time its action is as a rule more agreeable, having less tendency to cause headache, nausea, and constipation; it is also much less stimulant in its operation, and does not produce the full diaphoretic effects of opium. Since the sub-cutaneous method of administration has become general, the use of morphia to alleviate pain has been much extended. It is stated to cause less constitutional disturbance when given hypodermically than by the mouth. Moreover, in some rare cases it seems to give more effectual and permanent relief when injected at the seat of pain, than when introduced elsewhere. The smallness of the dose required and the rapidity of its operation, are two practical advantages of the hypodermic method. It may be employed to allay pain and spasms occurring in almost any condition of the system, as in the varieties of neuralgia and colic during the passage of renal and biliary calculi, in tetanus, in inflammation of various kinds, in short, pain from whatever cause arising. Dose, 1-10th to ½ gr. Very dangerous. 2s. per drachm.

Musk.—The dried secretion from the follicus of the prepuce of moschus moschiferus, native of Thibet and other parts of Central Asia. Musk is a stimulant and antispasmodic, hence it has been used in hysteria and epilepsy, and also to rouse the system in cases of an adynamic type as in typhoid pneumonia. Its price, however, is almost prohibitive. Dose: 5 to 10 grains. We need not say use it sparingly. 6d per gr.

Nux Vomica.—The seeds of the strychnos nux vomica, growing in and imported from the East Indies. The action of nux vomica is chiefly, if not wholly, due to the strychnine it contains. It acts as a bitter stomachic and often relieves in some forms of dyspepsia, as in phrosis. Nux vomica is much used in the treatment of paralysis, more especially when depending on lead poisoning and in other forms of local paralysis, such as atony of the bladder. It is also of service in giving tone to the muscular system in cases where debility has arisen after severe illness, such as rheumatic fever, also to give tone in impotence from nervous exhaustion. Its power as an aphrodisiac is often well marked. Dose of extract ⅙ to ½ grain; of tincture 5 to 15 drops. 2s 6d per drachm; tincture, 6d per ounce. Dangerous.

Oil of Cinnamon.—The oil distilled from cinnamon bark is a stimulant, aromatic, and carminative; useful as an adjunct in diarrhœa; may also be employed in flatulence. Dose: 1 to 3 drops. Use with care. 1s per drachm.

OIL OF CLOVES.—The oil distilled in Britain from cloves. Cloves and the oil are stimulant, aromatic, and carminative, employed in atonic dyspepsia, to allay vomiting in pregnancy, and to relieve flatulence; locally used to arrest the pain of carious teeth. 1s 6d per ounce. Use with great care.

OIL OF CAJUPUT.—The oil distilled from the leaves of the Cajuput tree growing in the Molucca Islands. A powerful topical and general stimulant and antispasmodic employed in flatulent colic, hysteria, and cholera, also in chronic rheumatism and low states of the system externally; when mixed with olive oil it is used as a liniment for chronic rheumatism and gouty parts. Dose: 1 to 4 drops. 1s 6d per ounce. Use with care.

OIL OF NUTMEG.—A concrete oil obtained from nutmugs by expression and heat. Nutmeg is an aromatic and gentle stimulant and carminative. In large doses it is said to possess well marked narcotic properties, causing drowsiness and even complete stupor and insensibility. Dose: 1 to 4 drops Dangerous. 1s 6d per oz.

OIL OF PEPPERMINT.—The oil distilled in Britain from the fresh flowering plant of mentha piperita. Oil of peppermint is stimulant and carminative. Dose: 1 to 4 drops. Use with care.

OIL OF PIMENTO.—The oil distilled from allspice. The properties are the same as cloves. Dose: 1 to 4 drops

OIL OF ROSEMARY.—The oil distilled from the flowering tops of rosemary. A powerful stimulant; useful in hysteria and nervous headaches. Dose: 1 to 4 drops. Use like the other, carefully. 1s per oz.

OIL OF RUE.—Distilled from the fresh herb. Oil of rue acts as a powerful topical stimulant and has been used in flatulent colic. It also appears to be antispasmodic and emmenagogue, and seems useful in hysterical affections and in epilepsy. Dose: 1 to 4 drops. With care. 2s per oz.

OIL OF SAVIN.—The oil distilled from fresh savin tops. Savin acts as an irritant, both internally and externally; it also appears to exert much power upon the uterus as an emmenagogue. In large doses it causes abortion, and its administration is attended with much danger. Savin should not be given in pregnancy. Dose: 1 to 4 drops. Dangerous. 2s per oz.

OIL OF SPEARMINT.—The oil distilled from the fresh herb when in flower of mentha viridis. Spearmint oil is stimulant and carminative, and is used as an adjunct to purgative medicines to correct flatulency. Dose: one to four drops. Use carefully.

OIL OF TEREBINTH, (oil of turpentine).—Oil distilled. usually by aid of steam from the oleoresin or turpentine of pinus australis, imported from America and France. In small doses it becomes absorbed, and acts as a stimulant, antispasmodic, astringent, purgative, and possesses great power of destroying worms in the elementary canal. In large doses it injures the kidneys and causes bloody urine. Dose : 5 to 20 drops. Dangerous.

PEPSIN.—The stomach of a recently killed pig, sheep, or calf, is cut open, and any adherent portions of food, &c., carefully removed, and the exposed mucous surface slightly and rapidly washed with cold water. The mucous membrane is then scraped with a blunt knife, and the viscid pulp thus obtained spread out on a plate of glass, and quickly dried. Pepsin has been given largely in cases of dyspepsia, especially when of the atonic kind, and has been asserted to be a very valuable remedy. Dose: two to five grains. 4s. to 6s. per oz.

PHOSPHORUS.—Prepared from phosphoric acid, or super-phosphate of calcium, made by acting upon bone ashes with oil of vitrol. Phosphorus is said to act as a powerful stimulant and aphrodiosiac. It has been employed on the continent in low fevers, cholera, &c. It has been used for headaches resulting from too prolonged mental occupation. Dose in the form of capsule or pill, 1-100th to 1-30th grain. Very dangerous. 6d. per oz.

PILOCARPIUS (nitrate of pilocarpine).—The nitrate of an alkaloid, obtained from extract of jaborandi. The properties are similar to jaborandi leaves. Dose: 1-30th to 1-6th grain. Dangerous.

PODOPHYLLIN, Resin of.—Is prepared in the following manner:—Mandrake root is exhausted by percolation with rectified spirits. The spirit is then distilled off, and the remaining liquid slowly poured into three times its volume of water. The deposited resin is afterwards washed on a filter with distilled water and dried. The resin acts as a drastic purgative, not unlike jalap or scammony resins ; it however, differs from them in its power of causing an increased secretion or flow of bile. That it frequently causes an emptying of the gall bladder is certain, but its operation in increasing the secretion of bile is doubted by some, for if many evacuations, they say, are caused by its action, the latter ones are of a mucous character rather than bilious. It is much used for congestion of the liver. Dose : ¼ to 1 grain. Dangerous. 9d. per drachm.

QUININE, Sulphate of.—The sulphate of an alkaloid prepared from the powder of various kinds of cinchona and Remijia bark. Quinine is employed in medicine as a tonic. In small doses it increases the appetite, especially of weak patients ; hence it improves their general health and muscular power. It also checks the sweating of extreme debility. As an antiperiodic, quinine acts as a specific in ague, malarious remittents, miasmatic, neuralgia, hepatic and splenic engorgements. Quinine is able to cure or relieve certain forms of neuralgia, which are not due to malaria. As an antipyretic, doses of 5 to 15 grains have a marked effect in reducing temperature in pyrexia, to whatever cause it may be due. It has also been employed in the continued fevers. Dose : tonic, 1 to 3 grains; antiperiodic, 5 to 15 grains. In divided doses, use it carefully, as serious consequences have accrued from large doses. 1s. per drachm.

QUININE, Valerianate of.—Is sometimes employed in medicines. It is said to be particularly useful in some forms of intermittent fevers, and spasmodic neuralgic affections. Dose: 1 to 5 grains. With care. 2s. per drachm.

QUININE AND IRON, Citrate of.—This salt possesses the combined properties of both iron and quinine, and is an elegant preparation. It must be remembered that the quinine is precipitated by alkalies. Dose: 5 to 10 grains. Safe in these doses. 6d. per drachm.

SALICIN.—A crystalline glucoside obtained from the bark of salix alba ; also from the bark of various species of populus and willow trees. Salicin is supposed to be tonic and anti-periodic, and has been recommended in intermittents as a substitute for cinchona. Dose: 3 to 20 grains. Safe in these doses. 6d. per drachm.

SANTONIN.—A crystalline neutral principle obtained from worm seed. Administered internally, santonin sometimes causes yellow or green vision, and again, even in a three grain dose, it stains the urine of a yellow colour. This effect may continue for two or three days, and is sometimes attended by irritation of the bladder. It is employed as an ánthel-mintic. Its small bulk and comparative tastelessness render it very suitable for children. It should be followed by a mild purgative. Dose, one to three grains for a child ; two to six grains for an adult. Dangerous in overdoses. 6d per drachm.

SCAMMONY, Resin of.—A resin obtained from dry scammony root by means of rectified spirits. A drastic purgative, generally causing much watery discharge, and often griping. Useful to give activity to other purgatives, which appear to diminish its violence. It is employed in cerebral and dropsical effusions, torpidity of bowels, and as a vermifuge for children. Dose, three to eight grains. Care in use.

SILVER, Nitrate of.—Is prepared by dissolving refined silver in a solution of nitric acid and water, and evaporating the clear solution, and allowing it to crystallize. Externally it is used to poisoned wounds, pustules, ulcers, venereal and other; also to diminish or destroy morbid growths. Occasionally it is rubbed on the skin to produce vesication. It is also used by oculists in the form of a lotion, of various strengths. Dangerous. 1s per drachm.

STRYCHNINE.—An alkaloid obtained from nux vomica. Strychnine is a very dangerous poison, with properties the same as nux vomica. Dose, 1-16th to 1-12th part of a grain. Very dangerous. Used in destroying rats, mice, rabbits and birds.

SULPHUR.—An elementary body found native as virgin sulphur. In small doses sulphur is absorbed into the blood and acts as a stimulant to the skin and different mucous membranes. Silver worn on the person of patients taking sulphur becomes blackened. In larger doses it produces a laxative or very mild purgative effect upon the bowels. Externally it is a slight stimulant, and has the power of destroying the itch insect, and all the vegetable parasites that infect the skin. Sulphur is a valuable remedy in mercurial ptyalism. Dose as a stimulant, 5 to 10 grains and upwards. As a laxative, 30 to 60 grains or more. Use carefully. 2d per ounce.

SPIRITUS ÆTHERIS NITROSI (popularly known by the name of sweet spirits of nitre), is prepared by the action of nitric and sulphuric acid on copper, while undergoing the process of distillation. Sweet spirits of nitre is a stimulant, diaphoretic, and diuretic. Used for the latter property in dropsies, also as a diaphoretic in slight febrile affections. Dose, ½ to 2 fluid drachms. Safe in these doses. 6d per oz.

TOBACCO LEAF.—The dried basis of Nicotina Tabacum, Virginia tobacco growing chiefly in tropical America. Tobacco, when internally administered, acts as a powerful sedative, especially affecting the heart. It is, however, seldom employed as an internal remedy on account of the dangerous depression sometimes induced.   Externally, tobacco acts as a powerful irritant.   The juice of the green leaves made into an ointment is good for piles.   Dangerous.   6d per oz.

THEA (Tea).—The dried leaves of Camellia Thea.   The appearance of tea leaves, is well-known.   The black and green varieties were at one time believed to be derived from different species.   It appears, however, that the differences between them are due solely to the mode of preparation. Green tea is made by rapidly drying the leaves, while the black teas consist of leaves which have undergone a process of fermentation.   Tea has been employed medicinally in the treatment of migraine, and some intermittent affections; as a stimulant in opium coma, in asthma, whooping cough, and other spasmodic disorders; generally, too freely.

VERATRIM.—An alkaloid obtained from veratrum viride, or green hellebore.   Veratrim causes topical irritation, as shown by the dryness of the fauces and vomiting.   After absorption it produces extreme depression of the heart, arterial and nervous systems   Veratrim is asserted to be a valuable agent in controlling the vascular system in cases of inflammatory disease, and especially in rheumatic fever, gout, and allied affections; the depression and slowness of the pulse appear to be characteristic symptoms of its actions.   Dose: 1-50th to 1-12th grain.   Very dangerous.   1s per drachm.

ZINC, Acetate of.—Prepared by dissolving carbonate of zinc in acetic acid, evaporating and crystallising.   It is chiefly employed as an external agent for the same purposes as sulphate of zinc.   Dose : 1 to 2 grains as a tonic; as a lotion or injection, 1 to 10 grains to the fluid ounce of water.   Dangerous. 6d per oz.

ZINC, Oxide of.—If given in large doses causes vomiting, but it is seldom or never used as an emetic.   In small doses it becomes absorbed, and acts as a tonic and astringent.   Its tonic effects are exerted chiefly upon the nervous system, as is seen in cases of chorea, epilepsy, hysteria, neuralgia, and whooping cough. It is also employed externally as a desiccant and astringent, upon excoriated surfaces and slight ulcerations, either as an ointment or alone, or mixed with starch and dusted upon the parts. Dose, 1 to 5 grains. Use very carefully. 4d per oz.

ZINC, Sulphate of.—In small doses sulphate of zinc acts something the same as the oxide, externally, in solutions of different strengths it is employed as a lotion or injection, as in ophthalmia, gleet, leucorrhœa, &c. Use it carefully. 3d per ounce.

ZINCI, VALERIANAS Valerianate of Zinc.—Prepared by mixing a solution of sulphate of zinc and valerianate of sodium, and separating and purifying the crystals which are formed. Valerianate of zinc is a nervine, tonic, and antispasmodic, and has been given with advantage in cases where the combined action of the metal and valerian seems desirable, as in hysteria, chorea, epilepsy, and various neuralgic affections, especially headache. Dangerous. Dose, 1 to 3 grains.

Dose for children :—The rule usually followed is Dr. Young's—which is as follows : Add 12 to the age of the child, and divide the age of the child by the sum. Thus, for a child of 3 years, it would be 3 divided by 3 + 12 = 3-15ths, or 1-5th of the dose of an adult.

POISONS.

GENERAL REMARKS.

With irritant poisons there is usually almost immediate action along the alimentary canal. The general symptoms are intense pain, vomiting, usually purging, and final collapse. It is important to discriminate the poison taken, the symptoms are so much alike. It is usually difficult to do this without the history of the case. The treatment should be immediate. The poison, if still in the stomach, should be removed as quickly as possible (diluent drinks, emetics, stomach pump); if in the intestinal tract, cathartics should be used; in collapse, external heat, and alcoholic drinks diluted.

The general symptoms with narcotic poisons are: Headache, giddiness, paralysis, coma, delirium, and usually convulsions. Death usually comes from failure of respiration. The first requisite in treatment is to maintain respiration. Flagellations, shakings, commands, galvanism, atropia hypodermically administered, and artificial respiration, are the general means to be employed. The temperature must be maintained. If any of the poison is in the stomach unabsorbed, it must be removed immediately.

ACID, ACETIC.—Symptoms and treatment similar to the mineral acids.

ACID, CARBOLIC.—Symptoms occur quickly. Generally the odour of the acid is noticeable, and white corrugated patches in the mouth. If possible empty the stomach with the stomach pump. Antidotes: Lime water, magnesia, mucilaginous drinks, olive or castor oil.

ACID, HYDROCYANIC.—Is one of the most intense and rapid poisons known. Its effects are the same whether it be inhaled, injected into the blood, or subcutaneously. It may cause death in two ways. A large dose proves fatal in a few seconds. The animal falls as if struck by lightning, with or without a cry. Its pupils are widely dilated. A smaller, but still fatal dose, causes death by aspnœa. The breathing is slow and gasping; the heart's action and pulse almost imperceptible; the pupils are dilated; consciousness is abolished; death is usually preceded by suffocative convulsions. Antidotes: The first measure to be adopted is artificial respiration, which must be kept up for some length of time. An auxiliary measure is the subcutaneons injection of atropia. Ammonia inhaled or injected into the veins.

ACID, MURIATIC, (spirits of salts).—Treatment same as sulphuric acid.

ACID, NITRIC.—Treatment as in sulphuric acid.

ACID, NITRO-MURIATIC.—Treatment as in sulphuric acid.

ACID, OXALIC.—Symptoms occur immediately with intense pain, vomiting of a brownish or greenish mucus. Sometimes the gastric symptoms are less prominent than the nervous symptoms. Antidotes: Lime, common chalk, whitewash. lime from ceilings of rooms, emetics. Do not give the alkaline carbonates.

ACID, SULPHURIC.—Antidotes: Immediate use of chalk, magnesia, whitewash, or soap in milk or water.

ACID, TARTARIC.—Antidotes: Magnesia, lime, soap.

ACONITE (Monkshood).—When an individual is fully under the influence of aconite, the pulsations of the heart are diminished in number. In fatal doses there is loss of sight, hearing, and feeling, followed by syncope, convulsions, and death. Antidotes: Empty the stomach, alcoholic stimulants, injection of ammonia into the veins; keep the patient quite on the back. Digitalis has been strongly recommended to maintain respiration.

AMMONIA.—Antidotes: Neutralize the poison by vinegar or other dilute acid, and give the general treatment required.

ANTIMONY.—Symptoms resemble cholera. Clear the alimentary canal by tannic acid and opium stimulants.

ARSENIC.—Acute arsenical poisoning may present at least two forms. In the one the symptoms are those of intense gastro-intestinal irritation. In the other the action of the poison seems to be concentrated upon the nervous symptoms, while the alimentary canal escapes. Treatment: Empty the stomach. If there has not been free vomiting, use as emetics mustard, sulphate of zinc; as antidotes, oxide of iron, magnesia, large draughts of oil or milk.

BELLADONNA.—Symptoms: Dryness of throat; dilated pupils; rapid breathing; collapse. Treatment: Empty the stomach with emetics or the stomach pump; maintain respiration; hot, then cold douche, flagellations, frictions, opium. Use catheter, if urine is retained; vegetable astringents.

CALABAR BEAN.—Symptoms: Depression of the heart, great muscular weakness, vomiting and purging. Treatment: empty the stomach, atropia in small doses, stimulants, frictions, heat.

CANTHARIDES (Spanish Flies).—Symptoms: Excessive pain and stricture in throat, violent genito-urinary symptoms. Treatment. Empty the stomach, milk and mucilaginous drinks, opium by the rectum; avoid oils, as they dissolve the active principle of the flies.

CHLORAL HYDRATE.—Treatment as in opium poisoning.

CHLOROFORM AND ETHER. — Symptoms: Asphyxia. Treatment: Plenty of air. Dash alternately hot and cold water upon the face and chest. Artificial respiration. Keep the feet higher than the head. In artificial respiration, act with the patient and not against him. Keep the tongue well forward. Dry heat and frictions to aid circulation. Continue efforts if need be for two hours. When poisoning takes place through swallowing chloroform, the stomach-pump should be used, and afterwards treat the same as with narcotic poisoning.

COPPER (Sulphate of).—Excessive vomiting of greenish or bluish matter, copper taste in mouth. Treatment: Eggs given quickly and repeatedly, milk, and opium.

DIGITALIS (Foxglove Leaves).—Symptoms: If the pulse is strong and slow with the patient horizontal, it becomes quick and feeble on his rising; dilated pupils, vomiting, intense headache. Treatment: Empty the stomach and bowels; give tannic acid freely, opium, alcohol; rest in horizontal position.

GAS, CARBONIC ACID.—Dash hot and cold water over the chest; electricity; artificial respiration.

GLASS SWALLOWED.—Crumbed bread, followed by an emetic.

GELSEMINUM.—Symptoms: Staggering gait, dilated pupils, blindness, power of speech lost, respirations irregular. Treatment: Emetics, alcoholic stimulants, heat, electricity, artificial respiration.

HEMLOCK (Conium).—A full dose of any preparation of conium given to a healthy man causes weakness of the legs and staggering gait, with affected vision and laboured, slow respiration. Treatment: Empty the stomach; heat, artificial respiration.

HENBANE.—Treatment the same as with belladonna.

IODINE.—Vomited matter usually bluish. Treatment: Starch or flour given freely in water.

IRON (Chloride of).—Treatment: Alkaline carbonates, lime water, magnesia, mucilaginous drinks.

LEAD (Acetate of, or sugar of lead).—Symptoms: Metallic taste in mouth, vomited matter often milky white. Burning pain in abdomen, stools black; nervous symptoms may be most marked; blue line on gums. Treatment: Empty the stomach with emetics of sulphate of zinc, or stomach pump, followed by large draughts of milk, and eggs, sulphate of soda, Epsom salts.

MERCURY, **Bichlorate of, (corrosive sublimate).**—Symptoms: Metallic taste in mouth, violent pain in abdomen, violent vomiting, scanty and suppressed urine. Treatment: Empty the stomach and give large doses of eggs.

OPIUM.—Large doses of opium' cause intense sleepiness, and there is great difficulty in awakening the patient; in still larger doses poisonous symptoms ensue, the sleep passing into a condition of stupor or coma, with gradually increasing slowness of respiration, feebleness of pulse, cold perspiration, and contracted pupils. Treatment: Emetics (20 grains of sulphate of zinc, ipecacuanha, mustard, common salt, followed by copious drinks of warm water. Maintain respiration. Cold then hot water dashed on breast. Atropia, hypodermically administered. Strong coffee.

PETROLEUM.—Empty the stomach with an emetic and use stimulants.

POISON IVY.—Dilute carbolic acid. Two drops of strong acid in wineglassful of sweetened water.

PHOSPHORUS.—Symptoms: Eructations of a garlic odour, violent gastric pain, vomiting, diarrhœa, vomited matters sometimes phosphorescent. Treatment: There is no antidote. Use sulphate of copper as an emetic. No fatty matter should be allowed. Magnesia in turpentine, and purgatives.

POTASSIUM, **Bromide of.**—Nervous stimulants. Opium.

STRAMONIUM.—Treatment the same as in belladonna.

STRYCHNINE.—In man strychnine causes twitching and rigidity of the muscles, followed by tetanic paroxysms, without loss of consciousness. In the intervals between the paroxysms the muscles are relaxed. Death may ensue from exhaustion between the fits of spasm or from aspnœa during a paroxysm, owing to protracted rigidity of the muscles of respiration. The fatal effects of an overdose of strychnine may be averted by the administration of chloroform or chloral. Tannic acid or vegetable astringents given freely.

SILVER, Nitrate of.—Symptoms : White discolouration of the lips and skin, afterwards becoming black. Vomited matters brownish or black. Treatment: Common salt is an antidote. Give large doses. Albumen, mucilaginous drinks.

VERATRUM VIRIDE (Green Hellebore).—Excessive vomiting, pulse exceedingly faint. Treatment: Stimulate vomiting by free draughts of warm water. The patient must lie flat on his back. Alcohol by the mouth and rectum; opium by rectum; ammonia, heat.

ZINC, Acetate and Sulphate of.—Symptoms: As with sulphate of copper. Treatment: Eggs beaten up in milk and water. Alkaline carbonates.

For Artificial Respiration, see Drowning (Index).

MEDICAL COMPOUNDS.

It has been said, "the world is full of extremes in religion, science, politics," &c.; but in no department of human knowledge is the statement more true than in medicine. Taking the regular doctors as the recognised exponents of the healing art, we find one class almost ignoring medicine; they are satisfied with looking at their patients, giving directions for their comfort, so that nature may not be hindered in her restorative work. This class of doctors pursue what is termed the expectant plan. With them we entirely disagree, for nature not only needs a fair field, but also a helping hand in her work of restoring the sick. Another class believe only in the minute doses of medicine. These, (the homœopaths), acting on their creed, " Similia similibus curantur—" like cures like,"—*i.e.*, that medicinal agents produce in the healthy body the same symptoms that they cure in the sick. This may be so with some of the poisons, but as far as our 20 years' experience goes, we know it is not so with our herbal medicines. We are always prepared to take a dose of any medicine that we prescribe, and do so very often, but never feel any the worse for it. If this theory were true we ought to have had all the diseases in the calendar. The faith of this school in infinitesimal doses is wonderful. An enthusiastic member told us he was now prescribing the millionth part of a grain of salt. It may be our dullness of perception, but for our lives we cannot see reason in the system. On the other hand the allopaths, whose creed is to cure by contraries, have taxed the mineral, vegetable, and animal kingdom to find innumerable and incongruous agents with which to combat disease. During the past 20 years the tendency with the most liberal physicians has been to contract their Materia Medica, weeding out the most dangerous agents, also those, which after repeated trials failed to show any curative power. It was said of a late celebrated doctor that when he began practice he had 20 remedies for every disease, but when he finished he had but 20 for all diseases. There is yet much room for improvement in the allopathic school. Our school (the eclectic botanic), desire to avoid these extremes and found a rational system without the contracting power of human creeds. We fancy some of our readers may say (as many have), what are we to do, seeing doctors differ so widely? We reply, take the hint given in the following well-known line:—"When doctors disagree, the people then are free." Use your freedom and your reason. Learn at least something about medicine before you swallow it. You would not go even to a well-known friend's house and eat anything he chose to give you without your knowing what it was. Of course it is very pleasant for a doctor to see strong faith in his patients, but we, in most cases at least, would prefer to see people of such an intelligent turn, that knowing their system and its peculiarities, they could doctor themselves and their families. This is the chief object we have in view in writing our book. In giving the following recipes, we might state that the reason (with which we agree), for compounding medicines, is that a stronger mixture may be had better designed to meet complications of symptoms so often presented in one case.   For instance, one person may be in good general health, and simply troubled with neuralgia.   In that case a simple medicine, such as gelsemine, might remove it; but another patient, in addition to neuralgia, may be suffering with dyspepsia, so to meet both symptoms you make a compound.   We hope this will be clear to everyone.   We earnestly request our readers to see that they get good ingredients and mix them carefully, and we can assure them that they will not often be disappointed with the result of our Botanic formula.

TINCTURES.

For the sake of saving our space, after giving a few with full particulars as to preparation, we will use the term "proof spirit," which meant two parts of spirit and one part of water, instead of giving the quantity of spirits and of water every time when a diluted spirit is wanted. The reason why some medicines require a stronger spirit than others is that they contain gums which are not soluble in weak menstruums. Some Botanic Chemists use for proof spirit half water and half spirit, but we prefer the stronger, as it is also the officinal or recognised standard. "Usual directions" will mean that the medicine will be steeped for one or two weeks, shaken up daily, pressed, filtered, and bottled for use. Tinctures requiring special treatment will be specified.

TINCTURE OF MYRRH (simple).—

Myrrh, in powder..................... One ounce.
Pure spirits of wine .... Twelve ounces.
Put the spirits and powder into a wide mouthed bottle,

shake up daily, then let it infuse from 10 to 14 days. Filter through filtering or blotting paper.*

TINCTURE OF MYRRH (compound).—

Myrrh, in powder .... Two ounces.
Cayenne, in powder .... One ounce.
Pure spirits of wine.................. One quart.

Prepare as last. This compound tincture is useful as a stimulant, antiseptic, and tonic. Good also for fits and spasms internally ; and as a liniment for rheumatic and other pains, externally.

TINCTURE OF BLACKROOT (Leptandria Verg).—

Blackroot, in powder .... Three ounces.
Pure spirits.......................... One pint.
Water .... Half pint.

Macerate, shake up daily, express and filter. Beneficial iu liver complaints and as a mild laxative. Excellent for that condition in children known as drum-belly, swelling of the mesenteric glands. Dose : from one to two teaspoonfuls one to three times a day. Children in proportion to age.

TINCTURE OF MANDRAKE ROOT (American).—

Mandrake in powder .... Three ounces.
Pure spirits .... One pint.
Steep 14 days, shake up occasionally. This is a useful medicine in liver complaints. biliousness, constipation, mesenteric disease, skin troubles, &c. Dose: 1 to 2 teaspoonfuls ; for children 10 to 30 drops two or three times a day.

TINCTURE OF PODOPHYLLIN is prepared by infusing 1 grain in 1 drachm of spirits. 1 in 30 is the proportion, and use same as mandrake.

---

* All Tinctures should be filtered through paper, either that specially prepared or blotting paper. Cork, and keep your bottles in a cool, dark place. Be sure and label them.

TINCTURE OF CAYENNE :—

    Cayenne in powder .... One ounce.
    Spirits of wine .... Fourteen ozs.
    Water........................... Six ounces.

Steep one to two weeks; shake up occasionally. This is one of the very best stimulants. From 10 drops to a teaspoonful in half or a whole cup of warm water sweetened may be taken whenever a natural stimulant is required. (See page 135.)

TINCTURE OF CRANESBILL.—

    Cranesbill root in coarse powder .... Three ounces.
    Pure spirits .... One pint.
    Water .... Half a pint.

Steep one or two weeks; shake up daily. Dose: from one to two teaspoonfuls in warm water sweetened, or in boiled milk. This will be found a good remedy in diarrhœa, dysentery, English cholera, and whenever an astringent medicine is needed.

TINCTURE OF GINGER.—

    Ginger in powder.................. Three ounces.
    Pure spirits of wine................ One pint.

Prepare as last. Dose: a half to two teaspoonfuls. In flatulence with pain in the stomach it will be found a grateful and useful medicine. In hot water sweetened it is much better than spirits. The tincture may be combined with any of the others as the case to be treated may indicate.

TINCTURE OF CINNAMON.—

    Cinnamon in powder .... Three ounces.
    Pure spirits .... One pint.
    Water .... Half a pint.

Steep and prepare as the others. Dose: One to two drachms. As a mild astringent and aromatic this tincture is very grateful. Given in mesenteric diseases, infantile cholera, diarrhœa, leucorrhœa, and profuse menstruation. May be combined to flavour and strengthen mixtures.

TINCTURE OF CATECHU COMPOUND.—

    Catechu Gum, broken .... One and a half oz.
    Cinnamon, in coarse powder .... One ounce.
    Pure spirits .... One pint.
    Water .... Half a pint.

Prepare in the ordinary way. Dose: from a half to two teaspoonfuls, in slippery elm tea or gum arabic tea sweetened. Good in gleet, gonorrhœa, dysentery, chronic diarrhœa, and whenever a strong astringent is required.

ANTISPASMODIC TINCTURE.—

    Lobelia (herb and seed, in powder) .... One oz.
    Skunk Cabbage (in powder) .... Half oz.
    Scullcap (in powder) .... Half oz.
    Cayenne (in powder) .... Half oz.
    Dilute (proof) Spirits of Wine .... One quart.

Macerate fourteen days, shake daily, express, and filter. Dose: from ten to sixty drops, or less or more.

    Highly useful in spasm, cramp, convulsions, hysteria, lockjaw, neuralgia, palpitatiom of the heart, &c.

TINCTURE OF SWEET-FLAG.—

    Sweet-flag (powder of root) .... Two ozs.
    Dilute (proof) Spirits of Wine .... Pint and half.

Macerate fourteen days, shake up daily, express, and filter. Dose: from a half to two drachms.

    Highly useful in offensive conditions of the stomach and bowels, mesenteric disease, ulceration of the mouth, throat, and internal viscera.

COMPOUND ACETATED TINCTURE OF BLOOD-ROOT.

    Blood-root (powder of) .... One oz.
    Lobelia Seed (in powder) .... One oz.
    Vinegar .... One pint.

Macerate fourteen days, shake daily, express, and filter. Dose: from one to two drachms in Bone-set or Chamomile tea, whenever an emetic is indicated.

TINCTURE OF BLOOD-ROOT.—

    Blood-root (in powder) .... Two ozs.
    Dilute (proof) Spirits of Wine .... One pint.

Macerate fourteen days, shake daily, express, and filter. Dose : as an emetic, from one to two drachms, combined with tincture of lobelia. As a nauseant and expectorant it should be taken in less quantity. As an external application to inflamed mucous surface it is unsurpassed by any known remedy. Highly useful in inflammation of the eyes, used alone or diluted with an equal quantity of soft or distilled water.

TINCTURE OF GOLDEN SEAL.—

    Golden Seal (in powder) .... Three ozs.
    Dilute (proof) Spirits of Wine .... One pint.

Macerate fourteen days, shake up daily, express, and filter. Dose : from ten to sixty drops two or three times a day in a little cold water.

This is an excellent tonic, and may be used with advantage in all cases of gastric debility, loss of appetite, disease of the liver, chronic diarrhœa, leucorrhœa, &c.

COMPOUND TINCTURE OF GOLDEN SEAL.—

    Golden Seal (in powder) .... One oz.
    Lobelia Seed (in powder) .... One oz.
    Dilute (proof) Spirits of Wine .... One pint.

Macerate fourteen days, shake daily, express, and filter. This may be made with equal parts of the alcoholic tinctures of golden seal and lobelia.

It is used in all cases of diseased mucous surfaces. Snuffed up the nostrils, or applied with a camel hair brush, in inflammation of the Schneiderian membrane, or chronic catarrh, it is most efficacious. It is also highly useful in ophthalmic cases.

TINCTURE BISTORT,—

    Bistort Root (in powder) .... Three ozs.
    Dilute (proof) Spirits of Wine .... Pint and a half.

Macerate fourteen days, shake daily, express, and filter. Dose :

from a half to two drachms. Most excellent in cases of
diarrhœa, choleraic disease, dysentery, relaxed condition of the
uvula, ulceration of the mouth, tongue, and stomach. May be
used alone or combined with other remedies.

TINCTURE OF QUEEN'S DELIGHT.—

> Queen's Delight (in powder) .... Three ozs.
> Pure Spirits of Wine .... Pint and a half.

Macerate fourteen days, shake daily, express, and filter. Dose :
from thirty to sixty drops.

Excellent in all cutaneous affections, scrofula, and
syphilis in its primary, secondary, and tertiary forms. It has
been presumed that this tincture is inert unless prepared from
the fresh root; but this is a mistake, its essential active
principle is in the oil, and where the root is well preserved its
medical virtues are retained.

COMPOUND TINCTURE OF BENZOIN.—

> Benzoin .... One oz. and half.
> Purified Borax .... One oz.
> Balsam of Tolu .... Half oz.
> Powdered Aloes .... Two drms.
> Pure Spirits of Wine (Alcohol) ..... One pint.

Macerate fourteen days, shake up daily, express, and filter.
Dose. from thirty to sixty drops, in old diseases of the air
passages, lungs, &c.

Most valuable as an external application to recent wounds,
ulcers, burns, and scalds. This is commonly known as
" Friars' Balsam."

TINCTURE OF ARNICA.—

> Arnica Flowers or Root .... Ounce and a half.
> Dilute (Proof) Spirits of Wine ...... One pint.

Macerate fourteen days, shake up daily, express, and filter.

Highly beneficial as an external application to glandular
swellings, inflammation, wounds, and ecchymosis or
coagulated blood, as in black eyes, bruises, &c.

TINCTURE OF CANTHARIDES.—

    Spanish Flies (in coarse powder)........... Half oz.
    Dilute (Proof) Spirits of Wine .... One pint.

Macerate fourteen days, express, and filter. Dose: from ten to fifteen drops three times a day.

    Highly useful in old gleets, chronic gonorrhœa, amenorrhœa, and incontinence of urine.

TINCTURE OF ASSAFŒTIDA.—

    Assafœtida (in small pieces)......... Two and half ozs.
    Pure Spirits of Wine (Alcohol) ...... One pint.

Macerate fourteen days and filter. Dose: from thirty to sixty drops. Excellent in hysteria, chorea, nervous excitement, convulsions, and epilepsy.

TINCTURE OF PRICKLY ASH BERRIES.—

    Bruised Prickly Ash Berries .... Four ozs
    Dilute (Proof) Spirits of Wine .... One pint.

Macerate fourteen days, shake up daily, express, and filter Dose : from one to two drachms every three hours.

    Highly useful in cases of debility, particularly in typhus and low fever cases generally. It is especially indicated in flatulency of the bowels, cholera, and rheumatism.

TINCTURE OF GENTIAN.—

    Gentian Root (crushed) .... Two ounces.
    Dilute (Proof) Spirits of Wine .... One and a half pint.

Macerate fourteen days, shake up daily, express, and filter. Dose: from thirty to sixty drops. Excellent tonic, useful in cases of debility, loss of appetite, &c.

TINCTURE OF CAMPHOR.—

    Camphor............................. Two ozs.
    Pure Spirits of Wine (Alcohol) .... One pint.

        Dose: from five to twenty or thirty drops.

    Highly useful in all cases where a stimulant is indicated; in flatulency, nausea, griping pains, spasms, &c.

TINCTURE OF OPIUM (Laudanum).—

> Turkey Opium (in powder) .... One and a half oz.
> Dilute (Proof) Spirits of Wine ...... One pint.

Macerate fourteen days, shake up daily, and filter. A full dose of opium is one grain, and this quantity is contained in about fifteen drops of the above preparation.

ANODYNE, OR CAMPHORATED TINCTURE OF OPIUM.—

> Turkey Opium (in powder) .... One drm.
> Benzoic Acid .... One drm.
> Camphor .... Thirty grs.
> Oil of Anise .... One drm.
> Dilute (Proof) Spirits of Wine .... One quart.

Macerate fourteen days, shake daily, and filter. Dose : from five to ten drops for a child ; for an adult from a half drachm to a drachm.

This is an excellent " palliative," and may be used with advantage in all painful cases where an " anodyne " is indicated.

TINCTURE OF PERUVIAN BARK. —

> Yellow Peruvian Bark (in powder) .... Four ozs.
> Dilute (Proof) Spirits of Wine .... Pint and a half.

Macerate fourteen days, shake up daily, express, and filter. Dose : from a half drachm to 2 drachms.

Exceedingly useful in intermittent fever, combined with other medicines, or taken in cold water, during convalescence.

TINCTURE OF RHUBARB.—

> Rhubarb (Turkey, in powder) .... Three and a half ozs.
> Cardamom Seeds (crushed) ...... Half ounce.
> Dilute (Proof) Spirits of Wine .... One quart.

Macerate fourteen days, shake up daily, express, and filter. Dose : as a purgative, from a drachm to half a fluid ounce ; as a stomachic, from a half drachm to a drachm.

TINCTURE OF ACONITE (Root of).—

> Aconite Root................ Two and a half ounces.
> Rectified Spirits .... One pint.

Macerate fourteen days, shake up daily, express, and filter.

Much prized by the Homœopaths in the prevention and treatment of measles, scarlatina, and diseases of a similar character.

Dose: In the milder forms of the disease, one globule every two, three, or six hours, alternated with Pulsatilla.

TINCTURE BELLADONNA.—

Belladonna Leaves .... One ounce.
Proof Spirit .... One pint.

Macerate fourteen days, shake up daily, express, and filter.

Equally prized by the Homœopaths, in the treatment of scarlatina. "It is" (Pulte says) "a specific for this disease, which is cured by its use alone, except in complicated cases." Dose: as the last.

TINCTURE DIGITALIS.—

Foxglove Leaves...................... Two ounces.
Proof Spirit.......................... One pint.

Macerate fourteen days, shake up daily, express, and filter.
Dose: 10 to 30 minims.

This preparation is used principally in the old practice in ascites and hydrothorax, and as a sedative in arterial excitement and disease of the heart. It was at one time held in high estimation, but has since fallen into disuse.

The tinctures, concentrated medicines, and most valuable pharmaceutical preparations, are not generally kept in stock by wholesale pharmaceutists; many of them, in fact, particularly the resinoids and principal oils, are not prepared in this country. We import principally from America.

Besides the tinctures already named, the following, from their known value, and our own experience, far exceed aconite, belladonna, and digitalis. Indeed we can truly say that their virtues are much more positive, and in every way safe.

TINCTURE GELSEMIUM.—

Gelsemium .... Two and a half ounces.
Proof Spirit .... One pint.

Macerate fourteen days, shake up daily, express and filter.

Invaluable in intermittent, remittent, typhus, typhoid, and nearly all other fevers. Also in puerperal fever, convulsions, peritonitis, painful menstruation, leucorrhœa, neuralgia, headache, gout, rheumatism, punemonia, &c.

Dose : from ten to fifteen or twenty drops, in a wineglassful or half wineglassful of water, every four hours.

TINCTURE OF VERATRUM VIRIDE.—

Green Hellebore Rhizome or Root...... Four ounces.
Rectified Spirit .... One pint.

Macerate fourteen days, shake up daily, express, and filter.

Most excellent in excessive arterial excitement, pericarditis, endocarditis, asthma, rheumatism, chorea, croup, scarlet fever, epilepsy, pneumonia, neuralgia, hooping cough, or wherever an inflammatory diathesis exists.

Add to a drachm of tincture an equal quantity of simple syrup. Dose: begin with eight drops every three hours, increasing the quantity one or two drops, until nausea or vomiting, or a reduction of the pulse to sixty-five or seventy the minute follow ; then reduce the quantity to one half in all cases. Females, and persons from fourteen to eighteen should commence with six drops, increasing one drop only, and decreasing as above. Children from two to five years of age should begin with two drops only, increasing one drop, and decreasing in the same way. Below two years of age one drop every three hours will be sufficient.

Its properties are expectorant, diaphoretic, alterative, nervine, emetic, and arterial sedative.

In pneumonia, typhoid fever, and many other diseases, it must be continued for from three to five or seven days ; it may be continued indefinitely, in moderate doses short of nausea, without the least inconvenience.

It is important to bear in mind that it is dangerous when given in too large doses. It is for this reason that we have recommended careful supervision during its administration. Should an over-dose be given, however, from ten to fourteen drops of Laudanum, in a drachm of Tincture of Ginger, will afford speedy relief.

It will be understood from the principal tinctures being simple that any of them may be readily formed into compounds, if necessary. Thus: equal parts of Tincture of Mandrake, Leptandrin, and Ginger, become a " compound tincture " by combination. The same may be applied to all the others.

Of the relative strength of Alcohol it will be sufficient to say that the specific gravity of ardent or " Pure Spirits of Wine " is 0·794, and of Dilute or Proof Spirit, 0·935. Ardent or Pure Spirit of Wine is one that is free from water; Proof or Dilute Spirit contains one-third distilled water. The former is termed " Alcoholic Tincture," and the latter " Hydro-Alcoholic Tincture."

The Resinoids, Extracts, Powders, Concentrated Remedies, Herbs, &c., recommended throughout the work, as well as very many others not introduced, are kept in stock at our establishments.

The foregoing tinctures are generally all that Botanic Doctors use; but as the British Pharmacopœia contains several that are not included, we will give them in addition. The uses of some of them will be found in our regular list of medicines (Page 153.) Space will only allow us to give their chief properties.

TINCTURE OF ALOES. –

 Socotrine Aloes, in coarse powder ... Half ounce.
 Extract of Liquorice .... One and a half ozs.
 Proof Spirit .... 1 pint a sufficiency.
Macerate fourteen days; shake up daily; express and filter.
Dose : 1 to 2 fluid drachms.   Lax. Emm.

TINCTURE OF ORANGE PEEL.—

 Bitter Orange Peel, cut small and bruised .. Two ozs.
 Proof Spirit .... One pint.
Macerate fourteen days; shake up daily; express and filter.
Dose : 1 to 2 fluid drachms.   Ton.

Preparations in which it is used.

Mistura Ferri Aromatica .... 1 volume in 32.
Syrupus Aurantii .... 1 volume in 8.
Tinctura Quininæ.

TINCTURE OF FRESH ORANGE PEEL.—

Bitter Orange
Rectified Spirit } of each .... A sufficiency.

Carefully cut from the orange the coloured part of the rind in thin slices, and macerate six ounces of this in eighteen fluid ounces of the spirit for a week, with frequent agitation. Then pour off the liquid, press the dregs, mix the liquid products, and filter. Finally, if necessary, add spirit to make one pint. Dose : 1 to 2 fluid drachms. Ton.

TINCTURE OF BUCHU.—

Buchu Leaves, coarse powder ...... Two and a half ozs.
Proof Spirit .... One pint.

Macerate fourteen days ; shake up daily ; express and filter. Dose : 1 to 2 fluid drachms. Diur.

TINCTURE OF CALUMBA.—

Calumba Root, cut small .... Two and a half ozs.
Proof Spirit .... One pint.

Macerate fourteen days ; shake up daily ; express and filter. Dose : ½ to 2 fluid drachms. Ton. Alt.

TINCTURE OF INDIAN HEMP.—

Extract of Indian Hemp................ One ounce.
Rectified Spirit .... One pint.

Dissolve the extract of hemp in the spirit. Dose : 5 to 20 minims. Ast. Ner.

COMPOUND TINCTURE OF CARDAMOMS.—

Cardamom Seeds, bruised .... Quarter oz.
Caraway Fruit, bruised .... Quarter oz.
Raisins, freed from seeds .... Two ozs.
Cinnamon Bark, bruised .... Half oz.
Cochineal, in powder .... Fifty-five grs.
Proof Spirit .... One pint.

Macerate fourteen days; shake up daily; express and filter.
Dose : ½ to 2 fluid drachms.   Arom. Car.

Preparations.

Decoctum Aloes Compositum .... 1 volume in 3½.
Mistura Ferri Aromatica .... 3 volumes in 16.
,,   Senæ Composita .... 1 volume in 14.
Tinctura Chloroformi Composita ..... 1 volume in 2.

TINCTURE OF CASCARILLA.—

Cascarilla Bark, coarse powder   .... Two and a half ozs.
Proof Spirit .... One pint.

Macerate fourteen days; shake up daily; express and filter.
Dose : ½ to 2 fluid drachms.   Ton.

TINCTURE OF CHIRETTA.—

Chiretta, cut small and bruised ..... Two and a half ozs.
Proof Spirit .... One pint.

Macerate fourteen days; shake up daily; express and filter.
Dose : ½ to 2 fluid drachms.   Ton.

COMPOUND TINCTURE OF CHLOROFORM.—

Chloroform .... Two fluid ozs.
Rectified Spirit.................... Eight fluid ozs.
Compound Tincture of Cardamoms ..... Ten fluid ozs.

Mix.   Dose : 20 to 60 minims.

TINCTURE OF CHLOROFORM AND MORPHINE.—

(CHLORODYNE).

		Contains in a 10-minim dose.
Chloroform	One fluid oz.	1¼ minim.
Ether	Two fluid drms.	¼ minim.
Rectified Spirit.	One fluid oz.	1¼ minim.
Hydrochlorate of Morphine	Eight grains	1-48 grain.
Diluted Hydrocyanic Acid ..	Half fluid oz.	⅛ minim.
Oil of Peppermint	Four minims	1-80 minim.
Liquid Extract of Liquorice	One fluid oz.	1¼ minim.
Treacle	One fluid oz.	
Syrup	A sufficiency.	

Macerate fourteen days; shake up daily; express and filter.
Dose : 5 to 10 minims.   Sed. Ast. Narcotic.

TINCTURE OF COCHINEAL.—

Cochineal, in powder .... Two and a half ozs.
Proof Spirit .... One pint.

Macerate fourteen days; shake up daily; express and filter.
Colouring liquid.

TINCTURE OF HEMLOCK.—

Hemlock Fruit, in powder .... Two and a half ozs.
Proof Spirit .... One pint.

Macerate fourteen days; shake up daily; express and filter.
Dose : 20 to 60 minims.   Narcot. Sed.

TINCTURE OF SAFFRON.—

Saffron .... One ounce.
Proof Spirit .... One pint.

Macerate fourteen days; shake up daily; express and filter.
Colouring.

TINCTURE OF CUBEBS.—

Cubebs, in powder .... Two and a half ozs.
Rectified Spirit .... One pint.

Macerate fourteen days; shake up daily; express and filter.
Dose : ½ to 2 fluid drachms.   Diur. Sed.

TINCTURE OF ERGOT.—

Ergot, finely comminuted .... Five ozs.
Proof Spirit .... One pint.

Macerate fourteen days; shake up daily; express and filter.
Dose : 5 to 30 minims.   Emm. Ast.

TINCTURE OF ACETATE OF IRON.—

Strong Solution of Acetate of Iron .... Five fluid ozs.
Acetic Acid .... One fluid oz.
Rectified Spirit..................... Five fluid ozs.
Distilled Water .... Nine fluid ozs.

Mix, and then add sufficient distilled water to make one pint.
Preserve in a stoppered bottle. Dose : 5 to 30 minims. Ton. Ast.

TINCTURE OF GALLS.—

Galls .... Two and a half ozs.
Proof Spirit .... One pint.

Macerate fourteen days; shake up daily; express and filter.
Dose : ½ to 2 fluid drachms.   Ast.

AMMONIATED TINCTURE OF GUAIACUM.—

Guaiacum Resin, in powder .... Four ozs.
Aromatic Spirit of Ammonia .... 1 pint a sufficiency.

Macerate fourteen days ; shake up daily ; express and filter.
Dose ½ to 1 fluid drachm.   Anti-rheumatic. stim.

TINCTURE OF HENBANE.—

Henbane leaves, or flowering tops.. Two and a half ozs.
Proof Spirit .... One pint.

Macerate fourteen days; shake up daily; express and filter.
Dose : ½ to 1 fluid drachm.   Sed. Nar.

TINCTURE OF IODINE.—

Iodine .... Half ounce.
Iodide of Potassium .... Half ounce.
Rectified Spirit .... One pint.

Dissolve the iodine and the iodide of potassium in the spirit.
Dose : 4 to 10 minims. Preparation, Vapor Iodi. Outward Use.

TINCTURE OF JABORANDI.—

Jaborandi .... Five ounces.
Proof Spirit .... One pint.

Macerate fourteen days ; shake up daily; express and filter.
Dose, ½ to 1 fluid drachm.   Dia.

TINCTURE OF JALAP.—

Jalap .... Two and a half ozs.
Proof Spirit .... One pint.

Macerate fourteen days; shake up daily; express and filter.
Dose : ¼ to 2 fluid drachms.   Car. Diur.

TINCTURE OF KINO.—

Kino	Two ounces.
Glycerine	Three fluid ozs.
Distilled Water	Five fluid ozs.
Rectified Spirit	Twelve fluid ozs.

Macerate fourteen days; shake up daily; express and filter.
Dose: ½ to 2 fluid drachms. Strong Ast.

TINCTURE OF RHATANY.—

Rhatany Root	Two and a half ozs.
Proof Spirit	One pint.

Macerate fourteen days; shake up daily; express and filter.
Dose: ½ to 2 fluid drachms. Ast.

TINCTURE OF LARCH.—

Larch Bark	Two and a half ozs.
Rectified Spirit	One pint.

Macerate fourteen days; shake up daily; express and filter.
Dose: 20 to 30 minims. Antibil. Stom.

COMPOUND TINCTURE OF LAVENDER.—

Oil of Lavender	1½ fluid drachms.
Oil of Rosemary	10 minims.
Cinnamon Bark, bruised	150 grains.
Nutmeg, bruised	150 grains.
Red Sandal-wood	300 grains.
Rectified Spirit	2 pints.

Macerate fourteen days; shake up daily; express and filter
Dose: ½ to 2 fluid drachms. Preparation, Liquor Arsenicalis.
Nerv. Car.

TINCTURE OF LEMON PEEL.—

Fresh Lemon Peel cut small........	Two and a half ozs.
Proof Spirit	One pint.

Macerate fourteen days; shake up daily; express and filter.
Dose: ½ to 2 fluid drachms. Flavouring.

ETHEREAL TINCTURE OF LOBELIA.—

 Lobelia, in coarse powder .... Two and a half ozs.
 Spirit of Ether .... One pint.

Macerate fourteen days; shake up daily; express and filter.
Dose: 10 minims to ½ a fluid drachm. Antisep. Relax.

TINCTURE OF HOPS.—

 Hop .... Two and a half ozs.
 Proof Spirit .... One pint.

Macerate fourteen days; shake up daily; express and filter.
Dose: ½ to 2 fluid drachms. Ton.

TINCTURE OF NUX VOMICA.—

 Extract of Nux Vomica .... 133 grains.
 Distilled Water .... 4 fluid ozs.
 Rectified Spirit .... 1 pint a sufficiency.

Macerate fourteen days; shake up daily; express and filter.
Dose: 10 to 20 minims. Ton. Ner.

AMMONIATED TINCTURE OF OPIUM.—

 Opium, in powder .... 150 grains.
 Saffron, cut small.................. 180 grains
 Benzoic Acid....................... 180 grains.
 Oil of Anise .... 1 fluid drachm.
 Strong Solution of Ammonia.......... 4 fluid ounces.
 Rectified Spirit .... 16 fluid ounces.

Macerate fourteen days; shake up daily; express and filter.
Dose: ½ to 1 fluid drachm. Sed. Nar.

TINCTURE OF PELLITORY.—

 Pellitory Root .... Four ounces.
 Rectified Spirit .... One pint.

Macerate fourteen days; shake up daily; express and filter.
Stim. Diur.

TINCTURE OF QUASSIA.—

 Quassia Wood, in chips .... Three-quarters of an oz.
 Proof Spirit .... One pint.

Macerate fourteen days; shake up daily; express and filter.
Dose: ½ to 2 fluid drachms. Ton. Stom.

TINCTURE OF QUININE.—

Hydrochlorate of Quinine .... 160 grains.
Tincture of Orange Peel .... 1 pint.

Macerate fourteen days; shake up daily; express and filter.
Dose : ½ to 2 fluid drachms. Ner. Ton.

AMMONIATED TINCTURE OF QUININE.—

Sulphate of Quinine .... 160 grains.
Solution of Ammonia................ 2½ fluid ounces.
Proof Spirit....................... 17½ fluid ounces.

Macerate fourteen days ; shake up daily; express and filter.
Dose: ½ to 2 fluid drachms. Ton. Stom.

TINCTURE OF SAVIN.—

Savin Tops, dried and coarsely powdered .. 2½ ounces.
Proof Spirit .... 1 pint.

Macerate fourteen days ; shake up daily; express and filter.
Dose: 20 minims to 1 fluid drachm. Emm.

TINCTURE OF SQUILL.—

Squill, bruised .... Two and a half ozs.
Proof Spirits .... One pint.

Macerate fourteen days; shake up daily ; express and filter.
Dose 10 to 30 minims. Expec.

TINCTURE of SENEGA.—

Senega Root .... Two and a half ozs.
Proof Spirit .... One pint.

Macerate fourteen days; shake up daily; express and filter.
Dose: ½ to 2 fluid drachms. Expec. Pec.

TINCTURE OF SERPENTARY.—

Serpentary Rhizome.............. Two and a half ozs.
Proof Spirit .... One pint.

Macerate fourteen days; shake up daily; express and filter.
Dose: ½ to 2 fluid drachms. Ton. Feb.

TINCTURE OF STRAMONIUM.—

Stramoniun Seeds, bruised .... Two and a half ozs.
Proof Spirit .... One pint.

Macerate fourteen days; shake up daily; express and filter.
Dose: 10 to 30 minims.   Nar. Sed.

TINCTURE OF SUMBUL.—

Sumbul Root .... Two and a half ozs.
Rectified Spirit .... One pint.

Macerate fourteen days; shake up daily; express and filter.
Dose: 10 to 30 minims.   Ner.

TINCTURE OF TOLU.—

Balsam of Tolu .... Two and a half ozs.
Rectified Spirit .... Sufficient to dissolve.

Macerate fourteen days; shake up daily; express and filter.
Dose: 20 to 40 minims.   Expec.

TINCTURE OF VALERIAN.—

Valerian Rhizone .... Two and a half ozs.
Proof Spirit .... One pint.

Macerate fourteen days; shake up daily; express and filter.
Dose: 1 to 2 fluid drachms.   Ner. Sed.

AMMONIATED TINCTURE OF VALERIAN.—

Valerian Rhizome................ Two and a half ozs.
Aromatic Spirit of Ammonia .... One pint.

Macerate fourteen days; shake up daily; express and filter.
Dose, ½ to 1 fluid drachm.   Stim. Ner.

MEDICINAL OILS.

We have already stated that the active medicinal pro perties of plants differ in quality, hence the necessity of the various preparations introduced throughout the work. The "Oils" in many cases are invaluable; unlike the "Tinctures," however, they are prepared to our hands, and we have nothing to do but to combine and use them agreeably with the cases indicated. Oils are *fixed* or *volatile*, that is to say, the former, after being given off, whether animal or vegetable, are permanent, whilst the latter pass off by evaporation. We select such only as are medically useful.

OL. ANISE.—

Highly useful in bronchial disease and coughs, particularly of infants. It can be taken on sugar, or combined with the Tincture of Mandrake, Ginger, Leptandrin, or indeed with any of them, agreeably with the disease indicated. Dose : 2 to 4 or 6 drops.

OL. CARAWAY.—

It is most excellent in griping pains of the stomach and bowels, particularly of infants. Dose : the same as the last.

OL. PENNYROYAL.—

Highly beneficial in flatulent colic, cramp, and pains in the stomach, amenorrhœa, and catarrh. Dose : same as Ol. Anise.

OL. FENNEL.—

Highly useful as a carminative, and may be used with very great advantage, particularly in the diseases of childhood. Dose . same as Ol. Anise.

OL. CINNAMON.—

Useful in griping pains, and in all cases where an astringent is indicated in connection with a stimulant and antispasmodic. Dose : same as Ol. Anise.

OI. WINTER GREEN.—

Aromatic and stimulant. Useful in all cases where these qualities are indicated. Dose : same as Ol. Anise.

OL. SAVIN.—

Stimulant and emmenagogue, used in amenorrhœa. Dose : from 4, 6, or 10 drops. Ten drops given three times daily on sugar is said to produce abortion.

OL. JUNIPER.—

Excellent in mucous discharges of the urethra and vagina ; also in dropsy and obstruction of the urine. Dose : from 5 to 15 or 20 drops.

OL. LAVENDER.—

Highly useful in nervous debility, headache, hysteria, chorea, &c. Dose : 1 to 6 drops.

OL. CUBEBS.—

Highly useful, used in the same cases as Ol. Juniper.

OL. SASSAFRAS.—

Excellent in obstruction of the urine, glandular enlargements, and diseases of the skin. Dose : from 3 or 4 to 10 drops on sugar. Good as an external application to wens and painful swelling of the joints.

OL. DILL.—

The plant from which this oil is derived is the Anethum Graveolens. It is a native of Spain, but cultivated in our gardens. It is most excellent in griping of the stomach and bowels, flatulency, convulsions, hooping-cough, and diseases of the chest. Dose : from one, two, or three drops on a little sugar, or a half dozen drops to a drachm of any of the tinctures indicated in the treatment for the diseases of children, afford immediate relief.

OL. RUE.—

Excellent in pertussis, hooping-cough, hysteria, amenorrhœa, and dysmenorrhœa. Dose : from one to five drops three times a day.

OL. Valerian.—

Highly useful in chorea, sleeplessness, and hysteria. Dose : from two to six drops.

There is nothing to add as regards the oils, except to say that they may be given on sugar, or with any of the tinctures, agreeably with the indications of cases treated, or the majority of them may be prepared and administered as essence.

ESSENCES.

For example:

ESSENCE OF CARAWAY.—

Oil of Caraway...................... One ounce.
Pure Spirits of Wine .... Nine ounces.
Mix, agitate, or shake well up.

The proportion of spirit and oil employed in this preparation is *one* of oil and *nine* of spirit. The same rule must be observed in the preparation of any one or more of the others. Dose in proportion; that is to say, for one drop of oil ten of the essence.

INFUSIONS.

Infusions are simply powders, leaves, or herbs put into a covered vessel, upon which cold, boiling, spring, or distilled water is poured and allowed to stand. They can be made strong or weak as required; generally speaking, however, one ounce of herbs or leaves is sufficient for 16 ounces of water.

When infusions are intended to be kept we must **add two
ounces** of pure spirits of wine to every quart. Delicate
infusions, such as red rose leaves, flowers of meadowsweet,
elder flowers, &c., if made in the proportions named, and the
spirit added as directed, or tincture of the same, if you can
get it, will keep any length of time if kept in a cool place.
The same may be said of all ordinary herbal infusions.

DECOCTIONS.

Decoctions are generally prepared from crushed barks,
roots, or seeds, and some few of the heavier plants. They are
gently simmered for a half-hour or hour, or more or less as
necessary. They can be preserved in the same way as
infusions, either simple or compound, for any length of time
if kept in a cool place, by simply adding the spirit or
tinctures.

Infusions, decoctions, and tinctures well prepared and
judiciously combined, meet the indications of almost any form
of disease.

MEDICATED WATERS.

These are prepared either by distillation or by triturating any of the Essential Oils with Carbonate of Magnesia. Thus :

CINNAMON WATER.—

Oil of Cinnamon .... Fifteen drops.
Carbonate of Magnesia .... Half drachm.

Triturate or well work up the two, adding very gradually one pint of distilled water. When the whole is thoroughly incorporated filter and bottle for use.

Rose Water, Spearmint Water, Mint Water, Pennyroyal, and all the fragrant waters, may be prepared by the same process.

SYRUPS (SIMPLE).

These are prepared by adding sugar to strong infusions, tinctures, or decoctions of herbs, as follows :—

SIMPLE SYRUP.—

Distilled Water .... One pint.
Lump Sugar .... One pound.

Gradually dissolve in a water bath, simmer for one hour, skim, bottle, and keep in a cool place. Used as a vehicle for more active medicines, particularly in the diseases of children.

SYRUP OF SQUILL.—

Acid Tincture of Squill .... Eight ozs.
Refined Sugar (in powder) .... One pound.

Dissolve in a water bath as the last, skim, and bottle for use.

Highly useful as an expectorant and emetic for respiratory or chest disease in children.   Acid Tincture of Squill is made by steeping two ounces of Squill Root in a pint of vinegar 14 days.

SYRUP OF ORANGE PEEL.—

Dried Orange Peel .... One ounce.

Boiling distilled water........ Three quarters of a pint.

Infuse in a covered vessel, and when cool prepare in a water bath with one pound of lump sugar.   Or as follows :—

Tincture of Orange Peel .... One ounce.

Simple Syrup .... Seven ounces.

Principally used as a vehicle for other medicines in diseases in childhood.

WORM AND TONIC SYRUP (for Children or Adults)—

Balmony .... One ounce.

Indian Pink Root .... One ounce.

Male Fern Root .... One ounce.

Senna .... One ounce.

Simmer in 2 pints water 20 minutes, strain, press, add 2 lbs. of lump sugar, ¼ lb. manna; let boil, skim, cool, and add of santonine 1 drachm, 2 ozs. tincture of mandrake, 1 oz. essence of ginger.   Dose : from 1 to 2 teaspoonfuls for children, to a tablespoonful for adults, in water, or neat, morning and night ; or if it does not open too much, three times a day, before or after meals half an hour.

SOOTHING SYRUP (for babies cutting their teeth, wind, and stomach trouble)—

Turkey Rubarb .... Half ounce.

Cinnamon Stick.................... Half ounce.

Valerian Root .... Half ounce.

Bicarbonate of Potash .... Quarter Ounce.

Simmer in 1½ pints of water half an hour, cool, strain, press through a cloth, add 1 pound lump sugar, simmer a few minutes, skim, and when cool add

Ess. Peppermint .... Quarter ounce.
Ess. Cinnamon .... One drachm.
Aniseed .... One drachm.

Dose : for infants under six months half a teaspoonful ; up to a year, three-quarters ; over, a small to a large teaspoonful, three to four times a day. (Note.—In boiling this syrup care must be taken, as it boils over very readily).

COUGH SYRUP—

Hoarhound .... One ounce.
Angelica Root .... One ounce.
Skunk Cabbage .... One ounce.
Lobelia Herb .... One ounce.
Slippery Elm .... One ounce.

Simmer half an hour in three pints of water, cool, strain, press through a cloth, return to vessel in which it was boiled with two pounds of brown or white sugar or syrup, simmer a few minutes, skim, and when cold add two ounces tincture camphor co. paregoric ; bottle. Dose : for a child, half to a teaspoonful 3 to 6 times a day ; adults, from 1 to 4 teaspoonfuls same number of times. Dose ought to be regulated by the effect it has on the stomach ; in some cases the large dose will sicken, if so take one that will not be too nauseating.

EXPECTORANT SYRUP.—

Saint John's-wort (herb, dry) .... Two ounces.
Sage (garden) .... One ounce.

Simmer in three pints of distilled or soft spring water down to a quart, express when sufficiently cool, filter, add two pounds of fine white sugar, and two ounces of syrup of lobelia ; simmer the whole in a water bath, in a covered vessel, for one hour ; skim, let it cool, and bottle for use. Dose : from a teaspoonful to a tablespoonful four or six times a day.

This is an excellent expectorant, and may be used with advantage in all inflammatory or irritable conditions of the bronchial tubes, pleura, and lungs. It is equally beneficial in hooping-cough, colds, &c., &c.

SYRUP OF LOBELIA.—

Acid tincture lobelia made by steeping one ounce herb and one of seed in a pint of vinegar 14 days. The syrup is simply weight for weight with sugar. Boil, skim, and cool.

SCROFULA SYRUP.—

Yellow Dock Root (dry and crushed).... Two ounces.
American Sarsaparilla (dry and crushed) Two ounces.
Sassafras Bark (dry and crushed) ...... One ounce.

Simmer in five pints of soft or spring water down to four, express when sufficiently cool, filter, add four pounds of fine white sugar, and two ounces of tincture of Stillingin; gently simmer in a water bath for two hours in a covered vessel, skim, let it cool, and bottle for use. Dose: from a teaspoonful to a dessert or tablespoonful four times a day.

This is a preparation that may be used with great advantage in all cases of scrofula and secondary syphilis, scald or scabbed head, eczema, &c.

PULMONARY SYRUP.—

Hoarhound (herb, dry).............. Two ounces.
Coltsfoot (herb, dry) .... Two ounces.
Sanicle, wood (herb, dry)............ Two ounces.

Simmer in three quarts of soft or distilled water down to five pints, and when sufficiently cool, express, filter, add five pounds of lump sugar, three ounces of tincture of pleurisy-root, two ounces of syrup of lobelia, and one ounce of antispasmodic tincture; simmer, for two hours, in a water bath, in a covered vessel; skim, and bottle for use. Dose: from a large dessertspoonful to a tablespoonful four and six times a day.

This is an excellent preparation in cough, pleurisy, and consumption, and may be used with equal advantage in all cases of respiratory disease.

SYRUP OF RHUBARB.—

Turkey Rhubarb (root, bruised) ...... Two ounces.
Boiling soft or distilled water .... One pint.

Infuse twenty-four hours, strain, filter, add one pound of

lump sugar, and one ounce of tincture of ginger; simmer in a water bath for one hour in a covered vessel, skim, and bottle for use. Dose: from one to two teaspoonfuls.

This is an excellent preparation, and may be used in all cases where a gentle laxative is needed.

SYRUPS, simple, compound, pulmonary, emetic, alterative, expectorant, and all other, may be prepared upon the same principle—that is to say, with strong infusions, decoctions, or tinctures. Two ounces of tincture, with 18 of simple syrup, make nearly all the syrups.

A water bath is on the same principle as the glue pot; put the vessel inside another in which is the boiling water.

GARGLES.

These preparations are employed in inflammatory and ulcerated conditions of the throat, elongated uvula, lose of voice, ulcerations of the gums, mouth, tongue, &c.

ASTRINGENT GARGLE.—

    Bayberry (coarse powder) .... One ounce.
    Boiling Water .... One pint.

Infuse twelve hours, strain, filter; and add Tincture of Myrrh (Simple) one ounce.

This is an excellent gargle, and may be used with advantage in all cases of ulceration of the tongue, gums, and mouth; also in elongated uvula, and aphonia, or loss of voice.

ANTI-FEBRILE AND INFLAMMATORY GARGLE.—

    Garden Sage .... One ounce.
    Cayenne (in powder) .... One drachm.
    Boiling Water .... One pint.

Infuse twelve hours, strain, filter, and add tincture of blood-root one ounce.

In inflammation and ulceration of the throat from scarlatina, quinsy, &c., this is one of the best gargles that can possibly be employed.

YEAST GARGLE.—

> Brewers' Yeast .... Two ounces.
> New Milk .... Half pint.
> > Mix, and sweeten with molasses.

In ulcerations of the throat, and offensive discharges from the mouth, gums, and teeth, this is most advantageous, but more particulary in cases of great debility.

STIMULATING GARGLE.—

> Sumach Berries (crushed) .... One ounce.
> Golden Seal (coarse powder) .... One ounce.

Gently simmer in a pint and half of water, for half an hour, in a covered vessel, and when sufficiently cool, strain, filter, and add one ounce of tincture of cayenne.

In old chronic ulcerations of the throat, this gargle will be found exceedingly useful.

LINIMENTS,

Are preparations employed in cases of rheumatism, white swelling, gout, stiff joints, glandular enlargements, muscular paralysis, quinsy, &c.

SOAP OR COMPOUND STIMULATING LINIMENT.—

> Castile Soap .... Two ounces.
> Oil of Sassafras .... One ounce.
> Pure Spirits of Wine .... Twelve ounces.
> Distilled Water .... Two ounces.

Mix and agitate until the whole are well incorporated.

This is an excellent preparation, and may be used with advantage in enlarged tonsils, or swelling of the throat, and glandular enlargements of any kind.

ANODYNE OR LINIMENT CUM OPII.—

Opium (in powder).................. Half ounce.
Camphor .... Two drachms.
Oil of Rosemary .... Half ounce.
Oil of Sassafras .... Half ounce.
Pure Spirits of Wine................ One quart.

Mix and agitate until the whole are well incorporated.

This is highly useful in rheumatism, gout, quinsy, white swelling, inflamed breast, and painful affections of every kind.

LINIMENT OF AMMONIA.—

Ammonia (liquor of, strong) .... One ounce.
Olive Oil .... Three ounces.

Mix and agitate.

This is a useful liniment in all ordinary cases. It is readily prepared, and many practitioners rarely prescribe any other.

SOOTHING LINIMENT OR COMPOUND NERVINE EMBROCATION.—

Opium (in powder) .... One drachm.
Camphor .... One drachm.
Castile Soap (scraped fine) .... One drachm.
Pure Spirits of Wine .... Two ounces.

Agitate together in a mortar until the whole are incorporated.

This is exceedingly useful in all cases where the inflammatory pains and irritation are very severe.

IRRITATING LINIMENT.—

Spirits of Turpentine .... One ounce.
Croton Oil .... Half ounce.
Olive Oil .... One ounce.
Sassafras Oil........................ Two drachms.

Agitate until the whole are well incorporated.

This is an excellent counter-irritant, and very useful in bronchial affections, old coughs, and chronic affections of the lungs. It should be rubbed in daily until the part vesicates or eruptions are formed upon the skin. Use with great care.

COMPOUND CAYENNE LINIMENT.—

Tincture of Cayenne .... One and a half ounces.
Tincture of Opium .... One drachm.
Oil of Rosemay .... One drachm.
Olive Oil .... Two drachms.
     Agitate until the whole are incorporated.

This is an exellent preparation, and may be used with advantage in neuralgia and rheumatic pains.

CHILBLAIN LINIMENT.—

Camphor .... Half ounce.
Chloral Hydrate.................. Half ounce.

Rub these up in a mortar till liquified, then add—

Morphia .... Ten grains.
Oil of Sassafras .... One drachm.
Spirits of Wine .... Four ounces.
Vaseline .... Two ounces.

Rub well together and apply to the chilblains two or three times a day.

BREAST LINIMENT.—

Linseed Oil .... One pint.
Spirits of Camphor............... Four ounces.

Mix, saturate a soft cloth and lay it on the breast; renew every four hours. This is excellent for inflamed breasts, and inflamed swellings of every kind.

DOMESTIC MEDICATED WINES.

These preparations are highly recommended by Dr. John Skelton, who says they have never been introduced in the form of medicines. Experience, however, backed by a knowledge of the recuperative powers of plants, has long convinced us that in the convalescent stages, as well as during the more severe paroxysms of fever, they are most efficacious,—that in fact there is no process of medication so simple and efficient.

MELLISSA (Balm Wine).—

Balm (herb, dry) .... Twelve ounces.
Water .... Two gallons.
Lump Sugar .... Four pounds.

Boil the water and infuse the herb in a covered vessel, let it stand until about blood warm, express, strain, add the sugar and two tablespoonfuls of brewer's yeast or barm ; mix well, keep it covered by the fire for forty-eight hours ; after which put into a two-gallon stone jar and let it remain forty-eight hours more, uncorked. It should now be corked tightly up, and kept in a cool cellar. It is important to bear in mind that the stone jar should have a spile or small tap, so that the wine may be drawn off without admitting the air, which would be done each time of using if it was drawn out from the top. Or in the absence of a stone jar it may be bottled as ginger beer in stone bottles, and used as required.

In all cases of low typhus, nervous debility, and during convalescence, this may be used with great advantage.

ULMARIA (Meadow Sweet Wine).—

This is most excellent in cases of intermittent and remittent fever, in accumulation of uric acid in the blood, or wherever the urine is surcharged with albumen or biliary deposit. In convalescence from diseases of this character it is most excellent, and may be used *ad libitum*. Prepared as the last, with the addition of one drachm of citric acid, which 'iould be put into the infusion with the yeast or barm.

COMPOUND TARAXACUM (Dandelion Wine).—

Dandelion (roots, green, cut thin) .... Two pounds.
Agrimony (eupatoria, herb, dry) .... Four ounces.
Sugar (lump) .... Six pounds.
Water .... Three gals.

Boil the roots gently for one hour, and draw the whole off upon the herb, cover up, and let it stand until about blood warm, strain, express, and add the sugar, with two tablespoonfuls of yeast ; mix, let it stand in a warm place, or by the fire, covered up, for forty-eight hours ; after which put the whole into a three-gallon stone jar, and let it remain forty-eight hours uncorked. It may now be corked up, and the " jar " fitted with a tap or spile, or be put into stone bottles as the mellissa, or balm wine.

This is most excellent in diseases of the liver, ague, or intermittent fevers. In convalescence following these diseases it may be used freely.

COMPOUND GINGER WINE.—

Ginger Root (coarsely ground) .... One pound.
Lemon Peel (crushed) .... Two ounces.
Sugar (lump)........................ Six pounds.
Water............... : .... Three gallons.

Gently simmer in a covered vessel for one hour, let it stand until about blood warm, strain, express, add the sugar and two tablespoonfuls of brewer's yeast or barm, mix well, let it stand, in a warm place, same time as the last, after which bottle, and keep in a cool place.

This is a pleasing aromatic stimulant, most excellent in cases of debility arising from a weak flatulent condition of the stomach. It may be used alone, in half-wineglassfuls, or wineglassfuls, three or four times daily, or mixed with a little hot or cold water.

CINCHONA WINE.—

Peruvian Bark (in powder) .... One ounce.
Pure Spirits of Wine .... Half-pint.
Port Wine .... One pint.

Triturate or mix the powder in a mortar with a small quantity of the wine, after which add the remainder of the wine. Macerate fourteen days, shake up daily, express, and filter for use. Dose : from one to two teaspoonfuls three or four times daily, in a little cold water.

GINGER WINE.—

Powdered Ginger	One and a half ounce.
Sherry Wine	Pint and a half.
Tincture of Ginger	One ounce.

Mix as the last, macerate fourteen days, shake up daily, express, and filter for use. Dose : from one to two teaspoonfuls in a wineglassful of hot water sweetened.

WORMWOOD WINE.—

Wormwood (coarse powder)	One ounce.
Sherry Wine	One pint.
Pure spirits of wine	Half a pint.

Mix as the others, macerate fourteen days, shake up daily, express, and filter for use. Dose : from a teaspoonful to a dessertspoonful or tablespoonful three or four times a day in an equal quantity of cold water.

This is an excellent tonic and stomachic, and may be taken with advantage, in all cases of impaired digestion.

COLCHICUM WINE.—

Colchicum (root, bruised)	Two ounces and a half.
Sherry Wine	One pint.
Best Gin	Half a pint.

Mix as the others, macerate fourteen days, express, and filter for use. Dose : from twenty to twenty-five or thirty drops three times a day.

This is an excellent remedy in acute rheumatism, and rheumatic gout.

DIET DRINKS.

The medicines of this class are designed to assist returning health after illness. They may be called convalescent medicines, correcting the stomach, liver, and bowels. They thus assist nature in her work of restoration. Besides, they also act as preventatives of disease. Dr. John Skelton (from whom we select a part of our formula) says that " the two great primary causes of disease are excessive heat and cold, either of which may induce or set up exhaustion at any time." Thousands of lives are annually lost for the want of this knowledge, and the means to regulate the circulation of the blood, which is the great factor in maintaining our health. These diet drinks will be found valuable as a beverage instead of the alcoholic drinks, to which so many resort as stimulants. In winter we would recommend those who are subject to colds to use the first.

DIET DRINK, No. 1.—

Infuse a teaspoonful of Composition Powder in one pint each of boiling water and milk, (or boiling milk alone, if there is a tendency to looseness). Stir, cover, and drink during meals, or any time through the day. This will be found very nutritious and gently stimulating. May be used by any one, especially those whose blood is poor and system weak.

CONVALESCENT DRINK (fermented) No. 2.—

Infuse four ounces of No. 1 Composition Powder in two gallons of boiling water, let it stand an hour ; strain carefully off upon four pounds of lump sugar. When dissolved, add two tablespoonfuls of brewer's yeast. Let it stand covered 24 hours, then bottle ; tie the cork, and keep in a cool place. This may be used as herbal beer at any time, either as it is or diluted with warm or cold water.

CONVALESCENT DRINK, No. 3.—

    Comfrey Root (dry and crushed) .... One ounce.
    Ginger Root (dry and crushed) .... One ounce.
    Columbo Root (dry and crushed) .... Two ounces.
    Two Lemons cut in thin slices.
    Boiling Water .... Two gallons.

Gently simmer the whole an hour. Let it cool to blood heat, then add one tablespoonful of yeast ferment, and bottle as last.

This is a good stimulant and tonic. Good for dyspepsia and general debility, and where there is weakness of kidneys and bladder.

CONVALESCENT DRINK, No. 4.—

    Poplar Bark (dry and crushed) ...... Two ounces.
    Pinus Canadensis (dry and crushed) .. One ounce.
    Cinnamon Bark (crushed) .... One ounce.
    Boiling Water .... Two gallons.
    Lump Sugar .... Four pounds.
    Yeast............................ A tablespoonful.

Ferment and bottle as last.

This is a good drink for feeble and aged people, especially where there is weakness of the back and loins.

CONVALESCENT DRINK, No. 5.—

    Dandelion Flower, fresh .... Two ounces.
    Agrimony Herb .... Three ounces.
    Culver's Root (in coarse powder) ...... One ounce.

Infuse in two gallons of boiling water. Let it stand covered for two hours; express, strain, and add two pounds of lump sugar and a spoonful of yeast. Stand it in a warm place 24 hours. Bottle and keep cool.

Where the liver is suspected or in recovery from an acute attack of jaundice, inflammation of liver, spleen, or internal organs.

CONVALESCENT DRINK, No. 6.—

 Wood Sanicle, dry herb .... Four ounces.
 Hoarhound .... Two ounces.
 Liquorice Root (in coarse powder)
 Mullen Plant .... Two ounces.

Prepare as No. 3, with brown sugar instead of white. This drink is highly recommended to those who are subject to chest disease, and as a preventative of the same may be used freely.

HERBAL BEER.—

This drink is becoming very popular in the colonies, where we are happy to see that the taste for ardent spirits is not nearly so common as in the Old Country.

 Hoarhound .... Two ounces.
 Nettles .... Two ounces.
 Ginger .... Two ounces.
 Quassia .... Quarter ounce.

Simmer in four gallons, strain upon brown sugar two pounds, add brewer's yeast two tablespoonfuls. Keep covered in a warm place for 24 hours. Bottle and keep cool. Especially good as a beverage in warm weather. An ounce of essence of lemon added will impart an improved flavour to this herbal beer.

COMPOUND POWDERS.

COMPOSITION POWDER.—

 Bayberry (powdered) .... Four ounces.
 Pinus Canadensis................ Two ounces.
 Ginger .... Two ounces.
 Cayenne and Cloves, of each ...... Quarter ounce.

This is Dr Coffin's celebrated mixture; the most of Botanic authorities vary it somewhat to suit their individual taste. The one we would recommend, as it is milder and pleasanter, is as follows:—

Bayberry Powder.................. Four ounces.
White Poplar .... Two ounces.
Ginger .... Two ounces.
Pinus Canadensis................. Two ounces.
Sassafras Bark Powder .... One ounce.
*Cayenne Pepper .... Quarter ounce.
Cloves........................... Quarter ounce.
Liquorice Powder................. One ounce.
Powdered Caraway Seeds .... One ounce.
Cinnamon .... Half ounce.

Dose: A teaspoonful in a cup of boiling water, stir, cover, let it stand 10 minutes, pour off the clear into another cup, sweeten, and add milk to taste. The amount of milk and sugar does not alter its medicinal quality; the object is to make it palatable. Please note that it is the infusion that is to be taken, not the sediment. We note this, as we were told of a case that reminds one of the Highland lady's mistake when she made tea for the first time. Infusing a quantity of tea she poured off the liquor and ate the leaves. Our assistant salesman was selling a tin of the Composition to a man in the country, when a lady, who was standing by, said. "Mr. ———, do you use that nasty stuff?" "Nasty do you call it? I think it is excellent. I not only take it myself, but give it to my horses. It saved the life of a valuable horse a short time since." She replied, "Well, you may take it, but you don't catch me buying it again." "But," said he, "are you sure you made it right?" "Of course, I made it according to the direction on the label." Thinking that she had made a mistake, he asked her to detail how she had prepared it. She said, "I put the teaspoonful into the cup,

---

* The quantity of cayenne pepper may be increased or lessened according to taste.

filled it with boiling water, stirred it, put in the milk and sugar, let it cool, poured out the clear, and drank the rest, and I declare I thought I was poisoned." The man, who was sitting on his horse at the time, nearly fell off in a fit of laughter at this ludicrous mistake.

COMPOSITION ESSENCE.—

To make this is perhaps too troublesome for private use, but we will give the recipe, as it can be made even in small quantities. Infuse, say, four ounces of the powder in a quart of boiling water, stir, cover, and let it get cold ; pour off the clear, stir up the sediment with another quart of boiling water ; let it cool again, pour off the clear again into the first lot, then put them in a clean enamel or tin-lined pan, pot, or basin ; evaporate slowly down to half a pint ; let it cool, then add two ounces of tincture of Composition, which is prepared like other tinctures, with two ounces of the powder to a pint of spirits of wine. To make this a clear, good-looking preparation, it will be needful to filter it through paper. Dose: One to four teaspoonfuls in a cup of hot water sweetened with sugar, three or four times a day if for the cure of a cold. A dose at bedtime will act as a preventive. The Composition powder or essence should be kept in every house, as a dose taken after exposure to wet and cold will act as the stitch in time and save trouble.

SWEATING POWDER.—

Powdered Camphor	Two drachms.
Powdered Ipecacuanha	One drachm.
Cream of Tartar	One ounce.
Powdered Opium	Half drachm.

Mix the powders well. Dose: from 5 to 10 grains in a cup of Composition tea. This is an excellent medicine where there is severe pain, and a perspiration desired. Good in acute rheumatism, pain in the joints, restlessness, nervous excitement, &c. It may be given every four to six hours when required.

CATHARTIC POWDER.—

Jalap, in powder .... One ounce.
Senna, in powder .... Two ounces.
Ginger, in powder .... Half ounce.

Mix well and take from a half to a small teaspoonful in a teacupful of hot water sweetened.

This is a good opening medicine. If taken in the morning, fasting, it will cleanse out the bowels in a few hours. If taken after meals it will be slower in its action.

A favourite aperient powder, and one often prescribed by the doctors is the—

COMPOUND LIQUORICE POWDER.—

Liquorice Root, in powder ...... One and a half ounces.
Powdered Senna .... One and a half ounces.
Sulphur .... Three quarter ounce.
Fennel Seeds, in powder........ Three quarter ounce.
Sugar .... Four and a half ounces.

Dose : from half to one or two teaspoonfuls in water when required.

EMETIC POWDER.—

Lobelia Herb and Seed in powder mixed One ounce.
Ipecacuanha .... One ounce.
Blood Root .... Half ounce.

Mix well, and give as a dose half a teaspoonful in Composition (half usual strength), Chamomile or Boneset infusion every 15 to 20 minutes till it operates. If the first dose acts too soon, that is within ten minutes, give another when it is desired to get the stomach well cleansed and the chest relieved of phlegm.

EMETIC POWDER, No. 2.—

Boneset Herb, in powder .... One ounce.
Lobelia Herb and Seed .... One ounce.
Cayenne........................... One drachm.

Mix two teaspoonfuls in a pint and a half of hot water sweetened, take in teacupful doses every ten minutes till the whole is taken. Most effective in breaking up colds on the chest, opening the pores, and calling up a healthy reaction.

A simple emetic powder is : Powdered Lobelia Herb, a teaspoonful in a cup of warm water sweetened, will generally produce a good emetic in from 10 to 3 minutes. If the system is weak it is not desirable to repeat it. If in bed, the patient may go to sleep, and awakening in a hour or two it will take effect. After the emetic has operated the first time, as it generally produces two vomitings it will be well to drink warm water, so as to cleanse the stomach well when it is thoroughly empty. A cup of digestive food made from the following powder will be beneficial.

DIGESTIVE POWDER.—

    Slippery Elm Powder .... Two ounces.
    Powder fine white Sugar .... Four ounces.
    Cinnamon (in Powder) .... Half teaspoonful.

Mix thoroughly. Dose : Two teaspoonfuls in a cup ; put in a tablespoonful of milk, beat up to a fine paste, then pour on equal parts of boiling milk and water. This is a good diet drink, highly nutritious for invalids and infants ; may be taken with meals or with cod-liver oil, the taste of which it will help to disguise. We have known infants raised to health on this mixture.

COMPOUND MANDRAKE POWDER.—

    American Mandrake (in powder) .... One ounce.
    Ginger .... One ounce.
    Cream of Tartar .... One ounce.

Mix well. Dose : A teaspoonful daily in a half teacup of warm water, sweetened.

A fine medicine in torpid liver, jaundice, scrofula, and heated condition of the blood. Used alone or in combination it will be found good for constipation, &c.

POWDER FOR INDIGESTION.—

Gentian (in powder) .... Half drachm.
Valerian .... Half drachm.
Bicarbonate of Potash .... Two drachms.
Cayenne .... 20 grains.

Mix well, and divide into 20 powders. Take one after meals when you rise from the table. Take it in a little cold water. Good for heart-burn, water-brash, indigestion, and similar ailments.

STOMACH BITTERS POWDER.—

Balmony (in powder) .... Two ounces.
Bayberry (in powder) .... Two ounces.
White Poplar Bark Powder .... One ounce.
Ginger .... One ounce.
Cayenne .... Quarter ounce.
Cloves .... Quarter ounce.

Mix well. Dose: A teaspoonful in a cup of boiling water. Cover, let cool, pour off, and drink the clear infusion, without sugar, three times a day. This is a first-class medicine, and has been well liked and approved for the last 50 years. For indigestion, want of appetite, tonic, &c., it will be hard to excel.

STOMACH POWDER.—

Balmomy .... One ounce.
Golden Seal .... One ounce.
Liquorice Root .... Half ounce.
Cayenne .... Thirty grains.

Mix until the powders are well incorporated. Infuse one ounce in a pint of boiling water, when cool, strain and bottle. Dose: a wineglassful three times a day.

An excellent medicine to promote appetite, strengthen the stomach, and assist digestion.

ALTERATIVE OR ANTI-SCORBUTIC POWDER.—

Queen's Delight or Stillingia .... One ounce.
Burdock........................... Two ounces.
Mandrake .... Half ounce.
Ginger .... Half ounce.

Mix until the whole are well incorporated. Infuse one
ounce in a pint of boiling water, mix well; when cool, strain
and bottle for use. Dose : one tablespoonful four times a day.

This medicine is particularly indicated in cutaneous
disease, scrofula, secondary and tertiary syphilis, old sores,
eruptions, irritation of the skin, &c.

DIURETIC POWDER.—

Buchu .... One ounce.
Queen of the Meadow................ One ounce.
Uva Ursi .... Half ounce.
Parsley Root....................... One ounce.
Ginger .... Half ounce.

Mix until the whole are well incorporated. Infuse two
ounces in a quart of boiling water, mix well; when cool, strain
and bottle for use, or it may be taken like stomach bitters.
Dose : a wineglassful four times a day.

This is very useful in obstruction of the urine, and weakness of the kidneys and bladder.

GRAVEL POWDER.—

Hemp Agrimony (root of)............ Two ounces.
Queen of the Meadow (root of)....... One ounce.
Marshmallow (root of) .... One ounce.
Ginger............................. Half ounce.

Mix until the whole are well incorporated. Infuse two
ounces in a quart of boiling water, mix well, and when cool
strain and bottle for use. Dose : a wineglassful four times a
day.

This is a most efficient medicine in cases of Gravel. It
breaks up and disunites all calcareous deposit in the kidney,
ureters, urethra, and bladder, and removes it by micturition.

It is a sure preventive wherever the predisposition exists, but when the stone is fairly formed, particularly if of oxylate of lime, little more can be done than to alleviate symptoms and prevent its further progress.

ANTISPASMODIC POWDER.—

Burdock Seed	One ounce.
Scullcap	One ounce.
Caraway	One ounce.
Lobelia (herb)	One ounce.
Ginger	One ounce.
Golden Seal	One ounce.
Cayenne	One drachm.

Mix until the whole are well incorporated. Dose: a teaspoonful in a tumblerful or half-pint of boiling water, at bed-time; also during the day, if necessary.

This is an excellent remedy in spasm, cramp of the stomach, bowels, and limbs; neuralgia or tic-doloreux, rheumatic pains, particularly of the head and face.

HEPATIC OR CURATIVE POWDER.—

Golden Seal	One ounce.
Black-root (Culver's Physic)	Two ounces.
Dandelion Root	One ounce.
Mandrake (American)	Half ounce.
Burdock	One ounce.
Ginger	Half ounce.

Mix until the whole are well incorporated, and infuse one ounce in a pint of boiling water; when cool, strain and bottle for use. Dose: a tablespoonful three times a day.

This is an excellent remedy for chronic constipation of the bowels, mesenteric disease, and disease of the liver, pancreas, and spleen.

NOTE.—Ulcerated conditions of the liver and mesentery may be known by the dark, yellow, and mottled skin, griping pains, relax and offensive condition of the motions.

In all such cases the powder should be taken in small doses as follows :—

Infuse about ten grains, or a quarter of a teaspoonful, in a wineglassful of hot water, and take twice or three times a day.

SPICE BITTERS.—

Bayberry	One ounce.
Golden Seal	Half ounce.
Prickly Ash	Half ounce.
Balmony	Half ounce.
Cinnamon	Half ounce.
Cloves	Two drachms.
Cayenne	Two drachms.
White Sugar (in fine powder)	Half pound.

Mix until the whole are well incorporated. Dose: one teaspoonful well mixed in a small teacupful of boiling or cold water, three times a day, and at bed-time.

This is highly useful in all the irregularities to which females are liable, and of great value in dyspepsia, loss of appetite, nervous debility, &c.

CORRECTIVE POWDER.—

Poplar Bark	Two ounces.
Bayberry Powder	One ounce.
Black Cohosh	One ounce.
Golden Seal	Half ounce.
Anise	Half ounce.
Cinnamon	Half ounce.

Mix until the whole are well incorporated. Dose: from a half teaspoonful to a teaspoonful, in a small teacupful of boiling water, sweetened with lump sugar, three times a day, and at bed-time.

This is indicated in amenorrhœa, or obstruction of the menses. It is well known to many females, particularly among the working class, and highly esteemed as a most valuable medicine.

RESTORATIVE POWDER.—

Balmony	Half ounce.
White Pond Lily	Half ounce.
Bistort Root	One ounce.
Cinnamon	Half ounce.
Tormentil	One ounce.
Cayenne	Half drachm.

Mix until the whole are well incorporated. Dose: same as the last.

Highly valuable in excessive menstrual discharges, menorrhagia, hæmorrhage from the uterus, flux, leucorrhœa or whites, and a lax or debilitated condition of the system.

PILE POWDER.—

Cranesbill (root of)	Two ounces.
English Rhubarb (root of)	One ounce.
Poplar Bark	Half ounce.
Bistort (root of)	One ounce.
Marshmallow (root of)	One ounce.
Ginger	Half ounce.

Mix until the whole are well incorporated. Dose: one teaspoonful three or four times a day in a teacupful of hot water, sweetened.

This is a most excellent remedy, and may be used with great advantage, whether the piles are external, internal, or bleeding.

PULMONARY OR COUGH POWDER.—

Marshmallow (root of)	Two ounces.
Polypody	One ounce.
Liquorice Root	One ounce.
Anise	One ounce.
Lobelia (herb)	Half ounce.
Scullcap	Half ounce.
Pleurisy Root	Half ounce.
Skunk Cabbage	One ounce.

Mix until the whole are well incorporated. Dose: one teaspoonful in a small teacupful of boiling water, sweetened, three times a day.

In cases of extreme debility it may be taken in new milk, boiled and sweetened, instead of water.

This is very useful in old coughs, debility, or weakness of the lungs, bronchial disease, and consumption. It may be used as directed, or combined with hoarhound, coltsfoot, sanicle, hyssop, ground ivy, or any of the herbal preparations indicated in pulmonary disease.

ANTI-CHOLERA POWDER.—

Angelica (root of)	One ounce.
Cranesbill	Two ounces.
Bistort	One ounce.
Sweet-flag (root of)	Two ounces.
Marshmallow (root of)	One ounce.
Cinnamon	One ounce.
Cayenne	Two drachms.

Mix until the whole are well incorporated. Dose: a teaspoonful in a cup of boiling water sweetened. Drink the infusion every hour or less as the case demands. (See article on cholera).

NEUTRALISING POWDER (BEACH'S MIXTURE).—

Turkey Rhubarb	Half drachm.
Bicarbonate of Potass	Half drachm.
Peppermint (fine powder)	Half drachm.
Boiling Water	Half pint.

Infuse in a covered vessel, and when sufficiently cool, strain, sweeten with lump sugar, and add a small wineglassful of the best pale brandy. Dose: one or two tablespoonfuls every quarter or half hour, or one or two hours, according to the symptoms. For children, in proportion.

" This is one of the most valuable preparations known for cholera morbus, cholera infantum (or summer complaint of children), diarrhœa, dysentery, &c. Its operation and effects seem to render it an almost infallible remedy."—*Dr. Beach.*

ENEMATA, OR INJECTIONS (CLYSTERS).

The use of injections in the treatment of disease is of very ancient date ; and when we reflect upon the position and character of the intestines, we can scarcely fail to see there are cases in which we cannot prudently do without them ; such as in putrid fevers, constipation and inflammation of the bowels, extreme debility, &c., and where the stomach can neither take food nor retain it when taken. Of the necessity of removing obstructive fæcal accumulations there cannot be two opinions ; nor of relieving the bowels of whatever has a tendency to increase putrefaction in malignant and low fevers ; nor of nourishing and sustaining the system in cases where the stomach refuses to act. To presume to reason upon their usefulness under such circumstances would be absolute folly, and yet there are professors who condemn them ; but we shall not be surprised at this when we remember the present wretched condition of medicine, and the darkness which obtains throughout the numerous sects and parties who practise it.

ULMUS OR SLIPPERY ELM INJECTION.—

Slippery Elm .... One drachm.
Sugar .... One ounce.

Mix until well incorporated, after which add a half-pint of warm milk and water and an ounce of olive oil, gently stirring the whole.

This injection is useful in the majority of cases, and it is rare that any other is required. In many cases, however, the "digestive food" answers every purpose, and as it is generally at hand there is no time lost in its preparation, all that is required is to mix a tablespoonful in a half-pint of warm water, milk and water, or milk, according to the indications of each particular case. Water answers every purpose where the object is simply to remove obstruction ; but where nutrition is required, or the action of any particular agent, it is necessary to use milk, beef tea, thin gruel, rice milk, and such preparations as the case appears to demand.

STIMULATING INJECTION.—

Antispasmodic Tincture	One drachm.
Digestive Food	Two drachms.

Mix in a half-pint of warm water, and sweeten with molasses.

This injection is indicated in all cases of fever of a low type, in colic pains, and spasmodic attacks of the bowels.

ANTHELMINTIC INJECTION,—

Aloes (powder)	Half drachm.
Common Salt	One drachm.
Slippery Elm (fine powder)	Half drachm.

~~Mix until the whole are well~~ incorporated, after which add a half-pint of warm water, sweeten with molasses, and stir briskly.

This is a most useful injection in cases of seat worms or ascarides, or where the colon or lower bowel is impacted with worms of any kind.

COMMON SOAP INJECTION.—

This is prepared by simply making a strong lather of soap and water, and where the object is simply to act on the lower bowel it may be used with advantage.

COMPOUND INJECTION POWDER.—

Ulmus Fulva (Slippery Elm)	Half ounce.
Black-root (Culver's Physic)	Half ounce.
Ginger	Two drachms.
Fine Sugar	Half pound.

Mix until the whole are well incorporated. Prepare as follows: one tablespoonful of the powder to half a pint of warm water.

This is a useful injection in all cases where the system is generally sluggish, and where it is necessary to act upon the liver.

POULTICES.

These preparations are exceedingly useful, and are indicated in a variety of cases. The following are sufficient for every purpose :—

SLIPPERY ELM POULTICE.—

Slippery Elm (in powder) .... Sufficient for size of
poultice required.

Mix with hot water or infusion of wormwood or other herb to form into a proper consistency, spread smoothly upon soft cotton cloth, and apply over the part affected. In order to prevent it sticking rub on some ointment on the part to be covered.

This poultice is most excellent in suppurative Abscess and old wounds of every kind. In inflammation, whether phlegmonous or simple, it may be applied immediately over the part affected; in abscesses and old wounds it should be placed between muslin cloths.

LINSEED POULTICE.—

Linseed (in powder) .... Sufficient.
Prepare as the last.

This is the common poultice for the hospitals, and in the absence of slippery elm it may be made to supply its place. It is used in almost all cases, either simple or compound, as occasion requires.

ANTISEPTIC POULTICE.—

Slippery Elm (in powder).............. Sufficient.
Vegetable Charcoal (in fine powder) .... Sufficient.

Mix equal parts with warm water or an infusion of wormwood,
and apply immediately over the part.

In old offensive gangrenous wounds this poultice is one of the best that can be employed. In the absence of slippery elm linseed meal may be used.

HEMLOCK POULTICE.—

> Hemlock (Conium Maculatum), herb, green Sufficient.
> Slippery Elm .... Sufficient.

Boil the herb, strip off the leaf or soft part, chop soft, and mix sufficient slippery elm with as much of the decoction as is necessary to give it a consistency.

This poultice is very useful in swollen or enlarged glands, whether of the neck or any other part.   In cancers or tumors, inflammation of the breast, orchitis, and indeed for glandular irritation or induration of any kind.

FERMENTATIVE OR YEAST POULTICE.—

> Slippery Elm .... Sufficient.
> Mix with brewers' yeast or barm, and new milk.

This is a most valuable poultice in all cases where it is desirable to hasten suppuration, or arrest the tendency to gangrene.

COMPOUND MUSTARD POULTICE.—

> Slippery Elm .... Sufficient.
> Mustard .... A fourth part.

Mix with water, and apply as hot as possible between layers of soft cotton.

This is one of the best forms of poultice for pleurisy, inflammation of the bowels, lumbago, or indeed for any kind of acute inflammatory attack.

COMPOUND BRAN POULTICE.—

> Wheat Bran .... } Equal parts.
> Slippery Elm .... }

Mix with hot vinegar to a proper consistency, and apply to the part affected.

This is excellent in severe rheumatic and gouty affections, particularly of the joints, and in synovitis or white swelling.

COMFREY POULTICE.—

Comfrey Root (in powder) .... Sufficient.

Mix with boiling water to a proper consistency, and apply immediately to the part affected, or between cloths.

This is an excellent poultice in cases of hernia or rupture, applied immediately after the protrusion is returned. If changed as necessary, kept in position, and rest enforced, it assists most readily to repair the break or loss of continuity. It was known by the synonym or name of "Knit-bone" by our Saxon forefathers, from the fact of its power of healing or uniting broken bones. Our modern scientific and over-wise modern physicians smile at this simplicity, but if they were to reflect, they might see at once that a broken bone depends for its re-union upon the integrity of the periosteum. It is because of its power in subduing the inflammatory condition of the membrane that the bone and broken part are so readily repaired.

HERBAL POULTICES.—

These are prepared with whatever herb or herb may be considered best fitted to meet the indications of disease. The leaves only should be used, and these green if possible; in which case they must be bruised in a mortar, and applied alone or mixed with slippery elm and boiling water sufficient to give the mass consistency.

PILLS.

These are simply combinations of medicinal substances. formed into small round masses, to the advantage of the patient, who thus escapes the taste of nauseous medicine.

APERIENT, OR ANTIBILIOUS PILL.—

Aloes (best socotrine) .... One ounce.
Gamboge .... Two drachms.
Mandrake (American) .... Two drachms.
Cayenne .... Four drms.
Oil of Peppermint .... Twenty drops.

Mix with sufficient gum acacia mucilage, and form into five
grain pills. Dose : two at bed-time, or less or more as necessary.
Excellent in constipation, bilious headache, &c., &c.

RHEUMATIC, RENAL, LEUCORRHŒAL, AND DIURETIC PILL.—

Solidified Copaiba .... One ounce.
Castile Soap (in powder) .... Two drachms.
Oil of Juniper .... Twenty drops.
Liquorice (Extract) .... One drachm.
Parsley Root .... One drachm or more.

Well work up the whole in a mortar, and form into five-grain
pills. Dose : from two to six daily.

Most invaluable in rheumatism, leucorrhœa, obstruction of
the urine, gonorrhœa, gleet, &c.

DIGESTIVE, OR COMPOUND LOBELLA PILL.—

Lobelia Seed .... One ounce.
Lobelia Herb .... Half ounce.
Anise Seed, in powder .... Half ounce.
Cayenne .... Two drachms.

Mix with sufficient gum acacia and treacle to bind the mass,
and make up into five-grain pills. Dose : one or more after
meals, as necessary. In delicate patients a two-and-a-half-
grain pill after meals will be sufficient.

Excellent in dyspeptic cases, pain or wind on the stomach,
&c., &c.

COMPOUND CARBON, OR ANTISEPTIC PILL.—

Charcoal (wood, fine powder) .... One ounce.
Calamus Aromaticus .... Two drachms.
Cayenne .... Half drachm.
Lobelia Seed........................ Half drachm.

Mix as the last, and prescribe in the same way.

Invaluable in offensive breath, water brash, dyspepsia, &c., &c.

COMPOUND MOTHERWORT PILL.—

Extract of Motherwort .... One ounce.
Scuttellarin .... One drachm.
Cayenne .... Half drachm.

Mix and form into five-grain pills. Dose: one every three or four hours.

Excellent in hysteria, palpitation of the heart, chorea, and disease of the nervous system generally.

HEPATIC PILL.—

Extract of Mandrake................ Half ounce.
Extract of Dandelion................ Half ounce.
Sanguinarin .... Twenty grains.
Oil of Caraway .... Ten drops.
Blood Root (pulv.)................. Sufficient.

Mix, and form into two-and-a-half-grain or five-grain pills. Dose: one or more at bed-time, as necessary.

Excellent in chronic disease of the liver, pancreas, spleen, jaundice, bilious and mesenteric disease.

CAYENNE PILL.—

Cayenne .... One ounce.
Oil of Spearmint .... Twenty drops.

Mix with gum acacia and treacle sufficient to form into a mass, and divide into five-grain pills. Dose: one or more after meals.

Excellent in flatulency, or debility of the stomach and intestines.

ALTERATIVE PILL.—

    Mandrake (American) .... Half ounce.
    Blue Flag .... Half ounce.
    Extract of Poke Root .... Half ounce.
    Prickley Ash .... Two drachms.
    Cayenne .... One drachm.
    Oil of Sassafras .... Twenty drops.

Mix, and form into five-grain pills. Dose from four to six daily.

Excellent in scrofulous, strumous, cutaneous, and syphilitic disease.

NEUROTIC, OR NERVE PILL.—

    Extract of Valerian .... Half ounce.
    Assafœtida .... Half ounce.
    Scutellarin .... Half drachm.
    Cayenne .... Ten grains.

Mix and form into five-grain pills. Dose: one every three or four hours.

Highly useful in chorea, neuralgia, or tic-doloreux.

ANODYNE, OR COMPOUND OPIUM PILL.—

    Extract of Opium (Turkey).......... One drachm.
    Extract of Liquorice............... Half ounce.

Mix, and form into five-grain pills. Dose: one at bedtime.

As an anodyne or opiate, this pill will be found most excellent; it should only be prescribed, however, where relief from severe pain cannot be obtained by other means. If preferred, the extract of hyoscyamus may be used instead of opium.

LOBELIA, OR EMETIC PILL.—

    Lobelia Seed .... Half ounce.
    Cayenne .... One drachm.

Mix into a mass with gum acacia and treacle, and divide into five grain pills. Dose: as an emetic, from four to six at bed-time in boneset, chamomile, or vervain tea.

Most excellent in cases where it is desirable to act on the system without excitement.

FAMILY PILL.—

Aloes (Socotrine)	Half ounce.
Extract of Butternut	Two drachms.
Extract of Liquorice	Two drachms.
Lobelia Seed	One drachm.
Oil of Caraway	Twenty drops.

Mix, form into a mass, and divide into five-grain pills. Dose: two at bed time, or one after meals.

This is an excellent pill for all family purposes, and may be used with advantage in every case where an aperient medicine is necessary.

DANDELION PILL.—

Best Rhubarb, in powder	One ounce.
Socotrine Aloes, in powder	One ounce.
American Mandrake, in powder	Half ounce.
Ginger, in powder	Quarter oz.
Gum Myrrh, in powder	Quarter oz.
Podophyllin Resin, in powder	One drachm.
Leptandrin	One drachm.
Cayenne	One drachm.
Oil of Peppermint	Half drachm.
Extract of Dandelion	About Two ounces.

Or sufficient to make into a stiff mass. Roll out in small pills about three-and-a-half grains. The dose of these will vary from one to four at bed-time, or when required. For a good family medicine it will be difficult to surpass this.

OINTMENTS.

These preparations act in the generality of cases from the protection which they afford to the part affected, equally as much as from their medicinal qualities.

HEALING OINTMENT.

Burgundy Pitch	Twelve ounces.
Beeswax (Yellow)..................	Eight ounces.
Lard	Four ounces.
Mutton Suet	Four ounces.
Olive Oil.........................	Two ounces.

Simmer until the first four are well melted, stir gently, add the oil, strain, express, well mix, and keep in a cool place.

It is necessary to bear in mind that the temperature affects the consistency of ointments, and that this may be met by adding or diminishing any one of the articles named.

Excellent for fresh or old wounds, sores, ulcers, &c.

COMPOUND SPERMACETI, OR MALLOW OINTMENT.—

Marshmallow (young green leaves) ..	Two ounces.
White Wax	Two ounces.
Spermaceti	Three ounces.
Olive Oil.........................	One ounce.

Gently simmer the leaves and spermaceti for one hour, strain, express, add the oil, well mix, and keep in a cool place.

This is an excellent ointment for chapped lips, sore nipples, fissures of the anus, &c., &c.

COMPOUND OINTMENT OF WOOD SANICLE.—

Sanicle (green leaves)	Two ounces.
Beeswax (yellow)	Six ounces.
Rosin (white)	One ounce.
Olive Oil	One ounce.

Prepare as the last.

Excellent in wounds of every kind, but more particulary for ulcers and old gangrenous sores.

CELANDINE OINTMENT.—

Celandine (gr'n. herb, Chelidonium majus) Two ounces.
Spermaceti .... One ounce.
Beeswax .... Four ounces.
Mutton Suet .... Two ounces.
Olive Oil .... Two ounces.

Gently simmer the first four one hour, strain, express, add the oil, well mix, and keep in a cool place.

Excellent in tetter, ringworm, scabbed head, pityriasis. lichen, &c.

COMPOUND DOCK, DISCUTIENT OR SCROFULA OINTMENT.—

Plantain leaves...................... One ounce.
Bitter Sweet (root of, crushed) .... Two ounces.
Yellow Dock Root (crushed) .... One ounce.
White Resin......................... Four ounces.
Olive Oil .... Four ounces.
Beeswax (yellow) .... Four ounces.

Simmer the whole gently for one hour, strain, express, well mix, and keep in a cool place.

This is an excellent ointment for discussing scrofulous and indolent tumours, glandular enlargements, swellings, &c.

PILE OINTMENT.—

Cranesbill (root, crushed, or coarse powder) One ounce.
Pinus Canadensis (ditto) .... Half ounce.
Beeswax (yellow) .... Six ounces.
Mutton Suet .... Two ounces.
Lard .... Four ounces.
Olive Oil .... One ounce.

Gently simmer the whole (except the oil) for one hour, strain, express, add the oil, well mix, and keep in a cool place.

This is a most excellent remedy for almost every purpose where an ointment is necessary. As an ointment for the piles, however, it is unrivalled.

EYE OINTMENT.—

>   Sanguinaria or blood-root, in coarse powder Half ounce.
>   White Wax .... Four ounces.
>   Olive Oil .... Two ounces.

Gently simmer the powder and wax for one hour, strain, express, add the oil, well mix, and keep in a cool place.

This is a beautiful ointment for inflamed and sore eyes, inflamed nipples, and painful sores of every kind.

SOOTHING OINTMENT.—

>   Red Poppy (flowers, dry) .... One ounce.
>   Elder Flowers .... One ounce.
>   White Wax........................... Six ounces.
>   Olive Oil .... One ounce.

Gently simmer the flowers and wax for one hour, add the oil strain, express, well mix, and keep in a cool place.

. This is a very soothing delicate ointment, and affords ready relief in rheumatism, painful tumours, swellings, inflammations, abrasions, &c., &c.

MARSHMALLOW OINTMENT.—

>   Marshmallow (tops and flowers, green).. Four ounces.
>   Lard or Vaseline.................... Four ounces.

Simmer till crisp, strain, and add one ounce of beeswax.

This is a good ointment for inflamed sores, swellings, &c. Use same as Healing Ointment.

TAR OINTMENT.—

>   Barbadoes Tar .... Half ounce.
>   Vaseline .... Two ounces.

Mix well. This is a good ointment for eczema, skin diseases, &c.

HERBAL HEALING OINTMENT.—

>   Vaseline or Lard .... Four ounces.
>   Marygold (flowers, green) .... Four ounces.

Simmer slowly till the flowers are crisp, taking care not to burn them, strain, and press, then add one ounce of beeswax and the same of burgundy. Melt, and keep in a stoneware pot. This ointment is an excellent application for healing wounds, sores, burns, &c. Apply on a soft cloth two or three times a day. It is not desirable to wash sores unless they are producing a quantity of matter. If so, wash with the healing soap. (See index.)

LOTIONS, WASHES, OR COLLYRIUMS.

Lotions are used pretty extensively in the old practice. Generally speaking, however, fomentations of hot herbs supply their place a thousand times better; nor do we know many forms of disease, apart from those of the eyes, where they are of any very great practical use.

WASH FOR INFLAMED EYES.—

Distilled or Rose Water .... One ounce.
Tincture of Hydrastis Canadensis ...... One drachm.
Tincture of Golden Seal .... One drachm.

Mix, and apply with a fine camel-hair brush night and morning.

COMPOUND BISTORT WASH FOR OPHTHALMIA, &C.—

Bayberry Powder .... Half ounce.
Tincture of Bistort .... One drachm.

Infuse the powder in eight ounces of boiling water, let it remain until cold, strain the liquor off clear, add the tincture, and use freely morning, noon, and night.

In inflamed mucous discharges from the ears, nose, vagina, urethra, or any other part, this is exceedingly useful.

ANOTHER WASH FOR INFLAMED EYES, &c.—

    Distilled or Soft Spring Water .... One ounce.

    Tincture of Myrrh (Simple or Compound) Two drachms.

                Mix and use as the last.

    It may be made weaker or stronger as circumstances require.

CHAPTER ON THE LAWS OF LIFE, HEALTH, ETC.

Before entering upon the most important part of our work, namely, the treatment of diseases, we think it needful to devote a few pages to lay before our readers some facts that, we trust, will be useful. While it is not absolutely necessary for even a person in practice to know all about the human frame, still it will help all to understand better how to prescribe for sickness, which, in most cases, is due to some or one of the organs not working according to nature. For this purpose we give a short chapter on anatomy and physiology. The first of these sciences consists in knowing the various parts of the body; the second in knowing the object and working of the organs and fluids of the system. As prevention is better than cure, the following pages will point out the means to do this. There are many who in health will refuse to give these things any consideration, thinking that they may never need medicine. This is a great folly, for "knowledge is power;" it will enable us to act in conformity with the laws of health, and thus ward off sickness, and if we are amongst the few who pass through this world of suffering with little or no trouble, we will still have the power of doing good to our less fortunate fellow-

creatures. Let us remember we may not always live in a city
where medical men are to be had at any time, and even there
emergencies may arise when some who have given heed to
these ways may be the means of blessing to their friends.
We can't know too much of a good thing.

ANATOMY AND PHYSIOLOGY.

Anatomy is simply a description of the body and its several
parts. The human system may for the better understanding
be classed into seven] divisions; 1. the bones; 2. ligaments;
3. muscles; 4. blood and lymph vessels; 5. nerves and centres;
6. organs; 7. skin and appendices. The bones number 200,
and are arranged as follows: in the spine, 26; in the head
and face, 22; the ribs, breast-bone, and a smaller one
beneath the root of the tongue, called the hyoid, 26; in the upper
extremities, 64; in the lower, 62. There are three very small
bones in the ear, and some developed in the tendons, with the
teeth and are not included in this number. Bones are divided into
four classes—long, short, flat, and irregular. The long ones
are the levers and supports of the body; the short ones give
strength and compactness to the joints; the flat for protection
of vital parts and attachments of muscles; and the irregular,
as the vertrebræ, for strength, muscular attachment, and
protection of the spinal cord. The bones that form the skull
and face are in adult life so closely united that a superficial
observer would conclude that these were but two, the skull and
lower jaw. Closer inspection, however, will show the line of
junction called sutures, the edges of which are serrated like
the teeth of a saw, so that the bones dovetail into each other.
The outside bones of the skull are six, and are named the
frontal or brow bone, the temporal, which contains the organs
of hearing, the sides and top of the head are formed by the two
parietal bones; while the occipital forms the back and lower
portion of the head, it rests upon the spine and transmits the
cord and its membrane. Inside the skull are the sphenoid
and ethmoid; they, with the occipital, unite to form its

floor, which has a number of openings in it for the passage of nerves and blood-vessels. The bones of the face are the maler and nasal, superior and inferior maxillary, into which the teeth are inserted; the bones of the upper extremity are the clavicle or collar bone, the scapula or shoulder blade; in the upper arm the humerus, in the fore arm the radius and ulna. In the wrist joint are eight short bones called the carpal, united to which are the phalanges or finger bones. In the body or trunk are the ribs, twelve on each side, the same number in male and female; ten of them are united all round, and two are called the floating ribs. The spinal column is composed of 24 bones, between which are round flat discs; each vertrebra has a circular hole through which the cord passes. On the upper and lower surfaces there are notches, which when united form the foramen, as it is called, through which the nerves pass out to the various parts and organs of the body. The spine rests on a bone called the sacrum, which in the child is formed of several segments, but in adult life it is one. The coccyx is the terminal part of the spinal column, composed of four small segments: the innominate bones so called from the difficulty of finding in them any resemblance to natural objects; those two called the hip-bones, with the sacrum and coccyx, form the pelvis. The femus or thigh-bone is the longest and largest in the body; it rests on the broad head of the tibia, which with the patella or knee-cap form the knee joint; the fibula, or as it is sometimes called the splint bone, lies to the outside of the leg, not as high up as the knee joint, it descends a little lower than the tibia, and is the outer bone in the ankle-joint. The small bones of this joint are seven in number and are called tarsal bones. The phalanges or toe bones complete the list, which being bound together by the strong ligaments and tendons, form the skeleton. Cartilages are pads or cushions placed between the articulating or joining ends, to prevent concussion or shock to the body.

The composition of bone in early childhood is about equal parts of organic and earthy substance. The former a gelatinous, and the latter mainly the carbonate and phosphate of lime.

From birth to death there is a very gradual increase of the earthy constituents, which renders strength and firmness up to a certain point, when a further preponderance causes brittleness, as in old age. A simple experiment will prove the above. If a bone (a long one is best) is burned in the fire, the gelatinous or animal matter will be separated and destroyed, leaving the earthy matter without adhesion. Again, if the bone is steeped in dilute muriatic acid sufficiently long, all the earthy matter will be dissolved, and you may wind it round your hand. The bones, like every other part of the body, except the nails, hair, and chrystalline lens of the eye, are supplied with blood-vessels and nerves, and are covered with a delicate membrane called the periosteum, from which parts of the bones lost through decay may be renewed.

THE MUSCLES,

which are about 500 in number, are the organs of motion, being formed of contractile tissue, and in direct communication with the brain. In the healthy state they are its obedient servants. This does not, however, apply to the involuntary muscles, which perform the digestive and assimilative functions, and the heart, which may be considered as one muscle, keeping up its contracting and relaxing, or systole and diastole movements from early foetal life to death. The muscles are said to have their origin in the fixed parts to which they are drawn in contraction and their insertion into the bone, or portion of the bone, designed to be moved. Their contracting power is caused by a stimulus from the nerve, which, when it is withdrawn, they relax. Their rapidity of movement seems to be marvellous, as in rapid speaking, playing musical instruments, such as the piano, where a large number of muscles are employed contracting and relaxing. The beautiful adaptation of the muscles to the bones gives the body its form and symmetry. In this short sketch we cannot go further into detail. We only wish to impress on the minds of our readers the fact that as they form the greatest part of our body, we should be careful to use and exercise them aright. This latter is essential to their truly healthy development, as instance the arm of the blacksmith.

The blood-vessels are divided into two—the arteries and the veins. The first carry the blood from the heart to the lungs, muscles, and bones, and other tissues of the body, leaving, if in a healthy condition, the material to renew the waste and add to the growth of the body in youth, and sometimes adult age. Having done this, it is then partly by the propelling force of the heart's action, and partly by capillary attraction, drawn into the veins, and conveyed to the heart, thence to the lungs, changed by giving off its poisonous carbonic acid gas, and taking in health-giving oxygen. The walls of the arteries are formed by three coats; the outer, strong and elastic; the middle, muscular; the fibres running round the tube give it a contracting power. The inner coat is a delicate serous membrane, smooth, to allow of a free flow of the blood. The veins, which have not the same pressure upon them, have also three coats, but are thinner, with little or no muscular action. Venous blood, with the exception of that returned from the lungs by the pulmonary veins to the left auricle, is unfit for the nourishment of the body until it is relieved of its carbonic acid, and replenished with oxygen.

The lymph vessels are connected with a system of glands which secrete lymph from the tissues. It is a clear, colourless fluid, which plays an important part in the healing of wounds. Included with these are the lacteals, which secrete the milk-like fluid from the intestines; that, with the lymph finds its way into the blood through the thoraci duct, the opening of which is at the root of the neck, where it terminates in a large vein called the subclavian.

NERVES.

Some suppose these to be hollow vessels, conveying a fluid from the brain and spinal cord to the muscles and tissues, but a microscopic examination does not justify this conclusion. Perhaps the best similitude of their important function is that of telegraph wires conveying the stimulus or vital force to every part of the system. The nervous system is composed of three parts—the cerebro-spinal, the ganglia, and the nerves. The brain and spinal cord are the first. The brain is con-

tained in the skull, where it is protected by its bony plates.
It is divided into the cerebrum, which consists of two lobes or
hemispheres united in the centre.   Externally it is covered by
the gray matter, which is composed of nerve cells.   There are
deep grooves or convolutions running in irregular lines all
over the surfaces.   This portion of the brain is the seat of the
special senses and will power.   The cerebellum, or little brain,
lies under and at the back of the cerebrum.   It is also in two
parts, united in the centre.   It is said to control and
harmonize the movements of the body and limbs.   There are
five cavities in the brain called ventricles.   At the base,
resting on the floor of the skull, are two important parts of
the brain, called the pons variola and medulla oblongata.
The pons is the bond of union between the parts of the
brain.   The medulla may be reckoned the beginning of the
spinal cord.   From it spring the nerves which control the
vital forces of life—breathing, swallowing, digestion, &c.
From the medulla the cord passes down the opening at the base
of the skull into the bony canal formed by holes in the vertebræ
or backbone ;   small openings in which allow for the
transmission of the costal nerves, comprising 31 pairs, which
convey the vital impulses to the muscles and parts of the
trunk, and unite with the nerves coming direct from the brain
to form phlexuses or network formations of nerves.   The cord,
when it reaches the bottom of the spine, terminates.   The
nerves that supply the leg are the great and lesser sciatic,
derived from the sacral plexus.   The great sciatic is the
largest nerve in the body, being at one point about three-
quarters of an inch broad.   It passes down the leg, lying
embedded among the muscles of the back portion.   It divides
into two branches called the popliteal.   One of these is
distributed principally to the superficial, and the other to the
deeper parts of the leg and foot.

The internal organs of the body are numbered from
above downwards.   The lungs, heart, diaphragm, liver,
stomach, pancreas, spleen, intestines smaller and greater, the

kidneys, and the bladder. The genital organs are not generally noticed in a sketch of this kind.

The lungs and heart are contained in the chest or thorax. The capacity of the chest will vary according to the size of the individual. The lungs are the right and left. The right lung is the largest, having three lobes, while the left has but two. The substance of these is elastic and spongy. It is generally supposed that the power of contracting and expanding is in the lungs, but this is not the case; they are simply passive. The diaphragm and the muscles of the thorax, by contracting press the breath out of them, and by relaxing allow the lungs to expand, and take in the air. The quick action of the above muscles enables us to cough and sneeze. It is interesting to know the great amount of air which passes in and out of the lungs in the course of the day. The quantity entering at each inspiration is about 40 inches per minute; 8000 per hour; 48,000 in 24 hours. Between the lungs, and partly covered in front by the left one, lies the heart. It is enclosed in a sack called the pericardium. The heart is a muscular organ, with independent nerve centres. Its power and rapidity of contraction are marvellous. In the normal condition of infant life it numbers about 150 beats per minute; in adults, 60. In 24 hours it contracts and dilates over one hundred thousand times. The working of this wonderful organ, propelling the current of life from before birth to death, shows the power of our Creator, and should satisfy and convince the fool, who says in his heart there is no God. The heart has four compartments, called auricles and ventricles. The former act as receivers of the blood as it comes from the veins. When the heart relaxes the valves of the left side open, and the venous blood flows from the auricle into the ventricle; it then contracts and sends the blood to the lungs. Being oxygenised, it is returned to the left auricle, then at dilation of left ventricle is received into it; and at contraction it is forced into the aorta, then to the arteries, then by the hair-like vessels to the most remote part of the system. The quantity of blood sent from the heart at each beat is about six ounces. This portion pushes the blood ahead of it, and so on the movement is continued, which is termed the circulation. The diaphragm is the partition between the chest and the abdomen. It is one vast muscle, attached to the ribs and backbone. The vessels and nerves from above pass through it. As we before mentioned, this is the chief organ in breathing. Lying under this is the liver, the largest gland in the body. It is divided into five lobes, attached by five ligaments. The office of this important organ is to secrete from the blood the bile, which is a necessary constituent of healthy digestion. On its under surface is the gall duct, which pours its contents into the duodenum, or first part of the intestines. As the liver is chiefly composed of blood in an unhealthy or imperfect condition, we do not think it is wise to eat this part of the animal body. The stomach lies under the liver, its largest part, the œsophagal entrance, lying to the right side, with the pylorus and outlet end to the left. It is a reasonable hint, especially to people with weak stomachs, to sleep on the left side, as this will facilitate the passage of the food out of the stomach. Still the muscular action of this organ in normal conditions is sufficient to accomplish this whatever end may be uppermost. As this organ stands first in importance, being figuratively called the kitchen of the mansion, we will endeavour to point out its delicate structure, so that our readers may be the more careful not to abuse it, for there is not an organ in the body so much abused as the stomach, not so much by what is eaten, as it will make its possessor feel uncomfortable if too much cramming is done ; but the greatest danger is in drinking. Liquids do not remain long in the stomach. They are absorbed by its innumerable glands, and as are their properties so will their influence be good or evil. Most of our readers have heard or read of the French Canadian who was shot in the stomach. The wound healed as a fistulous opening. He was employed as groom by a doctor, who introduced a speculum, and saw the condition of the stomach in its healthy state ; the various effects of the different kinds of food, and the time taken to digest them. As this is important, we will give the result of his investigation in tabular form when treating of indigestion. (See index).

Dr Beaumont, the gentleman above referred to, sounds the note of alarm to all who are encouraging a taste for alcoholic drinks. The healthy organ, when a glass of brandy or spirits has been thrown into it, takes on a similar appearance to that of a piece of meat dipped in hot water. From this fact it is concluded that a number of such drinks, will, so to speak, parboil the stomach. If it were not for the fact that nature has such repairing power, alcohol would not be as it is now termed, a *slow* poison, but facts constantly prove that nature's repairing powers cannot keep up with the folly and madness of the drunkard, who pours down his depraved throat this fire-water, which destroys the delicate sense of taste, congests, inflames, ulcerates, and destroys the secreting and digesting power of the stomach, hardens the liver, and at last morally hardens the heart, and even in this life has led to the combustion of the whole body. A case is on record of a female drunkard who could drink a bottle of brandy a day. It is not known how she ignited, or whether it was a case of spontaneous combustion, but what remained of her was found in the shape of fine ashes which covered the room in which she suffered vital cremation or living burning. Another story is told of how a poor drunkard ended his madness. He was in the act of lighting his pipe when the fumes of his poisoned breath caught fire. His mouth, throat, and internal parts were so saturated with it that he burned to death. Oh, ye moderate drinkers, beware lest this evil come upon you. Your only safety lies in abstinence, counting all spirituous drinks as drugs, which should only be resorted to in case of sickness. A word or two with regard to doctors who prescribe this. Some of the medical men now-a-days do think there is much virtue in such drinks, and prescribe them honestly. Others have confessed to their brethren that it was more a matter of policy than faith with them; so in order to please their patients, whisky, brandy, ale, and porter were given as stimulants, tonics, &c. It has been said that in some places a doctor could not get a practice who did not pander to this depraved taste. In view of the facts we have written concerning the human body, animated by the spirit of life from God, it will be admitted, as it has been in the past, that it is one of the most wonderful of His works. We cannot conceive how some men professing to be scientists can believe that blind chance could have produced such a wonderful mechanism, endued with such self-repairing power. These facts ought to make us careful to live in harmony with not only nature's laws, as they are called, but also the revealed will of God, who desires that his creatures should be happy, and so live in the flesh that if we do go the way of all the earth,* we may die in the sure and certain hope of a resurrection into eternal life. The thought occurs to us that no anatomist will ever describe the future immortal body, for it will be deathless, therefore scalpels, knives and saws will never divide it, as they have this mortal form.

SAMUEL THOMPSON'S THEORY OF LIFE, MOTION, &c.

As a rule rational treatment is based on rational theory, but as all rules have exceptions, so has this one. For instance, a doctor will often prescribe an article without knowing how it works. This is called empirical prescribing. Rational prescribing is when an agent is administered that is known to affect some organ, fluid, or part of the system in a given way. That true medical genius named above did not rest satisfied with guess-work. He therefore sought out the reasons for disease and different actions of herbs on the system,

---

* There are some who will not go this way. (See I. Corinthians xv. 51.)

reducing the whole to a well-considered theory, which might
be summed up in a sentence, viz :—In heat is the principle of
life ; death is the absence or loss of heat. Those who have
read Dr. Coffin on this subject will find Thompson's ideas set
forth in a very clear way, but there is one thing that must be
noticed by devout persons in both Thompson and Coffin, they
lose sight of the Author of life, as not only the great Cause,
but the Source and Sustainer of it. The illustration used very
frequently for human life is that of a locomotive. The
machine is complete in all its parts, the water in the boiler,
but there is no life till the great principle, heat, is applied
when the fire is lighted. The water is turned into the motive
power, steam, which conveys its power to the piston, then to
the wheels, and thus the machine is started into action. So, it is
said by Coffin, our stomach is the furnace, the food is the fuel,
the blood the water, which, heated, sets the human machine into
action. This illustration may be very good in its way,
but it falls immeasurably short of the truth. Of late years the
microscope has revealed the fact that the source of life is not
confined to one organ, or part of the body, but that living
minute cells constitute each section of it. Thus the heart is
a centre of life in itself, so also are the lungs, the brain, the
blood, liver, kidneys, and muscles. Doubtless they all
require heat to remain in health or life, but there is a
sustaining cause behind all, which we, as Christians, recognise
as God, the Fountain of life, for in Him we live, move, and
have our being. We do not say that Thompson, Coffin and
others denied this, but it is almost the same if it is not
acknowledged. Thompson summed up the theory upon which
he built in these lines :—

> " My system's founded on this truth—
> That man's air, water, fire and earth—
> That death is cold and life is heat ;
> These tempered well, your health's complete."

As far as we are concerned in this life, we are prepared to
admit the truth of his theory. Heat is the outward manifest-
ation of life, and there cannot be health if the heat of our

bodies is much below or above the natural amount, which in the ordinary Fahrenheit thermometer is 98 degrees. A rise to even 100 is indicative of trouble, while 102 betokens a condition of fever that should receive treatment at once; 104 is a high state of fever, 106 is a most dangerous condition; while it is affirmed that 107 indicates death in the subject. The falling below 98 is equally dangerous in the same proportion. In view of the above facts it must be apparent to all that our safety lies in maintaining the normal temperature of our bodies. To do this three things are needful. (1st.) Good food, pure air, and water. (2nd) Suitable clothing, exercise and baths. (3rd) Medicines when needed that will either raise, depress, or maintain the natural temperature. These we have pointed out in the Materia Medica, and now, as our space is limited we must curtail our theorising and close our present chapter by giving

THOMPSON'S COURSE OF MEDICINE,

which has been proved in many thousands of cases the best means of restoring the natural heat of the body. Those who have a cold will find it as true as life that this course will cure in one night. Presuming that our readers have not a steam-bath apparatus, which we will describe further on, the first thing is to heat two bricks in the fire When they are sufficiently hot get a cane-bottomed chair, or one with holes in it; put a folded cloth on the bottom, and under it a tin basin sufficiently large to hold the two bricks with water surrounding them, if this is not to be had a bucket will do. Pour into it a kettle of boiling water. The patient being ready, put one of the bricks into the water. Sit the patient on the chair, cover with blankets up to the neck, so that all the steam is kept in; now give a drink of Composition tea. If more steam can be borne, put in the other brick, lifting up a corner of the blanket for the purpose. In ten minutes to a quarter of an hour give another drink of Composition, a cupful at a time. When the patient feels faint it will be time to stop. Then let there be ready a bucket or basin of water with the chill taken off and a half to a fourth of vinegar added. Take off the blankets, sponge down with water and vinegar, rub dry with a coarse cloth, put on clean, well-aired under-clothing ; put to bed ; when settled there mix a teaspoonful of powdered lobelia herb in a cup of Composition tea, half usual strength ; stir well, let it infuse by the fire, pour off the clear, and give to drink every fifteen minutes till it operates. Another and perhaps a better way to prepare the emetic is by infusing one ounce of the herb in a pint of boiling water with one teaspoonful of Composition powder an hour, strain through a cloth and give in half teacupfuls every quarter of an hour till it has thoroughly cleansed the stomach. About two hours after a meal will be the best time to take this course of medicines.

When the bowels are confined it will be necessary to cleanse them by a good cathartic. A dose of the powder so named should be taken in the morning on the day it is intended to take the course as above described. In cases of sudden attack, where it would not be safe to delay, an injection ought to be used so as to cleanse the bowels thoroughly. In order to impress this most useful course upon the minds of our readers, we give the poetical direction, written in a somewhat crude manner, which sets forth the object and aim of the writer in a more condensed form.

First steep the coffee No. 3, (Composition Powder)
With No. 2, then use it free. (Cayenne included in No. 3)
To clear the cold and raise the heat,
Now place a hot stone at the feet ;

The inward warmth now oft repeat,
And change the stone when lost its heat.
The fountain above the stream keep clear,
And perspiration will appear.

Then take the emetic No. 1, (Lobelia)
Until its duty is well done.
The stomach cleansed, the head made free
From filth and pain both equally,

Then live awhile in sweet repose,
Then wash all o'er and change your clothes.
Again to bed both clean and white,
And sleep in comfort all the night.

Now take your bitters by the way (Stomach Bitters)
Two, three, or more times a day.
Your appetite, if it be good,
May be appeased by wholesome food.

Physic or drugs I would not choose
To have you first or last to use ;
For if you take them much in course,
They will disorder reinforce.

Should the disorder reinforce.
Then follow up my former course ;
The second time I think will do,
The third to fail I seldom knew.

The emetic No. 1's designed
A general medicine for mankind,
Of every country, clime, or place,
Wide as the circle of our race.

In every case, and state, and stage,
Whatever malady may rage,
For male or female, young or old,
Nor can its value half be told.

To use this medicine do not cease
Till you are free from your disease;
For nature's friend this sure will be
If you are taken sick at sea.

If anyone should be much bruised,
When bleeding frequently is used,
A lively sweat upon that day
Will start the blood a better way.

Let names of all disorders be
Like to the limbs joined on a tree;
Work on the root and that subdue,
Then all the limbs will bow to you.

So as the body is the tree,
The limbs are colic, pleurisy;
Worms and gravel, gout and stone:
Remove the cause and they are gone.

My system's founded on this truth—
Man's air and water, fire and earth;
That death is cold and life is heat,
Their temporal weal your health's complete.

NOTE.—The steam bath is not mentioned as a part of the above treatment, the hot brick or stone taking its place. This may be done when the patient cannot sit over the steam, but a good steaming is best when it can be given. To sum up the botanic course in a few words, we direct: 1. A purge to cleanse the bowels. 2. Composition to raise the inward heat and clear off canker. 3. A vapour bath, to open the pores of and cleanse the skin. 4. An emetic, to cleanse the stomach. 5. A dose of bitters and some gruel, slippery elm preferred. The purge may be taken at morning or noon, and the other at night. When there is no time to wait for the bowels to move, use an injection suited to the case.

HYDROPATHY.

While it is true that some men exaggerate the benefits of water in the treatment of disease, affirming that it is the alpha and the omega of all successful treatment, (we think this is narrowmindedness of a very pronounced type), still we are willing to acknowledge the great medicinal] value of the various modes of applying water, not only in curing, but also in preventing disease. Hydropathic books, such as Smedley's, Kirk's, and others, which were written to set forth the virtues of the water treatment, are like all other human books, too one-sided. They abound with examples of the success of their treatment, but prudently omit the unsuccessful cases. While we, as authors, think it wise to cast the mantle of charity over our own failings, we ought to guard against the common evil of exaggeration. The author's father, who died at the early age of 34, of consumption, was induced to test the merits of this system. He entered one of the first establishments, where he was steamed, packed, scrubbed, douched, &c., for the space of a month or so, with the result that he came out much worse than he was before entering; he took his bed immediately and lasted only six weeks after Another young man entered Smedley's celebrated institution with a severe cold on the chest; in two weeks he was carried out for his funeral. Doubtless these are only exceptions, still they ought to exclude immoderate boasting Failures such as we have given are having a beneficial effect on the more progressive hydro-pathists, who are adopting our Eclectic System and giving internal medicine along with their water treatment This is a hopeful sign, not only with them, but with the older medical sects. We cannot afford to despise anything which has been proved good and useful in relieving human suffering, as in our treatment we shall recommend the various kinds of baths that we think will benefit our patients and readers. We give the following, which for the sake of easy reference we shall number, and strongly recommend as both preventive and curative :—

WATER AND BATHS.

No. 1, MEDICATED BATH.—This is simply made by boiling or infusing the herb or medicine in a half to a whole gallon of water, emptying into a flat bath or pan. Let the body be stripped before the fire if it is cold, and washed all over with it, then dried with a bath towel. In this way sulphur and other baths may be given.

No. 2, PLUNGE OR LOUNGE BATH.—To plunge into cold water, whether fresh or salt, first thing in the morning, is a powerful means of toning the system, and therefore good for nervousness, debility, relaxed habit of body, indigestion, disease of the liver, inactivity of the skin, or a relaxed condition of it. Salt water, or salted water, is in general the best.

No. 3, COLD SHOWER BATH.—To stand under a shower bath for a half to two minutes. on rising from bed, is as good for similar complaints as the plunge, and especially for determination of blood to the head, and may be taken at night for sleeplessness : or for this latter the hands and face, neck, and head may be washed well with cold water. A temporary shower bath may be contrived by one person holding a cullender or large strainer over the head, whilst another pours into it a jug of water. Stand in a tub to catch it.

No. 4, COLD SPONGE BATH.—We usually order this to be either natural or artificial salt water. It should be done quickly with a sponge or flannel cloth all over the body, followed with a brisk rub with a dry towel. Very delicate persons in winter may raise the temperature of the water to that of the surrounding air. We have found this of immense service in raising the tone of the system in general, and especially in nervous debility debility of the womb, dyspepsia, &c.

No. 5, WARM BATH.—This, as a general rule, should be taken in the evening ; for. as it relaxes the energies of the system, if it be taken in the morning the person is very liable to take cold after it, or feel unfit for the daily occupation. To make a warm bath for children obtain a large washing-tub. Pour in not and cold water sufficient. The warmth should be comfortable to an ordinarily warm hand. If a salt bath, add sufficient coarse salt to make it taste as salt as sea water. Then lay, or sit the child in it, and rub him all over for three to seven minutes. Take him out, dry him well, and wrap up warm. This is of great service in fevers, dysentery, diarrhœa, and cholera. For the latter the temperature of the bath should be as high as it can be borne ; for fevers not so warm. Adults should take warm baths for from ten to twenty minutes.

No. 6, COLD COMPRESS.—This consists of a piece of linen or cotton of the proper size for the purpose, folded four or six ply, dipped into cold water, wrung out tightly, and applied to the part affected. Over it should be bound a similarly folded dry cloth to keep in the moisture and steam that is generated by the heat of the body. It is still better if a piece of oilskin, or sheet gutta-percha, of suitable size, be put betwixt the wet bandage and the dry one. To allay heat and reduce inflammation and swelling it is excellent ; also to relax contracted sinews. For the head in fever, or any other part much inflamed, the heat of which it is desirable to reduce quickly, the wet bandage may be applied alone uncovered.

No. 7, HOT STIMULATING COMPRESS.—This consists of a flannel bandage, prepared in the same way as the above-mentioned cotton one, dipped into hot water, and cayenne pulverized sprinkled on the surface, to be applied next the skin, covered over with a dry flannel bandage, in the same way as for the cold compress. This is of great service as an external stimulant and counter-excitant for relieving inflammation and irritation seated in parts below where it is applied.

No. 8, FOOT BATH AND HIP BATH.—(See warm bath.) Apply it to the feet, or as high as the hips. Salt, mustard, or cayenne are usually prescribed in the warm foot and hip baths. In hysterics, headache, faceache, nervous and general debility, the warm foot bath is very valuable ; also whenever there is a determination of blood to the head, inflammation in the throat, or other parts adjacent. The foot baths should be continued for ten or fifteen minutes; the hip bath about the same time. This latter is more particulaaly applicable to female complaints.

No. 9, SHEET BATH.—Obtain a light sheet, or table-cloth or towel if for a child. Let it be suitable to the size of the patient. Dip it into cold or lukewarm water, wring it tightly out, spread it on a double blanket, and then lay the patient naked in it. Roll it quickly round him, and inclose it completely with the external blanket, tucking it well in at the neck and feet, so that no part of the moist sheet is protruding out. Cover over with other blankets, &c., tucking them well in to keep out the air. As the patient gets warm and begins to perspire, sponge the face with a little cold water from time to time. Medicine to help to produce perspiration, or cold water for the same purpose, may be given whilst the patient is in the sheet. This application is second only to the vapour bath for producing perspiration and allaying fever. For children it is superior, because so much more readily applied. The patient should remain in it for two, four, or six hours, until a free moisture is produced upon the skin. The hotter the skin of the patient when the sheet is applied, the happier will be the effect produced by it. When the patient is taken out of the sheet, he should be sponged over with cold salt water, or vinegar and water, and rubbed dry briskly with a towel, the same as when taken out of the vapour bath.

No. 10, SEA BATH.—The virtues of this bath are well-known. Sometimes when other treatment fails, sea bathing will cure. When the weather is sufficiently temperate, it may be indulged in; but in the case of children and delicate persons, the water may be brought in doors, and the chill taken off it in very cold weather. We have found it particulary useful in cases of seminal weakness.

No. 11, SULPHUR BATH.—This can be prepared by simply throwing a handful of the flour of sulphur into a basin or pail of tepid water. Sponge it on the body, and let it remain on ; that is, dry without wiping it off.

No. 12, HOT AIR OR TURKISH BATH.—A very good and simple way to get all the benefits of this oriental bath is to cover over with blankets, and put some methylated spirits into a saucer, and set fire to them. If too much heat is evolved, a piece of tin put on the saucer will, by covering some of the surface, lessen the flame and heat. After perspiring sufficiently, wash down as in the vapour bath. (See Thompson's course.)

VAPOUR BATH APPARATUS.—We have had made to order a very simple and useful contrivance for giving the vapour bath. The boiler is made of strong tin or galvanized iron, round, about 10 inches in diameter and six to eight high. A tapering spout. half-inch opening, at one side of the top to allow a rubber tube to slip over. Opposite to the spout, put a tap to regulate the supply of steam. The tap may be screwed in or a separate hole made for a cork to allow of filling the boiler. The rubber tube should be about six feet long, the end of it taken under the chair, put into a cup on its side, or a receiver, which is simply a tin with a perforated top. holding some herbs through which the steam passes up to the patient. It will be needful to have the top to slip off so as to get in and out the medicines when a medicated steam bath is needed. We can supply the apparatus complete for 15 shillings.

HOW TO PROMOTE HEALTH, HAPPINESS, AND LONG LIFE.

There are but few to whom the way to these great blessings is not open; still through a violation of nature's laws on the part of some of their progenitors or the individuals themselves, diseases and deformities may exist that no human skill can ever remedy. In such cases there remains to be obtained in God's appointed way the glorious and certain hope of an immortal body, which cannot be invaded by sickness, deformities, or death. A careful study of the New Testament will make this plain. The ancient proverb, "Man know thyself," comes to us with the force of a most reasonable command, if we desire to live long and be happy. Our bodies, though wonderfully adapted to resist disease and renew their energies, are at the same time but frail tenements and require reasonable care to ward off the many dangers that threaten them. A minute knowledge of the delicate and wonderful mechanism of the human body is not, as we have before stated, requisite, still it will enhance the admonition to watchfulness if we know just so much of it as to impress us with the fact that in a moment by a simple mistake it may be either thrown out of harmony or destroyed. In the promotion of health the first responsibility rests with the parents or guardians of youth. Since it has pleased our Creator to bring us into the world the most helpless of his creatures, with them it may be said that the moulding of our life depends. The first thing that parents (or those that are likely to be), and in fact all should do, is to cultivate a happy and contented disposition. A little reflection will convince everyone that discontent with our condition, unless we are not using reasonable diligence to better it, is a folly that can scarcely be exaggerated. Sensible and observing parents are cognisant of the fact that like begets like. As a rule, a merry heart (says the wise man) is a continual feast, and if we could see the effects of it in ourselves which we admire in others, it would doubtless lead us to the acquisition of this treasure, which few of the rich men of the earth possess. God has implanted in the breast of average parents sufficient love to cause them to take care of their offspring while in infancy, still a want of the first principle of training causes untold mischief, not only to the children themselves, but society at large. Let the mother see to it that her own system is kept in thorough good order, as it is through her that the child is first supported. Good wholesome food, though it may be very plain, with strict temperance in drink, will benefit both mother and child. If the mother is weak, a good vegetable tonic, with pure milk, will be found much better than beer, wine, porter, or whisky. It is not a delusion, as some characterise it, that the first appetite for stimulants which ruins millions is drawn from the mother's breasts. Don't let your children cry much, as they would not do so if they were happy. Keep them clean and give them fresh air when weather permits. If you can afford it get a perambulator, at any rate do not injure your older children by making them twist their sides carrying about a baby. As a rule no solid food should be given before eight months old, as the salivary glands do not secrete fully before that time. We cannot emphasise too much the influence of the parents' example. It should be as near perfection as it is possible, for the foundation of the character is laid here. A humorous writer says "to train up a child in the way it should go, you must travel that way yourself," example not only being better than precept, but the latter is almost void without the former. Time and space alone forbid us from giving numerous examples of the blessings brought about by a strict observance of the above rule and the fearful consequences of neglect.

There is one principle which more than any other enables us to carry out the perfection of our characters—that is faith in God, and a realization of the purpose of our being. Not only for this short fleeting life are we created, but for a brighter, more glorious, and eternal existence in the perfection of God. The Apostle Peter, in his short but inspired discourse to the convention in Jerusalem, explaining the conversion of the Gentiles, said: "God made no difference between us and them, purifying their hearts by faith;" and the wise man says : " Keep thy heart with all diligence, for out of it are the issues of life." A good heart then, or a love of the good and beautiful, is the essential of a happy and prosperous life even in this world, while it is indispensable to that which is to come.   Next to carefulness in following the right path, we should avoid running after the fashions and pleasures or vanities of the world, which are destructive to health and happiness.   Smoking narcotic tobacco is one custom which we would condemn.   We often see a boy with a pipe in his mouth.   Where has he learned this filthy habit ?   Probably from his father, who may be hypocritical enough to thrash his son for doing what his own example has taught him.   Or see the young lady putting a vice round the most important organs of her body in the shape of tight-laced stays.   Let every mother who wishes her daughter to grow up healthy, and in time gave birth to healthy children, not only persuade, but, if needful, use her authority to prevent this outrage on the female form.   Some customs have been so much exposed, and so far banished, that we need only mention them to warn against a revival, viz., low-bodied dresses, where the chest is exposed, and thin shoes, or more properly slippers, used on damp streets.   Late parties, balls, theatres, &c., have not only sent thousands to an untimely grave, but have augmented the sum of human suffering in the weak offspring of mothers, who never took to heart the Apostle's warning that " she that liveth in pleasure is dead while she liveth." As we have already extended this chapter as far as our limits will reasonably allow, let us, for the sake of impressing it on the mind and making it better remembered, give a few numbered directions, realising the fact that it is more easy to give advice than to take it.

1. Begin and continue the practice of early rising.   The old scale of sleeping hours are not too stinted.   For infants and young children as much as they can ; for a man, six or seven hours ; for a woman, eight hours, or one less may

do ; while for a fool, nine or more will identify him as such. The morning is the time when freshness and beauty reign. Therefore rise early and enjoy it.

2. Keep the body clean inside and out with water. Read chapter on Hydropathy for direction.

3. Wear clothing suited to the season and climate in which you live. Change your under garments once a week, when you should also take a bath and wash the body thoroughly. Keep your feet clean. If they sweat much wash them every night, and renew your socks or stockings.

4. Keep as far as possible and reasonable from danger. Do not walk under buildings in course of erection. Many have lost their lives by so doing ; nor take part in street brawls, unless you are trying to rescue the innocent from violence. People are often shot down in street riots, some of them being only lookers on, who should have been in their houses.

5. Avoid all intoxicating drinks, for they are evil, and that continually. Some may say that Paul recommended Timothy to take a little wine for his stomach's sake, and often infirmities. Very good, but as you are not Timothy, and probably have nothing the matter with your stomach, we would not recommend it, as many better remedies have been found since Paul and Timothy's time for the stomach.

6. Observe regular habits in eating, sleeping, and exercise, which latter should be in the open air, and not less than two hours per diem. Ladies and invalids should throw open the windows if they cannot get out and exercise in this manner, if possible, unless their state of health forbids it. Never sleep in a close room, nor in a draught. Let the beds and clothes be well aired through the day, and above all do not remain with wet feet and clothing.

7. Strive to keep a peaceful and contented mind. Remember that all things work together for good to them that love

God. If you do not love Him, then a knowledge of His love should be the first thing you seek—love as revealed in Christ Jesus. Do this, and you cannot fail to be happy now and for ever.

8. Always be complete master of your passions, they were given for your control, and to become their slave is to sell yourself to the devil for nothing; therefore be not soon angry, for the wrath of man worketh not the righteousness of God. A great man speaking to his oppressed countrymen said, " Be of good cheer, brethren, God permits evil, that by fighting it we might find favour in His sight; " in other words trials develop the moral excellencies of man.

9. Be careful what kind of physic you swallow, for much of it is not fit to be thrown to the dogs. If a doctor is going to give you mercury in any of its forms, unless it be the 1000th dilution of the homœopaths, tell him that you perfer keeping the disease you have, to taking stuff that may and often does create a worse. We deny that mercury can cure disease that other harmless remedies cannot.

10. If you are a parent, or if not, don't put off the study of at least the first principle of medicines till you or some of your beloved ones are sick. Always be ready to take the stitch in time which will often save the other nine. For this purpose keep a family medicine chest and make yourself acquainted with the properties of each medicine; this will give you confidence in using them. Under this head we would recommend the friendship of a doctor in whom you have confidence, for it is not always desirable nor safe for a man to be his own doctor any more than his own lawyer. It is best, however, to prevent the need of either by walking discreetly.

11. Watch against avarice in your heart, as you would against a plague. Remember that in the eyes of the great God the avaricious man is an idolator and worse, as it starves thousands and shuts up the bowels of compassion against the cry of suffering humanity. " The gold of the miser shall eat his flesh as doth fire."—Jas. v. 3.

12. Let these words of divine truth be branded on your heart : "The wages of sin is death, but the gift of God is eternal life through Jesus Christ our Lord."—Rom. vi. 23.

DISEASES OF CHILDREN.

It is a fact that holds good in both vegetable and animal kingdoms that young life is easier destroyed than that which is more advanced. Up to a given point our bodies become stronger and better able to resist disease ; then beyond this point they become more susceptible to it and less able to resist and throw it off. So in the first year of human life the mortality is very much greater than in after years. This is lamentably so in some of our large cities, where the statistics show that about one half of the children born die before they reach the first year. This very large mortality is brought about by the condition of society, which confines the greater portion of the population to the narrow streets, lanes and ill-ventilated houses in which the poor are often compelled to pass their lives. It is a matter of thankfulness to us that in the colonies the poorest are not so unfavourably circumstanced ; still, even here, there is much room for improvement in the homes of many in our larger colonial cities.

In the treatment of children there is one difficulty peculiar to those of tender years, they cannot tell us what ails them, so that we have to fall back upon our experience of the outward manifestations for our diagnosis (or conclusion of the trouble), which affects them. Some of these are pretty plain, indicating to the eye of experienced mothers the more common class of infantile troubles, but there are diseased conditions not so easily detected. It is our purpose in these pages to help parents and guardians to determine the name and nature of the sickness that may be on or coming on their children, as well as the most important part of administering such medicine as will with the Divine blessing restore them to health. In examining young children, who are often refractory, we must be patient with them till we have done this part of our work thoroughly. First inspect or look over the outside, then the tongue and throat. This is not an easy matter, but its importance must be manifest to the reflecting. In the absence of a proper tongue depressor, a tea or dessert spoon handle will answer the purpose. Take the child to the light, hold its head back, put the spoon on the tongue and depress it so as to allow you to see into the child's throat, for it is here we sometimes find a focus of trouble. The temperature of the body is an important point in diagnosis, and if people can afford a clinical thermometer it can be easily understood how to use it. The sounds in the chest are also an important means of indicating trouble. To understand these aright requires practice ; it is not, however, so difficult but that intelligent people may acquire some practical knowledge of healthy and unhealthy sounds heard in the chest. (For information on this point see Chest Affections, index.)

As the health of the child depends so much on the health of its mother, especially during its uterine development, it will not be improper here to give the rules laid down for her guidance in that excellent little book " Skelton's Family Medical Adviser."

1. Endeavour to obtain as much exercise in the open air as you can without fatiguing yourself.

2. Use good nutritious food, but simple and not too much, nor late suppers.

3. Use no alcholic drinks, but take toast and water daily if thirsty.

4. Take no mineral drugs, nor indeed vegetable physic either if you can do without it.

5. Wear no bones in your stays, and be sure not to lace tight.

6. Hold no society with tale-bearing women, whose chief delight is in raking up the horrible.

7. Be careful not to overstrain the body by over-reaching.

8. Drink no more coffee nor tea than is sufficient for the meal.

9. Beware of passion ; never quarrel nor look upon unpleasant sights of any kind.

10. Keep as many beautiful figures and pictures in your bedroom as possible.

11. Take care, as the time approaches for your confinement, to be provided with a good midwife and nurse, raspberry leaves, burnet, elder flowers, and composition powder.

12. A skilful woman is far preferable to a man-midwife. Be sure the bowels are not confined.

13. Drink freely of raspberry leaf and composition tea during labour. Remember that heat expands and cold contracts.

14 In cases of doubtful labour, cross-birth, or extreme difficulty, bear in mind that no surgeon dare refuse to attend.

15. In cases of flooding, which rarely or never happens if the directions given have been attended to, apply cold water cloths to the uterus and lower part of the abdomen, and give freely to drink infusion of burnet and elder flowers. Make a quart strong, into which put a tablespoonful of composition powder, sweeten and give to drink till the flooding is arrested. Simp'y bear in mind that the blood is the great agent of life. * A Mrs Wotton, a skilful London midwife, told us that she had succeeded in saving the patient's life when all other means failed

---

* An injection of cold vinegar has stopped severe flooding.

16. During and after delivery, the patient should be kept as warm and quiet as possible, and a little gruel given as often as the stomach will admit.

17. The nurse should be careful in washing the infant not to injure the skin nor scratch it with her nails. The water should be slightly tepid or warm, the body wiped dry with a fine soft cloth, loosely wrapped in flannel, and put to the breast as soon as possible.

18. Don't physic the baby, and remember not to stuff its poor little head under a heavy weight of bed-clothes. Remove everything offensive from the room as speedily as possible, side up, as they say in Yorkshire, and when things are comfortable call the husband into the room, that he may enjoy the delight of seeing his treasure and thank Heaven that he is a father. NOTE.—This may apply only to the first.

19. Remain confined to the room no longer than is necessary. Keep a fire in it in winter; if cold or wet don't leave the room for a day or two or more after getting up, and longer in winter than in summer.

20. In going out after confinement for the first time be sure and wrap up well. Keep the feet warm and dry. Take a little composition tea before leaving the house and some again on returning. Keep the baby from draughts or exposure to the cold, don't lay it open to the gaze of old women or young ones on the street, if you meet them. Having now introduced the child in its entrance into this life, let us speak of the troubles that are likely to befall it in its early days.

MOTHERS' MARKS (Nevia Materna.)

These fortunately are of rare occurrence. When they do occur they are a source of grief to the parents, especially if on the face. The removal of them involves a surgical operation, which, although not dangerous, requires caution. Where a competent surgeon can be had it will be best to either take the child to him or get him to call ; the difference is only one of expense. If the parents wish to do it themselves, the simplest way to do it is to thread a darning needle with a white cotton crochet thread, pass it through the base of the tumour or elevation, tie it on top, cut off the ends, put through another thread at right angles, tie in the same way, on the top, put in four to six, or as many as necessary; now put on a slippery elm poultice between muslin cloths, renew every six hours till the part festers and comes off; then dress with healing ointment. There is another way which some may prefer, as it does not hurt the feelings so much. Get a piece of caustic potash in the stick, wrap a paper round it, as it melts with the heat of the hand rub it gently on the top of the tumour, taking care not to let it get on to the surrounding flesh. When the tumour begins to look discoloured, stop, dry it, then apply a slippery elm poultice as before, till the growth has turned into a sore. When it looks clean apply the healing ointment. The same treatment will do to remove wens and small tumours. Deformities of various kinds we might treat upon but we cannot afford space, especially as the assistance of a surgeon is almost indispensable, at least in severe cases.

RUPTURE, OR HERNIA.

Umbilical or navel hernia is the most common form. It often happens after the part of the cord which is left at birth comes away, that a weakness of the skin and muscles underneath will allow a part of the intestines to protrude This should be attended to at once. A kind of truss must be. made to fit over the opening. Get a piece of cork about half an inch thick and broad enough to cover and overlap the edges half an inch; now cut a hole into it three-eighths of an inch to allow for the shape of the navel; pare the edges of the cork on the upper side only; cover it with a piece of soft chamois or wash leather; leave the hole depressed, but covered to let the navel into it, then fasten it to the belly with strips of adhesive plaster, and over all a bandage round the body. See that it is kept in its place till it drops off, or you may remove it in the course of a week, and if healed, put over a poultice made in the form of a round cake, about the size of a crown piece, of powdered comfrey root and cold water ; renew it every day for a week or two, then if all is well no further trouble may be feared.

INGUINAL HERNIA.

This form of hernia is different to the former. The cause is a weakness of the muscles, and other tissue of the abdomen. It is not generally known that the testicles are developed in the abdomen, from whence they descend into the scrotum or bag shortly before birth. In their passage through the inguinal canal it sometimes happens that through weakness in the parts a portion of the gut will come through. The first thing to be done when this is discovered, (which is noticed by the swelling of the bag, and sometimes a doughy feeling when pressed, or if gas has been generated a springy one), is replacing the parts ; to do which the child must be laid on its back with its legs raised, and the parts manipulated till they are back in the abdomen. If this cannot be done without, rub into them or bathe them with ether, which will render the passage much easier. A truss or some similar contrivance must be applied to keep up the intestines and the canal closed. A piece of cork sewed into a bandage, and fitted so as to press over the part above, and the side of the bag will answer the purpose. The treatment of females is the same.

IMPERFECT ANUS AND VAGINA.

Sometimes the new-born infant may have one or both of these mal-formations. If it seems but a thin membrane that closes them, the finger gently pushed may suffice to remove it. If it is very firm, then it will be necessary to procure the aid of a surgeon, as it would be dangerous for an inexperienced person to use a bistoury, which is the instrument required for this operation.

APHTHÆ OR THRUSH.

This is probably one of the first disorders to which infants are subject. In certain parts so few escape that some may think it is almost unavoidable. This is not so, for with proper care and favourable circumstances it is very unlikely to occur The causes that lead to it are impurity of air, improper nourishment, &c. The symptoms of it are so well known that it is scarcely needful to notice them. The small ulcers on the tongue, mouth, and throat, plainly show it. The disease is generally free from danger in the first stages ; but if neglected a train of symptoms will follow, which it may be difficult to remove—fever, vomiting, diarrhœa, hiccough, &c., followed by dark livid spots, with sometimes a fatal termination. Taken in the first stage it is easy to remove. Make a medicine as follows :—

THRUSH MEDICINE.

Raspberry Leaves	One ounce.
Agrimony	One ounce.
Yellow Dock	Half ounce.
Ginger	Quarter oz.

Crush the root, and put in a clean enamelled or tin-lined saucepan ; simmer ten minutes, strain and press through a fine cloth ; sweeten with lump sugar. Give a teaspoonful six times a day every two or three hours , if very bad, two hours. Pour out some of it, say the half, into which put a teaspoonful of borax. Mix well, and put a piece of soft cloth round the forefinger. Dip it in the wash, and rinse out the mouth several times a day. Keep the child warm, clean, and in ordinary cases nature will do the rest. If the case is a severe one, it will be needful to give the infant emetic syrup to cleanse the stomach, then the soothing syrup. If, however, the first directions are attended to, there will be little fear of it becoming fatal.

HICCOUGH.

Wherever hiccup or biccough is found, the mother should examine carefully the condition of herself. It has its origin in many CAUSES. Sometimes it arises from an impurity of the milk, at others from acidity of the infant's stomach, or whenever the mother suffers from indigestion, or has taken indigestible food or stimulating drinks of any kind, the unpleasant symptoms appear. It will often be found sufficient simply for the mother to alter her mode of living, for so closely connected is the child's life with hers, that she cannot possibly suffer without the infant being affected. It sometimes happens, however, that the weakness has been inherited from the father; if he has suffered from indigestion of long standing, or other disease, the child will often be found to suffer also.

The following medicine may be prepared and given with the greatest advantage :—

INFANTS' SOOTHING SYRUP, No. 1.—
English Rhubarb Root, dry, cut small One ounce.
Cinnamon, bruised................ Quarter ounce.
Aniseed .... Two teaspoonfuls.

Boil the whole gently in three-quarters of a pint of water for half an hour ; strain, press, sweeten well with honey, and give from a quarter, half, or whole teaspoonful of this mixture, according to age, from four to six times a day, when the symptoms are most troublesome.

The syrup here recommended is harmless, simple, and effective, and will keep in this form for some time, if preserved in a cool place. It may be increased in strength, and given in larger doses with advantage, where the bowels are confined, to older children and adults also.

SNUFFLES, OR STOPPAGE IN THE NOSE.

The nostrils of infants are often stopped up, or plugged with a thick accumulation of mucus, the result of cold, irritation, or inflammation. A little lard or fresh butter rubbed in night and morning, or a bit of soft rag dipped in warm milk applied inside the nose, and a little balm or pennyroyal tea, will generally be found sufficient. After this has been done for a few nights, if it still continues, give a warm bath. The above treatment rarely fails to remove it in the course of two or three days.

COLIC, GRIPES, WIND OR FLATULENCY.

Children are often troubled with gripes, pains in the bowels. and wind in the stomach, the causes of which are irritation and inflammation. It is generally accompanied with restlessness, crying, hiccoug' drawing the legs up towards the chest, and purging of greenish matter. It will be necessary to relieve the bowels of the irritation as soon as possible; for this purpose give freely of the Soothing Syrup, No. 1, or a medicine made as follows :—

INFANTS' SOOTHING SYRUP, No. 2.—

    Spearmint .... Half ounce.
    Ladies' Mantle .... Quarter oz.
    Cinnamon Powder.................... A teaspoonful.

Pour half a pint of boiling water upon the whole, mix, sweeten well with lump sugar, let it stand an hour, strain clear, and give a teaspoonful three or four times during the first hour, gradually diminishing it as the pains subside.

If the bowels are swollen and hard, add half a teaspoonful of powdered mandrake to the mixture, and prepare with it ; or what is better, add a teaspoonful of tincture of mandrake after the medicine is prepared.

TINCTURE OF MANDRAKE.—

    American Mandrake, powdered.... Quarter ounce.
    Ginger, powdered................ A teaspoonful.

Put into a wide-mouthed bottle, add four ounces of spirits of wine, shake it daily for a week, after which clear it through filtering paper, and keep it in a bottle ready for use.

The mother should bear in mind that as the child receives his nourishment from her, its stomach sympathises with every thing she takes, and this should induce care and caution in the kind of food taken ; for where there is disorder in the mother, there must also be disorder in the child.

VOMITING

Is also very common with infants, and should be

attended to.   When the milk comes off in an unaltered state, or very little changed, it may be expected to arise from an overloading of the stomach, or from the richness of the milk itself, in which case the infant should not be allowed to remain at the breast until it gives over of its own accord, but the mother should regulate the supply by considering the quantity the child can digest comfortably.   When vomiting arises from an irritable stomach and constipation, it will be wise to relieve the bowels by gentle laxatives.   For this purpose give the Soothing Syrup, No. 1 or No. 2, with the tincture of mandrake added.   Prepare also and give a medicine as follows :—

INFANTS' EMETIC SYRUP, No. 1.—

Ipecacuanha .... Quarter ounce.
Vervain .... Half ounce.
Cinnamon Powder .... A teaspoonful.

Boil the whole in a pint of water for ten minutes, let it cool, strain clear, sweeten with honey, and give a teaspoonful every ten or fifteen minutes until vomiting takes place.

A little Soothing Syrup, No. 2, may be given after the stomach is cleared.   Keep in mind this truth, " the stomach is the centre of sympathies," and if it be disordered, the whole body will be disordered also.   Therefore, simple vegetable emetics are at all times safe and certain with infants.

LOOSENESS OF THE BOWELS

Is frequently brought on by overloading the stomach, or by keeping the child in a close, ill-ventilated room, want of cleanliness and general attention, cold, &c., or by giving, as is often the case with some mothers, fat rancid bacon to suck ; but whatever the causes may be, the remedy is clear enough. First give a little of the Soothing Syrup, No. 1, to relieve the irritation ; and if the child is sick at the stomach, give the Emetic Syrup, No. 1, after which prepare—

INFANTS DIARRHŒA SYRUP, No. 1.—

Burnet Herb	Half ounce.
Wild Mint	Quarter ounce.
Cranesbill, or Herb Robert	Half ounce.
Ginger	Teaspoonful.

Simmer the whole in a pint of boiling water for ten minutes, mix well, strain, sweeten with lump sugar, and give a teaspoonful four or six times a day.

If the looseness continues after having given the medicine two days, give Emetic No. 2, and follow on with the same medicine for another day, adding six drops of tincture of mandrake during the day; and should it show no signs of stopping, prepare and give a medicine as follows:—

INFANTS' DIARRHŒA SYRUP, No. 2.—

Cranesbill Root.....................	One ounce.
Marshmallow Root	Half ounce.
Cinnamon	Quarter ounce.

Bruise and boil the whole in a pint of water down to half a pint, strain, sweeten well with lump sugar, and give a teaspoonful six or eight times a day.

Keep in mind that the medicines here recommended can do no harm, inasmuch as they cure by removing the causes, whilst in themselves they are as harmless as the mother's milk. Never forget to keep the infant clean, dry, and warm, and give it, when its health is returning, plenty of nursing in the pure open air.

SORES BEHIND THE EARS

Arise from a vitiated condition of the blood, full habit of body, want of cleanliness, infection, or from transmitted scorbutic disease. They are simply manifestations of nature seeking to rid the body of impurity.

TREATMENT.—Wash the sores with tepid water and glycerine or healing soap every night and morning. Make a decoction of raspberry leaves and lobelia thus:—

Raspberry Leaves .... One ounce.
Lobelia............................ Half ounce.

Simmer in one and a half pints of water ten minutes, cool, and strain through a fine cloth, and bathe the sores with a piece of soft rag; when they are dried with a very soft cloth apply the healing ointment or vaseline on a thin rag over the sores. For an internal medicine give the following :—

Sarsaparilla Root .... One ounce.
Clivers .... Half ounce.
Dock Root .... Half ounce.
Burdock Root...................... Half ounce.
Ginger Root .... Quarter ounce.

Simmer the roots in a pint and a half of water down to a pint, or for half an hour; take off the fire, put in the clivers, stir, and let it cool, strain, sweeten with lump sugar, and give from a teaspoonful to a dessert spoonful four to six times a day, according to age. If the bowels are confined put in a few drops tincture of mandrake or give infants' soothing syrup.

CONVULSIONS OR FITS

Are very common with children, and are always connected with other forms of disease. The causes are various; such as internal irritation, congestion, acidity of the stomach, teething, inflammation, fever, constipation of the bowels, water on the brain, determination of blood to the head, worms, &c., and often from the application of mercurial precipitate, or zinc ointments, for the purpose of removing ringworms, sores behind the ears, and other eruptive diseases. In treating convulsions it will be necessary to know the causes from whence they arise. The most common cause is derangement of the stomach. When this is suspected, give an emetic of lobelia fluid extract, if you can get it, 12 drops in a teaspoonful of warm water; if not, an infusion of the herb, half ounce to the cup of boiling water, given in teaspoonful doses every five minutes till vomiting takes place. Keep the child on the left side, and prepare a warm bath with some bitter infusion—

mugwort, wormwood, or best of all, valerian—four ounces of these to the gallon. To get the strength out of them, simmer them a few minutes in some of the water, then pour into the bath. This treatment will usually relieve the attack. If the bowels have been confined, relieve with a simple injection, into which put half a teaspoonful of powdered gum assafœtida to four ounces injection, or give the soothing syrup, made stronger, if needed, by adding tincture of mandrake. To prevent the recurrence and cure, make a medicine thus :—

Skullcap .... Half ounce.
Valerian .... Half ounce.
Peletory of the Wall .... Half ounce.
Antispasmodic Powder .... Quarter oz.

Simmer the first three in a pint of water ten minutes ; take off the fire, stir in the antispasmodic powder ; cover, let cool, strain through a fine cloth ; sweeten, and give a teaspoonful every hour if the fits continue, or four to six times a day. If the fits arise from water on the brain, carry out the treatment recommended under that head.

As fits are often caused by worms, it may be safe to give the treatment for them. As we have said, try and find out the cause ; seek to remove it, and the convulsions will cease.

NOTE.—In very young infants, when it is desired to make them vomit, the mother may wet her nipple with the fluid extract of lobelia. This plan is useful when there is tightness of the chest, cough, &c.

In the *Medical Times*, an eclectic journal, the following is given as a remedy when these symptoms are present : No fever, no great quickening of the pulse, the convulsions occurring every half hour or hour, preceded by restlessness and moaning ; give from two to five drops of acetic ether in syrup just before the attack occurs or immediately after. If the attack cannot be anticipated, we would only try this after the other means have failed ; but it is not likely they will.

SCALD, OR SCABBED HEAD

Is very common in infancy, for children's heads are full of fine
blood vessels, and as the blood is thrown with more force
where there is disorder, the least disarrangement in the
circulation often manifests itself by eruptions of various kinds.
The head should be kept cool, lightly covered, and the hair
never suffered to grow too long ; be well washed daily with
warm glycerine-soapy water, as well as the body, afterwards
using a little cold water.   The head is sometimes covered in
this disease with thick dry brown scabs, from which is discharged matter of a thin watery kind, so poisonous and
penetrating, that if any of it fall upon the neck and shoulders
it will fret and eat away the skin.   It is by no means difficult
to remove, if proper attention and the means are applied.
The hair should be cut close, and the head washed, as already
stated, morning and night, after which a lotion, made as
follows, may be applied cold :—

> Dock root, common, fresh, bruised .. Four ounces.
> Lobelia seed .... Half ounce.

Boil the whole in two quarts of water for twenty minutes,
strain, let it cool, put it into a stone bottle, and add an ounce
and half of tincture of myrrh.

After washing the head, as recommended, and drying with
a soft towel, moisten it all over for about five minutes with the
above lotion.   Prepare an ointment made as follows :—

> Dock-root, green, well bruised...... One ounce.
> Blood-root, dry, and well bruised.... Quarter ounce.
> Bistort ,,   ,,   ,, ... Quarter ounce.
> Lobelia herb, crude................ Two teaspoonfuls.
> Mutton suet .... One ounce.
> Lard .... Six ounces.

Gently simmer the whole over a slow fire for an hour, then
strain and squeeze the ointment through a coarse cloth.

Let it cool, and after washing and wiping the head
thoroughly dry, rub a little into the parts affected, night and
morning.   Keep the bowels open by giving Infants' Soothing

Syrup, No. I, strengthened, if necessary, with tincture of mandrake.

INFANTS' ANTI-SCORBUTIC MEDICINE, No. 2.

Dock-root, crude, dry................. One ounce.
Queen's delight, in powder .... Quarter ounce.
Clivers .... One ounce.
Fumitory .... One ounce.
Alterative Powder .... A tablespoonful.

Gently simmer the whole in a quart of water, down to a pint and a half, strain, sweeten well with lump sugar, and add a tablespoonful of tincture of stillingia (Queen's delight.) (See Index).

Give of this mixture a teaspoonful four times a day, if the child is twelve months old; or more or less in proportion to the age. Should the stomach require it, give Infants' Emetic Syrup, No. 1 or No. 2, as necessary, No. 1 is the best for children very young at the breast. No. 2, if over twelve months. Give a warm medicated bath occasionally of clivers, and as much exercise daily in the open air as possible. Always remember to raise the perspiration immediately after the bath, by giving warm ground ivy tea.

RICKETS

Are generally found in children between the ages of nine months and three or four years. There is generally protrusion of the breast-bone ; flabbiness of the flesh, and often distortion of the spine and limbs. The countenance is pale, the cheeks sallow, with cough, debility, hardness of the bowels, difficulty of breathing, and a disinclination to motion, softness of the bones. The causes that lead to this condition are generally hereditary. Weak mothers in the older countries, who have to work hard upon indifferent nourishment, and live in unwholesome houses and neighbourhoods; the same may apply to the father. There is little to be expected from medicine alone, as long as the unfortunate conditions which are the remote cause continue. What is termed hygiene is the best remedy.

Good food, rich in the bone-forming elements, such as oatmeal, wheatmeal, beans, marifinila, milk, eggs, &c., exercise in the open air, with careful nursing, not allowing the child to stand on its legs, if it has this tendency, till it is strong enough to support its weight.   If there is a tendency to bow legs, or to become knock-kneed, means ought to be taken to straighten the legs by in the first place bandaging them together at bed-time; keep the bandage on all night.   If knock-kneed use splints put outside the legs, and bandage them so as to draw out the knees.   In the morning a cold bath, with sea or salted water. Give it quickly, dry with a moderately coarse cloth.   Don't let the children eat all day, but at regular times.   Give them principally wheatmeal or brown bread and good milk.

Look well to whatever symptoms are present, and give a suitable medicine to regulate the bowels.   For this purpose the soothing syrup and tincture of mandrake, if required, will do.

For a general tonic we would recommend—

Gentian Root .... Half ounce.
Dandelion Root .... Half ounce.
Unicorn Root .... Half ounce.
Ginger .... Quarter oz.

Simmer in one pint; strain, sweeten, and bottle; add half an ounce of tincture of orange peel, and two drachms of hypo-phosphate of iron, and give from a half teaspoonful to two, according to age; up to one year, a teaspoonful.   Shake up the mixture before giving it.   Some, realising that rickets are always more or less accompanied by weakness of the bones, have recommended bone flour, prepared by grinding to the finest powder bones well dried.   We think it would be well to try this remedy; about a small teaspoonful in the food once or twice a day.   We keep this in stock.   The regular and general prescription is the chemical food—the only objection to it is the injury it causes to the teeth.

TEETHING.

The development of the teeth is a natural process, and in ordinary cases is attended with little or no pain.   Some

mothers, who have had large families, have testified that they
never had any trouble with their children's teething. The
order and time of their appearance is as follows :—About the
seventh month the first tooth may be seen in the front of the
lower jaw ; this may be followed by one next to it ; then two
will appear in the upper jaw ; these, with two more on the
sides, are the eight incisors ; then follow the two canine
upper and lower, four ; the four molars, grinding, or back teeth,
on either jaw, complete the first or milk set, 20 in number.
These generally last from four to six years, being gradually
replaced with the permanent set. which, alas, is not very
permanent This much of general information on the teeth
must suffice, but our inquiry now is what can be done to
encourage the development and relieve the symptoms which
sometimes occur in teething 1st. We would strongly
protest against doing two things, which are far too frequently
resorted to, giving narcotic physic either in the shape of
laudanumised cordials or teething powders, which generally
contain that preparation of mercury called calomel—a white
powder which is supposed to have a wonderful power in
reducing inflammatory conditions Then another of the same
colour, morphia These, with the sugar of milk, are, if not
the only, at anyrate the chief ingredients of the teething
powders, which, given to the poor babies make them sleep ;
and fond mothers think them harmless, but the number of
infantile deaths, falsely attributed to teething, prove the
delusion We feel confident that the simple remedies, such
as the Soothing Syrup and Soothing Drops are far better than
these narcotised cordials, infants' preservatives, royal mixtures,
dentition powders, teething powders, &c.

The second folly, we are happy to say, is falling into
disuse, and the sooner it is obsolete the better—that is
lancing the gums This is sometimes called helping nature,
but our opinion is it is interfering with her. When the time
comes the teeth will find their way through the soft gum even
as they did through the hard bone. The great object is to

attend to the general health, first of the mother, from whom the child draws its nourishment, also that of the baby. See that the stomach and bowels are kept right. In the form of medicine, if required, use only the simples we have mentioned, and all things being equal, you will have little trouble with baby's teething. If the infant is brought up on the bottle, we would recommend the slippery elm digestive food, with good milk. If the milk is vomited in lumps put in a little salt. If the stomach is very weak five to ten grains of pepsin added to the pint of milk, or milk and water, kept warm for from three to five hours, will predigest it.

We may here give a few hints on the care of the teeth in childhood and adult life. The great bulk of mankind pay little attention to these most useful members till they begin to ache. Then they will seek to cure the pain with nostrums, which often augument the evil; when the tooth is too troublesome, the offending member is often extracted. This ought to be a warning to take more care, but it is generally soon forgotten, till one after another is gone, the sufferer hoping to get a new set when the bulk of the original ones are out. We heard an eminent dentist in Chicago tell the class of students, of which we were a member, not to be deluded with this hope, as it was just as easy to run a race with a wooden leg as to masticate your food with artificial teeth.

First, then, we would recommend parents to see that their children use the brush to their teeth, after the permanent set has been acquired, night and morning, or especially at bedtime, when any fragment of food between the teeth may be removed. Salt and water, into which a few drops of Condy's Fluid (or solution of permanganate of potash), sufficient to colour the water, will form a good tooth and mouth wash. Let the teeth of children be examined occasionally, and if any signs of decay are seen, then take them to a dentist for advice. If it is desirable to get them stopped, have it done, as a decaying tooth becomes a cause of infection to the others. If they ache cannot be stopped, have them drawn.* The green colour which appears on the front teeth of some people, is caused by an over secretion of two glands, situated at the junction of the upper front gum and inner lip. To remove this is not an easy matter; but perseverance will do it in this way: Get a small piece of wood, shaped at the end after the fashion of a front tooth, cover it with a bit of cloth, dip it in bicarbonate of soda (baking soda), rub with this every night and morning for about five minutes, dipping and rubbing, and you will soon remove this disagreeable colour. As a dentifrice, we would give the following mixture, which we are certain will not disappoint you :—

Tincture of Myrrh .... One ounce.
Soap Liniment .... Half ounce.
Oil of Wintergreen .... Twenty drops.
Spirit of Roses .... One drachm.

Mix and use with the brush, or, if a powder is preferred, take—

Blood Root, in powder .... Half ounce.
Orris Root, in powder .... Half ounce.
Soap Root, in powder .... Half ounce.
Precipitated Chalk .... Half ounce.
Bistort Root, in powder................. One ounce.
Otto of Roses .... 6 to 10 drops

Pass through a sieve, and use as above.

CROUP

Is a disease which often proves fatal in a few hours, if not properly treated. Numbers of children are annually carried off by it, and yet it is by no means difficult to cure, if taken in time. It is most prevalent in cold wet seasons, and in low marshy districts ; and is brought on by cold or obstructed perspiration, and generally begins in the night. Damp houses, wet feet and clothes are some of its most prevalent causes. It

---

* Some mothers regard this as barbarous advice, but we ask, is it humane to have the child tormented, and the whole family worried, on this account ? If the permanent set of teeth are not coming in regularly, or are superfluous, get a dentist to correct them.

may be known by a peculiar kind of croaking noise, connected
with the attack, quickness of the pulse, and great difficulty of
breathing.   The face is flushed, with more or less fever, and
the cough, which arises from the inflamed windpipe, has a
sharp peculiar ring with it.

In treating this complaint the first thing is to regulate the
temperature of the room.   If there is a fireplace in it, kindle one;
if not, take the child where there is one.   Heat is an important
means of cure.   As soon as possible get a warm bath, immerse
the feet and legs up to the body; also the arms up to the
elbows.   Wipe dry, wrap in warm flannel, put to bed, and
give every opportunity for free breathing.   Put a hot bottle to
the feet, and the cough syrup in the infusion of ground ivy, or
cough powder, or composition.   If you have neither, give it in
warm water or ginger tea.   Dr. Coffin recommends the acid
tincture of lobelia from a tea- to a tablespoonful in an infusion
of cayenne, half to a teaspoonful of the cayenne to the cup of
boiling water.   Let it stand covered a few minutes.   After
stirring, pour off the clear.   Sweeten and give a tea- to a
tablespoonful with the acid tincture, repeated every half hour
till vomiting takes place.   Put a hot flannel compress, sprinkled
with cayenne, on the neck, and renew it as often as cold, every
half hour.   In severe cases look well to the stomach of the
child, and give suitable remedies if disordered.   As a daily
medicine the pulmonary or cough syrup should be given in
doses to suit the age of the child.

HOOPING COUGH

Is a contagious disease, generally confined to childhood.   It
seldom proves fatal under proper treatment, except in weak
constitutions, and relaxed rickety habits of body.   It commences
with difficulty of breathing, thirst, fever, &c., and often
continues a long time despite the most active exertions   It is
accompanied by a thick husky cough, presenting all the
appearance of a common cold.   The tongue is generally shrunken
up, and darker than when in health.   In the first or early
stages of the disease the cough is dry and harsh.   This is

changed as it advances to a convulsive cough, accompanied with a peculiar sonorous sound, which has been called " hooping," arising from contraction and inflammation of the larynx and parts connected with the air passages, producing sometimes complete suffocation. The paroxysms or fits last about five minutes, more or less, and are generally very distressing.

The cause of this trouble is the same as croup. It is considered more infectious. The old idea was that it had a certain term to run, but this has been proved fallacious. When the affection is first noticed. a warm bath may be given, and the patient put to bed in new flannel, if possible ; a hot bottle to the feet, wrapped round with a cloth, damped with vinegar, and the following syrup prepared :—

Lobelia Herb .... Half ounce.
Hyssop .... One ounce.
Ground Ivy .... One ounce.
Yerba Sanita .... Half ounce.
Cloves .... Quarter ounce.
Stolkham Tar .... A teaspoonful.

Simmer the whole in as much water as will cover them, strain, add a pound of honey ; let it boil gently for five minutes, skim carefully, cool, and keep in a cool place, and give from a half teaspoonful, for a young infant, to a table-spoonful, according to age The limit of the doses may be determined by the effect on the stomach Do not give sufficient to cause vomiting. In the preparation of the mixtures we would remind parents that the medicines are grouped into classes. A careful reading of their properties will enable them to make up mixtures of such things as they have, when the things enumerated in the mixtures recommended are not to be had in time. The indication in all throat and chest affections are expectorants, stimulants, and tonics. From an American Journal we have a strong recommendation for sulphur fumigation. The directions are to burn a pound in the bed-room for six hours, with windows and doors fastened ; stop the burning before the children are put to bed in the room. It is affirmed that two or three of these fumigations will cure. Sometimes a visit to the gas-works, and good inhalation of the tar, has done much good. A few drops of carbolic acid put into a cup of boiling water, and the steam inhaled, also gives relief. A change of air will sometimes be effective when all other means fail.

The latest remedy for whooping cough is the sweet chestnut leaves. Make a strong decoction, and give from a teaspoonful to a wineglass four times a day, according to age. We prepare the fluid extract, which is a very convenient way to give it.

INFLAMMATION OF THE CHEST

Is a very common complaint with infants, and like other forms of inflammation, arises from cold or obstruction. It begins with tightness upon the chest, fever, restlessnes, cough, dfficult and short breathing, &c., and if not attended to, often terminates in death. We need not remind our readers that the above symptoms call for prompt treatment. Stimulants and expectorants are here indicated. Each botanic doctor has his favourites ; as the simplest and probably the best medicine, we would recommend :—

Pennyroyal Herb .... Half ounce.
Balm .... Half ounce.
Ginger Root .... Quarter ounce.
Hyssop .... Half ounce.
Pleurisy Root, in coarse powder ...... Half ounce.

Infuse the whole in a pint of boiling water one hour, strain, sweeten, and give, if an infant, a teaspoonful every hour. If the fever is high, drop 10 drops of tincture of aconite into the mixture. This will bring out a perspiration and lower the fever. As an application to the chest, make a strong infusion of lobelia, blood-root in powder, and balm. One ounce of each infused by the fire one hour ; strain, press, and fold a soft cloth about four ply ; wet it with the infusion, wrap it round the chest, cover with a calico binder ; renew this every hour, making the infusion warm each time. Congestion of the lungs or chest is simply a preceding stage of the same trouble; treat it in the same way. Pleurisy is another form of chest affection, but in the infant it is not easy to distinguish one from the other. The one treatment will do for all. Keep the room well ventilated, at an equal temperature; and the hot bottle at the feet wrapped in a vinegar cloth. If this treatment is carried out faithfully there will not be much to fear as to the results, except in some few cases, when all that human skill and care can do may fail. Some of our readers may think our treatment too complicated or troublesome. They may desire something simpler. This is not unreasonable, as all cases are not alike in severity, and a simple treatment will be sufficient in ordinary cases. This being so, we prescribe the following :—

Pleurisy Root, in powder .... Half ounce.
Composition .... One teaspoonful.
Lobelia, in powder .... Half teaspoonful.

Infuse in a pint of boiling water; stir, let stand one hour, pour the clear, sweeten, add sugar and milk to make it palatable, and give from a teaspoonful every hour, gradually lengthening the time between the doses as symptoms improve. This treatment will do for old or young, increasing the dose according to age. Attend to the bowels and give a light diet. For a cooling drink, balm tea or wine will be found beneficial.

NOTE.—If the infant is very young, and the condition of the chest, i indcated by the difficulty of breathing, requires it, an emetic may be produced by the mother putting the lobelia fluid extract on her nipple. Don't lose time by doubting which you will try first. Take the first treatment; if it does not suit try the second, or any of the expectorants, sudorifics and stimulants. Read up the herbs and you will find the benefit in the increased confidence you will acquire.

WATER ON THE BRAIN.

We have already spoken of water on the brain in connection with convulsions or fits. The following are the principal causes of the disease :—Concussion, general weakness of the brain, relaxed condition of the body, excrescences within the skull, exposure to cold southerly winds and rains, watery state of the blood, &c., &c. It generally attacks children between the ages of twelve and eighteen months, or even up to three or four years, and may be known by the disproportionate size of the head, the motion which the child makes with one or both hands, pain in the crown of the head or over the eyes, sickness, dulness, general heaviness, and irregularity of the pulse. The skin is either flushed or pallid, and the child is often delirious and convulsed.

Treatment : An elastic bandage should be applied round the head to keep up a gentle pressure. A hot bath to the lower parts. Put the child in up to the navel for ten minutes ; wipe dry, dress in warm underclothing, put the hot bottle to the feet, produce and keep up perspiration ; then give the medicine indicated, sudorifics, diuretics, and stimulants. Prepare the following :—

Peletory of the wall .... Half ounce.
Agrimony .... Half ounce.
Broomtops............................. Half ounce.
Cinnamon .... Quarter oz.
Ginger .... Quarter oz.

Simmer in one and a half pints of water for 15 minutes ; strain, sweeten, and give in sufficient doses to keep up perspiration, and stimulate the kidneys. Under a year a teaspoonful every hour. The dose may be increased up to a tablespoonful for older children. In severe cases it will be needful to give injections and emetics every day, or every other day. An injection may be prepared by putting a teaspoonful of lobelia powder into a cupful of the mixture. Let it come to the boil, cover, and when milk-warm, strain, sweeten with a teaspoonful of treacle, and inject half of it into the bowels. Try and keep it in a few

minutes. In all probability this will cause vomiting, which is
desired. If it does not, give some of the emetic powder, or
put the fluid extract on the nipple. This, which is a
modified Thompsonian course, has cured many even hopeless
cases. If the child is old enough, the vapour bath should not
be neglected. The father may give it one on his knees, as
Thompson did, (see page 13.) In addition to the elastic bandage
on the head, a cold compress may be put on in the form of a
linen or cloth cap, wet with vinegar or vinegar and water will
been found beneficial. There is one word for this, as for many
other complaints, that is, perseverance.

SCARLATINA, OR SCARLET FEVER

Is a dangerous disease, most prevalent with the young. It is
contagious, malignant, and inflammatory, and often carries off
whole families. The disease commences in the same way as
all other fevers, with cold and heat alternately, shivering, &c. ;
after which the skin presents a red spotted appearance, at
first covering the breast and neck. It may be distinguished
from the measles by the fact of the spots being larger,
irregular, and gradually running into each other, and finally
assuming a general scarlet rush over the whole body. It is
generally accompanied with an affection of the throat,
difficulty of swallowing, great thirst, hot skin, &c., and as the
disease advances, headache, which often becomes intense ;
the sleep is broken by sudden twitchings of the limbs,
convulsive starting and very often delirium. When the disease
is violent and not properly managed death takes place at a very
early period. The causes are numerous, independent of contagion ; unwholesome food, filthy and damp houses, uncleanliness, putrid animal and vegetable effluvia, &c. It is hard,
sometimes, to account for the appearance of this trouble,
especially in the colonies, where the conditions of life
are more favourable than at home. We have seen it originate
in a family where none of the above-named causes were
found. While we would avoid anything approaching
to superstition, may we not acknowledge that the sense

of the common verdict is applicable here, that it is a visitation of God; that (the young may die while the old must.) However, our concern is most with the remedies. We have reason to be thankful that the mildest form is the most common, which, if treated properly, is easily cured. Before giving the treatment, we have just a word or two with regard to precaution against infection. There are two extremes to which people go, the one is being too careless, and the other too much afraid. While in America, we noticed on several house doors a red card, printed with these words, "Scarlet fever." This was no doubt a good city bye-law. It is well to let people know, but it is very unchristian for the relatives of the afflicted to refuse to visit the sick because there is contagious trouble in the house. This is true of some who call Jesus their Master, but who seem to forget His teaching, " I was sick and ye visited Me not." We have known of this mean fear carried so far as to cause its possessor to refuse a shake of the hand, (lest the contagion should be communicated), even with a housemate of the stricken one. With proper precaution there is no need for this barbarous conduct. If you meet your relative do not shun him, for remember your turn may come to need sympathy. If you are afraid of carrying infection wash your hands in carbolised, or chloride of lime, water, burn some sulphur and stand over the fumes, and you need not fear. If you go to visit the sick, you need not inhale their breath. When you come out or before you go in, smell freely of camphor, a piece of which may be carried in a perforated box, or loose in the pocket. Fumigate your clothes; take a vapour or warm bath, and you will have an approving conscience that you have done your duty in visiting the sick. These remarks will apply to all contagious diseases. Avoid extremes.

Scarlet fever is a dangerous and variable disease. It is divided into three varieties, which may be compared as bad, evil, and worst. The mildest form, which happily is the most common, is called scarlatina simplex. It is ushered in like nearly all fevers, with lassitude, shivering, headache, heats and colds, sometimes vomiting, quick pulse. From about the third or fourth day the characteristic red spots appear about the neck and chest, spreading over the body till it is covered with the scarlet or red-coloured eruptions. There are generally no throat symptoms in this form, or if any, very slight. The colour begins to change about the fifth day. The second, scarlatina anginosa, has similar symptoms, with the addition of severe throat affections, which inflame, swell, and stiffen the neck; and the whole system seems more under the control of the poison. The third or worst form, is called scarlatina maligna. The fever is more intense, the eruption of a darker hue, pain in the head of a severe throbbing nature, and the throat almost in a putrid state.

From the symptoms present we see that there is a poisoned condition of the blood. Our energies, then, must be directed to the elimination of this morbid matter. The medicines indicated are sudorifics, stimulants, antiseptics, and diuretics. If the patient is an adult, give a Thompsonian course (see index); if a child, a hot bath up to the thighs for 10 minutes, wipe dry, put on clean underclothing, with a hot bottle to the feet; give an emetic of lobelia, suitable to the age of the patient (see powders). After the emetic, sponge the body with vinegar. Prepare the following medicine :—

Raspberry Leaves	One ounce.
Sumach Berries	Half ounce.
Pennyroyal	Half ounce.
Vervain	Half ounce.
Horehound	Half ounce.

Gently simmer the whole in a quart of water, take off the fire, stir in a quarter ounce of fever powder, let cool, strain, and take, for an adult, half a teacupful every two hours. If the throat is sore put on a poultice of German camomiles, scalded with vinegar; cover up with oiled silk or gutta-percha tissue to keep in the steam, and flannel to retain the heat; renew the poultice every two hours or oftener if it gets cold; keep the bowels moderately open. If the first course of medicine does not have the desired effect, repeat it, and follow up the treatment. If the throat becomes very sore use a gargle made thus:—

Golden Seal........................ One ounce.
Gum Myrrh, in powder.............. Half ounce.
Prickly Ash Bark .... Half ounce.
Sumach Berries .... Half ounce.
Cranesbill Root, dry and crushed .... One ounce.

Simmer the whole in a quart of water twenty minutes, strain, add an ounce of chlorate of potash and two ounces compound tincture of cayenne. If the patient can gargle, it will be better, if not the mouth and as much of the throat must be washed out with it as possible. In the absence of this gargle, or as a substitute for it, if it does not seem sufficient after a fair trial, a solution of three grains of the permanganate of potash to the ounce of water has been strongly recommended. It often happens that after the disease has subsided a kidney trouble appears; they become congested, inflamed, and in severe cases disorganised. In this condition diuretics must be withheld, and the skin stimulated to do the work of the disabled kidneys. Of the sudorifics we would recommend the jaborandi leaves. Give the infusion in sufficient quantity to keep up a good perspiration, till the inflammatory condition of the kidneys has been overcome.

NOTE.—We may have something further to say on operation for desperate cases of scarlet fever and croup. (See index).

SMALL-POX.

In the colonies we may be thankful that this much dreaded disease has been kept outside, or nearly so, as only a few cases have occurred, and that in recent arrivals who were quarantined, and thus the disease kept from spreading. There can be no doubt but our sparse population, and other fortunate circumstances, has much to do with our immunity from it. May these continue, as the disease is one that strikes terror to the human heart. The dispute as to the advantages or otherwise of vaccination, is still unsettled, and is likely to be for all time. Our own opinion is that as long as it is kept out of the colonies there is no need for vaccination, but as the law requires it, we think it as well to comply; see that it is vaccination, and not simply inoculation. Taking matter from one child to another has been the cause of much mischief. Diseases, such as syphilis, consumption, or tuberculosis, the cause of consumption, as well as other skin diseases, it is affirmed even by doctors, have been transmitted in this way. If it is true Dr. Jenner did discover a means of lessening this great scourge. It was vaccination with the cow-pox lymph, or matter that he advocated. If the Government compel people to get their children vaccinated, let parents see to it that it is this kind and not the human matter it is done with.

Small-pox has been truly called " the scourge of the human race," and is supposed by some to have been known in all civilized countries from time immemorial. The disease is divided into two kinds—distinct and confluent. In the former the eruptions are single and separated ; in the latter they run together. The latter is the more dangerous, arising from the fact of the greater degree of putridity or virulence in the body. The symptoms are so well known that few with any experience can possibly mistake them. There is a dull, listless, and drowsy appearance, with loss of appetite and great weariness, sometimes three or four days before the eruptions begin to present themselves. The pulse is quick, with chilliness, succeeded by fever. At first the pocks or pustules present the appearance of flea-bites on the face, arms, and breast. There is redness in the eyes, pains in the limbs, and sometimes fainting and vomiting. From the appearance of the pustules, generally about the fourth day to the eleventh, they pass through different stages, first filling gradually with a whitish matter, which changes as it advances to a yellow tint. In more violent cases they turn brown, with little black spots in the middle. This is an unfavourable sign, particularly if the tongue be covered with a thick brown crust, and cold shiverings, with delirium and grinding of the teeth is often followed by unconsciousness and death.

Although this is not a disease peculiar to children, yet it often attacks them, and being less able to resist it, they are in greater danger than adults. The treatment for a child is similar to that for scarlet fever; the warm bath, hot bottle or brick wrapped in a cloth, and infusion of equal parts of composition and fever powders. Fever powder, which we shall refer to often, as we have found it so good, is prepared as follows :—

FEVER POWDER.

Lobelia Herb, in powder	One ounce.
Crawley Root, „	One ounce.
Skunk Cabbage, „	One ounce.
Pleurisy Root, „	One ounce.

Mix well. This powder given in half teaspoonful doses in warm water, sweetened, will usually bring out a perspiration in half an hour; or a teaspoonful in a pint of boiling water; steep one hour, strain, sweeten, and give as much as the stomach will bear till the patient is in a perspiration; lessen the quantity then so as to keep open the pores. When this has been taken, the composition (made pleasant) alone will suffice till the eruption is well out. Now make a medicine as follows :—

Saracenic, or Eve's Cup	One oz.
Wild Sage	One oz.
Marigold Flowers	One oz.
Clivers................................	One oz.
Vervain	One oz.
Bayberry Bark, in coarse powder..........	One oz.

Gently simmer the whole in a quart of water; strain, and for children, if they will not take it without, sweeten it, and give according to age; the adult dose being a wineglassful every two hours till the crisis has been passed, which is generally the eighth day. Keep the bed clean. Be sure that the clothes are dry and warm when put on. To quench the thirst, which is sometimes very great, dissolve half a teaspoonful of cream of tartar in a cup of hot water, sweeten, add a few drops of essence of lemon, and give freely; keep the room warm and well ventilated. Sponge the body twice daily with tepid water, and the healing or glycerine soap. To prevent pitting, a mixture of cream and fine oatmeal gruel is painted on the face and hands often; give a light farinaceous diet, digestive food, see to the bowels. If obstinate, an injection should be given. This treatment, for an adult, with a Thomsonian course, will answer well. If the patient is too weak to sit over the steam, the hot brick and vinegar cloth will answer the purpose. During the last stage, when the parts of the skin are being thrown off, cover them with an ointment, made by simmering an ounce of green, or half an ounce dry marigold flowers in four ounces of vaseline; spread on soft rags, and cover sores.

CHICKEN-POX.

Chicken-pox is by no means a dangerous disease, although it is common to children. It is generally preceded by slight fever, similar to that of small-pox and cow-pox, and the eruptions make their appearance about the third day, in small, dark-coloured inflamed spots, about the breast and back. A small vesicle or pimple rises in the centre, with a whitish transparent covering. About the second day after the eruption, the spots appear like small bladders filled with a thin clear fluid, which change, and become turbid and hard. About the fourth day, they assume a crusted appearance, begin to break, and about the eighth or ninth day gradually fall off altogether. There is not much treatment needed in this eruption. Keep the child in a warm ventilated room; give a tea of pennyroyal, agrimony, and marigold flowers, half ounce of each to the pint, sweeten; wash with the healing soap; keep the bowels open, and do not let the child out till the skin is in its normal condition.

COW-POX, OR VACCINATION.

Cow-pox is an eruptive disease originating and belonging to the cow. It is, in fact, a form of small-pox. The symptoms are not so severe, however, but have a striking resemblance to it, so much so that even the observant may mistake the one for the other. Jenner's theory, in introducing vaccination, was that this is a much milder form of the pox than the small or human kind. So he argued if the cow-pox was induced by vaccination, persons so affected would either escape or have small-pox, in a mild form. Like all human theories this has been proved erroneous numberless times; not only so, but the artificially-given complaint has ruined many constitutions, not so much from the animal as from the human lymph. Treatment same as small-pox, modified according to the symptoms of the case.

RINGWORM

Is an eruption of the skin, generally appearing in circular patches about the head, neck, face, and shoulders ; of a reddish colour, studded with minute pimples, which break and renew themselves continually. The disease requires care and attention ; for if neglected, it will most likely spread until all the upper part of the body becomes affected. To cure it is an easy matter. Wash the head with carbolic soap, dry, and rub in an ointment of blood-root; or paint with iodine tincture, or carbolic acid and glycerine, equal parts. Any poison of a kind that will not injure the parts will destroy this form of disease; still it is not safe to use them when the above will cure with a few applications.

INFLAMMATION OF THE EYES.

This complaint is a serious disease, and generally results from the want of knowledge in the treatment of several maladies to which children are liable. Cases of this kind are often met with after small-pox, measles, chicken-pox, scarlatina, &c. Some residue of the virus or poison is left in the body, which settles in the eyes, in consequence of which the parts become congested. Congestion produces suppuration, and the vessels thus surcharged break into one another, producing the unsightly appearance and painful discharge, often destroying the whole of the eyelids, and sometimes the sight altogether. There is another form of this, called in text-books, muco-purulent ophthalmia, which is usually the result of gonorrhœa in one or both of the parents, especially the mother. The appearance at birth, or manifested soon after, of the thick yellow discharge from the eyes, shows the nature of this grave affection. Little can be done, but keep them clean, which is no easy matter. For a babe we would recommend a tea of raspberry leaves and gum myrrh, one ounce of the leaves, half an ounce of gum myrrh in powder. Infuse in a pint of water one hour, strain, and after wiping off the matter bathe the eyes with a soft rag every hour or less as needful. If the baby is very young, it will be better for the mother to take medicine. The compound decoction of sarsaparilla, with the alterative pills, if required, will be beneficial. For inflammation of the eyes, not of the above type, make an eye-wash with

Marshmallow Roots .... One ounce
Raspberry Leaves .... Half an ounce
Gum Myrrh, in powder .... One drachm

Infuse as before, strain, and use three to six times a day, with a small soft sponge. Do not use the same lot of mixture twice. Once or twice a week, according to the strength of the child, give a medicated vapour bath of burdock, common dock, and yarrow, a handful of each. Simmer them in a quart of water ten minutes, throw them into the can or basin, and steam over them for fifteen minutes; wipe down with the vinegar and water, dry, put to bed, give composition to keep the perspiration up for some time. The antiscorbutic mixture, given for sores behind the ears, or scald head, will answer for this purpose. This may be alternated with any other purifying mixture. The way to cure is through the blood, assisted with local applications. A poultice of slippery elm, put on at bed-time, has been found beneficial. If an ointment is required, the vaseline and marigold preparation, recommended for small-pox, will be found an excellent ointment for inflamed sore eyes.

MEASLES

Is an inflammatory disease, generally communicated, it is

supposed, by contagion. It may be distinguished from small-pox, cow-pox, and chicken-pox, by the peculiarity of the symptoms, which are : a discharge of watery humours from the nose and eyes, sneezing, coughing, &c., with a copious supply of red spots generally covering the whole surface of the body, which become fainter as the disease subsides, and finally fall off in thin mealy scales. If improperly managed, it leaves a virus behind, which vitiates the blood, and forms scurvy, running at the ears, scald head, scrofula, sciatica, white swelling, dropsy, and consumption.

Treatment : Keep the patient in a warm, well-ventilated room, give the pulmonic syrup in a weak infusion of composition and pleurisy powder, alternated with a tea made of marigolds and agrimony, or pennyroyal. Keep in for some time after the disappearance of the eruptions.

It is sometimes difficult to distinguish the difference of these eruptive troubles. The Americans tell of an old quack who was called to see a family of three children who were ill. The first, he said, had the scarlet fever ; the second had the measles ; the third one had 'em mixed.

WORMS.

Children are often troubled with worms, of which there are three kinds—the Tænia, or " tape-worm," Ascarides, or small " seat-worm," and the Teres, or " round worm." They are not the cause of disease, but simply the effect of a bad condition of the body. There is nothing more tedious or troublesome to parents whose children are thus afflicted, and which, despite the efforts to remove, still infest the body. The first things to be considered in the removal of worms are the symptoms and condition of the patient. Sudden startings in the sleep, twitching of the muscles, grinding of the teeth, itching and scratching of the seat, rubbing and picking the nose, paleness of the features, griping pains, and tainted breath, are sure signs that the digestive organs are greatly disarranged, and that worms of one kind or other infest the body. The thing to be done is to correct the stomach

and digestive tract. I the skin does not look healthy, a
course of medicine once a week will be advisable. Make a
medicine as follows :—

Pink Root .... One ounce.
Senna .... Half ounce.
Extract of Butternut .... Quarter ounce.
Gum Myrrh, in powder .... A teaspoonful.

Dissolve in hot water ; infuse one hour, strain, sweeten with
treacle, and give from a tablespoonful to a wineglassful two or
three times a day. If there is irritation at the rectum, some of
this may be injected. Make it a little stronger with a pinch
of powdered aloes. This will destroy the parasites and give
relief. There are numerous remedies for worms. You may
try any of those you fancy, till you get the right. (See index.)

Tansy flowers powdered, mixed into an electuary with
treacle, is a good vermifuge. A teaspoonful for a child above
three years, less for younger ones, will, if given the first thing
in the morning, soon clear the stomach and intestines of the
pests.

CHOLERA INFANTUM.

We have already referred to similar troubles under the
head of colic, gripes, wind, and looseness of the bowels.
These may be said to be the milder forms of this disease,
which, in some of the more northern parts of the colonies,
carry off many dear ones; while in America, where the
summers are extremely hot, the mortality of children is often
alarming for two or three months in the year. The causes
are, a high temperature, which rises above the inward heat of
the body—so to speak, raises the stream above the fountain—
which is always a dangerous condition, especially if the pores
of the skin are not kept open and free perspiration maintained,
bad sanitary surroundings, eating unripe fruit or unwholesome
food, &c. The symptoms are, prostration, face pale, dark
appearance of the lips, eyes turned up and partly closed ; the
pulse is weak and irregular, vomiting and purging of thin,
watery, clay-coloured stools; the surface of the body has a

cold, clammy feeling. The symptoms, which may develop very quickly, point out the gravity of the case, which ought to receive our most earnest care and treatment. If the child is not too exhausted, let the stomach be cleansed with a simple emetic, for it is here the trouble often begins. Infuse half an ounce of ground ivy in a teacupful of boiling water, cover, let it stand ten minutes, strain off about half, sweeten with lump sugar, and give freely every five minutes in teaspoonful doses for about an hour ; then strain off three tablespoonfuls more of the infusion, into which put five drops of antispasmodic tincture and a teaspoonful of syrup of lobelia, sweeten with lump sugar, keep warm by the fire, give a teaspoonful every ten minutes till the whole is taken. This will act as an emetic, clear the stomach of the choleraic matter, and waken up the action of the intestines. This treatment is first, and if neglected, our efforts to stop the purging may be fruitless. Having thus relieved the stomach of its irritating contents, we must now give a medicine to relieve the intestines. For this purpose a grain of the compound powder of leptandrum (in a little of the infusion, without the lobelia and tincture), which is composed of—

COMPOUND LEPTANDRUM POWDER.

Leptandrum	One drachm.
Podophyllin	Twenty grains.
Ginger	Half drachm.
Hydrastis	Half drachm.

Rub well together. The ordinary adult dose is from two to three grains immediately after meals, taken in a little roast apple, or jam.

Continue to give the infusion ; see that the child is kept warm and the room well ventilated. For a food give the digestive powder or food (see index) ; prepare it with boiling milk, and give it as the stomach will bear it. The dose given above is for a child from 12 to 18 months, if older or younger, regulate the dose to suit the age. For an astringent medicine give the Diarrhœa Mixture No. 2 ; if the child is over two years the mixture may be strengthened by the addition of one ounce of tincture catechu. Should the disease have passed into its third stage it will not be safe to give the emetic, as the exhaustion may be too great.

Prepare a medicine thus:—Burnet herb, half an ounce; infuse in half a pint of water 15 minutes to half an hour, strain, sweeten with lump sugar, and add tincture of cranesbill root two teaspoonfuls, or cholera drops one teaspoonful. Give in small doses every half hour or 15 minutes. While this medicine is preparing we would recommend (if the child is not too far gone), a bath of slightly tepid water, about 65 degrees, the chill only taken off; immerse the child up to the neck, now pour on its head cold water as it comes from the tap in ordinary weather for two or three minutes. The child may gasp, but it will do good. Take it out of the bath, wipe dry, wrap in warm flannel, and give the medicine. The above treatment modified is strongly urged by Dr Skelton, whose experience was as vast as his practice was successful. He warns parents or practioneers not to sit doubting, nor listening to the croaking of foolish people, but to begin at once and use these harmless and effective remedies. Dr Coffin's mixture for this, and the milder forms of the trouble, is as follows:—

Turkey Rhubarb Root .... Quarter ounce.
Cinnamon Bark .... Quarter ounce.
Ginger Root .... Quarter ounce.
Peruvian Bark .... Quarter ounce.

Boil in a quart of water twenty minutes, strain, add half a pound of lump sugar, cool, and give from a tea- to a tablespoonful every two or three hours, according to symptoms. We know of this mixture saving a child's life in Dunedin, after a doctor said it would die soon.

CYNOSIS, OR BLUE DISEASE.

This is a rare trouble, but it may happen at any time, therefore we may be justified in giving its symptoms, causes, and treatment. While the child is in the womb there is an opening between both ventricles of the heart, called the foramen ovale (oval opening). This, in the course of nature, should close about birth; a failure in doing so causes the symptoms, which are, imperfect circulation, blue colour of skin, coldness, difficulty of breathing, partial stoppage of the pulse, fainting, convulsions, and wasting.

The treatment:—Medicine can do litttle or nothing for this condition; we can only relieve the symptoms and give nature every chance and help, hoping for a whole or at least a partial closure of this abnormal opening. If fainting or convulsions, give a mixture of antispasmodic tincture, half drachm; oil of spearmint, four drops; shake up, and give two drop in about six of soothing syrup; if the bowels are confined give more of the soothing syrup, with a few drops tincture of mandrake added.

If a gentle stimulant is required, that is, when the blue colour and coldness are the only symptoms, mix tincture of ginger, a teaspoonful; oil of cinnamon, four drops; give two or three drops in a little syrup. As a diet the digestive food may be given with advantage; keep the child warm and comfortable.

INFANTILE JAUNDICE OR YELLOW GUM.

This can hardly be called a disease, but its appearance two or three days after birth occasions the mother and nurse some anxiety. The yellowness of the skin, and possibly the unnatural colour on the napkins are its only symptoms. The cause is bile in the blood. We would not recommend any medicine for the infant; let the mother take two grains of co. leptandrum pd. an hour before noon and at 7 p.m. This in a few days, will remedy the trouble. If the yellowness still continue give two drops of the tincture of fringe-tree bark three times a day to the baby, or let the mother take a teaspoonful three times a day.

DIPHTHERIA.

This is probably the worst form of disease that attacks the young, especially in the colonies. Whole families of children have bean carried away by it. The reason for its great mortality is the want of intelligent and vigorous treatment at the first discovery of it. The symptoms by which it is ushered in are similar to scarlet fever; some hold that it is only a modification of that disease. There is a feeling of weariness, headache, chills, the tongue is furred, a deep redness at the back of the mouth, the glands of the throat are enlarged, the skin dry and hot, the pulse is quickened. The second stage is marked by the formation of a bluish white patch or patches on the mucous membrane of the soft palate, tonsils or sides and back of the throat. The third stage is when this false membrane degenerates into ulcers. The first step in the treatment, if it can be had, and the patient is in the first or second stage, is a full Thompsonian course. The vapour bath may be given in bed by the hot brick and vinegar cloth, but the emetic and injection must not be omitted. The course may be repeated every other day. A hot stimulating poultice should be prepared and applied to the throat, wormwood, mugwort, ragwort, an ounce of each. Boil the herbs in one and a half pints of water in a covered vessel half an hour, ring out the herbs, sprinkle a little cayenne over them and apply as hot as possible; renew every half hour by heating the liquor and dipping the poultice in it. A local steam bath to the throat may be prepared by boiling for five minutes one ounce each of ragwort, wormwood, and cudweed. Throw boiling hot into a bowl or jug, over which place an inverted funnel, and let the patient inhale the steam for a quarter of an hour, four times a day. Keep up the perspiration by combining diaphoretics stimulants, and diuretics. A good combination will be—

Yarrow .... One ounce.
Horehound .... One ounce.
Tansy .... One ounce.

Simmer 10 minutes in a quart of water, take off the fire, and stir in diuretic powder, one ounce: cayenne, half a teaspoonful; let cool, strain through a fine cloth, and give according to age, from a teaspoonful to a wineglassful every two hours.

As a solvent for the false membrane many other things have been tried and recommended ; sulphur, sulphuric acid, sulphurous acid, chlorate of potash, tincture of iron, pepsin, papoid, &c. Some of them have succeeded in many cases and failed in others. The one that has had the most success is the sulphur. The best way is to blow it through a quill on to the parts. Some prefer to paint on a strong solution ; others, if the patient is able, recommend gargling. The internal treatment of the sulphur cure is—

Precipitated Sulphur Powder .. One and a half drachms.
Chocolate Powder .... One drachm.
Essence of Cinnamon........ Half drachm.
Water .... One ounce.
Glycerine .... Two ounces.

Rub up the powder and mix all together, and give a teaspoonful every hour ; decrease as patient improves.

Some doctors recommend a kettle of limewater to be kept on the fire boiling while the danger lasts. One in Wanganui, New Zealand, thought he had found a specific in the steam of the blue gum ; but sometimes all will fail. If our readers should have to treat this disease let them give the course of medicine, and if they have nothing at hand but sulphur, use it. If the child is young give it a hot bath up to the hips of mustard and water ; keep up the perspiration , use your judgment, calmly trust in God, and do the best you can, for life and death are in His hands Having now, we think, pointed out the common troubles that are peculiar to children, we must close this division of our work. Trusting that parents who do us the honour of reading our book may see the wisdom of trying our simple remedies, we would recommend such to keep in stock at least some of the principal medicines enumerated. Remember they cannot do harm, but used judiciously, may save many a dear one from an early grave.

DISEASES OF ADULT LIFE.

There is one condition present in nearly all diseases, that is called inflammation. Some will challenge this statement, but it is true nevertheless. This condition may not appear visible, but it is argued that all pain is caused by it and obstruction to the circulation either of the blood or some of the other fluids of the body. The word itself denotes to set or be on fire, and the burning pain generally felt justifies in some measure the name Seeing the importance of this subject, it will not be unprofitable to spend a little time on its elucidation.

SKIN DISEASES AND INFLAMMATIONS.

The abnormal condition known as inflammation is what may be termed one of the phenomena of nature. Its manifestations are easily discerned, but the process proper that brought them about still forms a matter of dispute with those who have thought and read much on the subject Perhaps the best and shortest explanation that can be offered is that it is an effort of nature to throw off some poisonous or effete matter from the parts inflamed This is clearly proved in the healing process of those wounds known as contused, where the flesh has been torn or badly bruised, then the four manifestations by which inflammation is universally known, heat, redness, pain, and swelling, soon appear Heat is caused by an increase of blood to the part, redness is due to the same; while pain and swelling are caused by an engorgement of the small blood-vessels and capillaries, which press upon the twig ends of the nerves, and thus cause pain and swelling. Inflammation may continue from an hour to several days, in an acute form; while in the chronic it may last for an indefinite period. It has but three terminations First by resolution, in which it disappears, leaving no trace behind; second by suppuration, when the parts in which the circulation has been destroyed are reduced into liquid matter called pus or humour, in Scotland bealing), is expelled from the body; third, gangrene or mortification, in which a part or the whole of a limb or organ may become disorganised beyond the possibility of repair. This termination most frequently takes place at the extremities, and where the system is in a moderately healthy condition, Nature usually forms a line of demarcation between the dead part and the living, and if allowed to remain long enough the mortified portion would separate ; but as this would not leave a suitable stump, amputation is resorted to for the purpose of giving the unfortunate patient the most useful limb possible. Inflammation may take place in any portion of the body, in extent from the size of a pin's head to the entire surface, and one or more of the internal parts. The general indications for treatment are, first, rest ; second, equalise the circulation ; use cooling and soothing lotions to the inflamed parts. This may be all that is needful in slight cases, where healing by resolution may be expected. Where pus is forming, if it causes pain and points to the surface, it may be well to puncture or lance ; then apply a poultice to cleanse the wound, which, when clean, should be covered with a good healing ointment till the new skin is formed. In cases where the last and most to be dreaded termination of inflammation is threatening to occur, the most active measures must be taken to prevent it, if possible The condition of the stomach, bowels, and kidneys must be seen to, and such remedies given as will help them to perform their functions in making new blood and expelling old worn-out tissue from the system. The best poultice for the part is a mixture in equal parts of slippery elm and charcoal, mixed with brewer's yeast, renewed every two to four hours till symptoms are subdued. In order to simplify our work, we think it best to deal first with local inflammations, as heading the list of those diseases that affect the different parts of our bodies Beginning with the skin, we find it subject to various kinds and degrees of inflammation.

ERYSIPELAS, OR ST. ANTHONY'S FIRE,

Is an inflamed condition that has a tendency to spread, and is sometimes contagious. It is divided into different forms, according to the degree of its severity, or the cause that produced it. Where it appears as a red remaining blush without fever, it is called erythema ; when the skin reddens, swells, and sometimes blisters, it is erysipelas proper; if it sinks to the deeper tissues and ulcerates, it is called phlegmonous ; if the swelling is soft and doughy, putting on pressure, it is œdematous. The symptoms which generally precede an attack are chill, fever, lassitude, shivering, headache, coated tongue, followed by hot skin, quick pulse, thirst, pain in the back and limbs, the skin becomes red or purplish, and a severe smarting, tingling, burning sensation, with stiffness, is felt. Swelling now begins. If in the face, the features may be unrecognisable, and the eyes closed, watery blisters, resembling scalds or small blebs ; sometimes the throat may swell and be painful. When the deeper tissues are affected matter may form, and the outer part slough off. In its worst form, when the head is attacked, delirium, followed by coma comes on, and the patient may die of effusion on the brain.

The causes of this distressing and sometimes fatal disease may be classified as intemperance, exposure to cold, especially after being in a heated place, want of cleanliness and attention to the skin, violent mental emotions, disordered digestion, wounds, and primary retention of waste products in the system.

Treatment : The purest air, water, and food, light, nourishing, and farinaceous, must be had. See that the stomach, bowels, and kidneys are in good order. Bed-clothes and garments must be first changed and kept clean. Persons having cuts or abrasions of the skin, and women near confinement, should not come too near, nor should those attending serious cases visit and handle anyone with skin broken, without first taking every reasonable precaution, such as washing, changing clothes, and disinfecting, according to the severity of the case they have been attending.

Medicine : Having, as far as possible, attended to the above directions, now make a decoction of the following :—

Burdock Root .... One ounce.
Bitter Sweet Bark .... One ounce.
Elder Flowers .... One ounce.
Sassatrass Bark .... One ounce.
Capsicum Pods or Chilies .... A teaspoonful

Bruise, and simmer the roots in one quart of pure water half an hour, then put in the flowers, let it stand till cold, strain and press, and give a wineglassful three or four times a day. This mixture may be strengthened by the addition of two ounces of the blood tincture (see index.) While this is being prepared, if the patient is not in a very feeble state of health' a full Thompsonian course may be given, which in many cases will expel the disease at once, or greatly modify its attack, and render its cure quicker and more certain (see index.) Various lotions have been recommended to be used before the blistering takes place. Equal parts of tinctures of lobelia and blood-root, to four parts of vinegar, makes a very good one ; a decoction of smartweed, &c. These lotions are put on with a saturated cloth and kept moist. At bedtime, if the pain is very severe, a poultice of slippery elm, the surface of which is covered with the breast liniment (see index), will give relief and assist the cure. Mashed craneberries have been strongly recommended. If they can be obtained fresh, use them fresh ; if not, should you wish to try them, you can get them preserved at our place. In order to keep down fever, or when the eruption suddenly disappears in the skin, the fever powder or fever tincture in full doses should be given to promote sweating and cause a determination to the surface. The eclectic treatment is based upon the same general principles. It is preferred by many on account of it being less troublesome to administer. In some cases it will suit the patient better. It may be alternated with the herbal. In any case it is good to fall back on one if the other does not fulfil indications after a reasonable trial. If there is fever, give a purgative of

Podophyllin...................... One and a half grs.
Leptandrin .... Four grains.
Cream of Tartar .... Twenty grains.

Mix and divide into two powders, and give one every six hours till the bowels move freely. Afterwards keep them open with a decoction of the following :—

Black Root .... One and a quarter ozs.
Wild Indigo .... Quarter ounce.

Steep in a pint and a half of boiling water, and give a dessert spoonful as many times as may be required. If the stomach should be sour, give a teaspoonful of magnesia carb. powdered chalk, or carb. soda. If the pain is severe, the parts may be steamed over a decoction of boneset. Tansy, wormwood, hops, poppy leaves or heads, made as decoctions, usually are beneficial. When the inflammation is very great,

Tincture Chloride of Iron .... One drachm.
Sweet Nitre .... Two drachms.

Mix and give 25 drops in a wineglassful of the infusion of maiden hair and elder flowers As a cooling wash, a solution of borax and sugar of lead ; mix two drachms of each in a pint of rain water, and a cloth saturated kept over the parts when not broken. If so, a poultice of slippery elm, mixed with hop yeast, must be applied. If erysipelas arises from wounds, to keep it from spreading paint the edges with comp tincture of cayenne and apply the elm poultice. Keep the inflamed parts always covered. Where there is a constitutional tendency to this disease, a patient continuance in the blood mixtures recommended above, with attention to the general health—avoidance of spirits or any intoxicating liquors, and all exciting causes—a permanent cure will almost invariably reward the diligent. The reader will find in our Materia Medica and compounds many agents which may be useful in curing erysipelas.

SALT RHEUM (Eczema).

This i a disease of the skin, not unlike the former in its chronic form. It may be detected by the following symptoms :

It appears generally about the hands and face, although other parts may be affected: the arms, groin, and chest in very bad cases are often covered with it. In its simple or dry form there is an inflamed elevated skin covered with dry scales, which, if rubbed or fall off, are soon replaced. There is considerable itching, tingling, and smarting, although in some cases there is little or no feeling. This kind of eczema is called psorisis. It is very tedious and difficult to cure; perseverance, however, and right treatment will succeed, especially if the patient is young and temperate. The most common form of eczema is an eruption on the skin of small watery vesicles crowded together on different parts of the body, but especially on the arms and legs. It is accompanied with severe itching, smarting, and a secretion of thin acrid matter, which, in a few days, turns to yellow or green scabs. It is caused by an impure condition of the blood through the retention of waste products, improper treatment of acute skin diseases, mineral drugs, as arsenic, mercury, working in mineral salts, acids, &c.

TREATMENT.—Make an infusion of—

Wild Pansy Herb .... One ounce.
Senna .... Half ounce.
Boiling Water .... One quart.

Take a half teacupful of it two to four times a day, four times unless it operates too freely on the bowels. In this, as in all acute skin diseases, a medicated bath should be given. To prepare, take burdock herb, dry, three ounces; simmer in a gallon of boiling water; when sufficiently cool, throw into a flat bath or the nearest thing to it. Sponge all the body over with this, wipe dry, then paint a liquid on the parts affected, composed of one part of liquid tar (wood) and three parts of rosewater. If this treatment does not show good results in the course of a week or two, it will be time to vary it somewhat. Make a medicine to take thus—

Barberis Aquifolium............... Two ounces.
Burdock Root, crushed .... Four ounces.

Simmer in one pint or as much water as will cover them for one hour, strain, and reduce to half a pint ; dissolve six drachms of iodide of potash, take a teaspoonful of this mixture in a wineglassful of the wild pansy and senna infusion. If the bowels are too much relaxed omit the senna. In making the infusion, if the affected parts are secreting the watery matter, instead of the tar liquid use a lotion of fluid extract pinus canadensis and white extract of witch hazel ; paint over twice daily till secretions stop Use the tar liquid again, or an ointment of vaseline, two ounces ; extract stramonium, one drachm. As this is a complaint that sometimes defies all treatment, it will be well to be patient, and if need be, try the various blood medicines, ointments, washes, &c., till you have got the best. Look after the general health, especially the kidneys, as it is principally through them that the blood is cleansed of its impurities. Try a Thompsonian course once a week ; it will do good.

HERPES OR TETTER.

This is another eruption to which the skin is liable. It is divided into various kinds, according to the part of the body on which it is found, and the form it takes. Causes are, obstructed circulation, derangement of the cutaneous nerves, liver complaint, debility, &c It consists of small patches of vesicles filled with water, which change into yellow matter, break and form scabs, these, in turn, fall off, and leave the skin somewhat inflamed The trouble is not difficult to cure, providing reasonable care is exercised and proper medicine taken. We would recommend, first, a vapour bath, with the full Thompsonian course once a week, omitting the emetic after the first, then a medicated local bath to the parts, of burdock same as recommended in eczema. Make a portion warm and apply with a soft sponge or rag to the parts every night, using the healing soap and tepid water to remove scabs or matter, if any. The celandine ointment then should be rubbed in, also in the morning. Take as a daily medicine

the alterative powder. If this mixture fails take fluid extract
of clivers, a dessertspoonful three times a day ; or the medicine
recommended for eczema. Keep the bowels open, attend to
general health, &c.

NOTE.—There is one form of herpes which is simply
ringworm, for the treatment of it see page 300.

MILIARY FEVER.

This disease is like the last in the form and manner of the
eruption, but is always accompanied by fever and profuse
perspiration (of a sour smell), with cough. It sometimes
assumes a severe form and becomes fatal. Its causes are
given, as bad ventilation, sleeping or working in hot rooms,
low state of vitality, want of attention to the skin, excessive
sweating, rheumatic tendency, &c. The symptoms are, small
vascular eruptions, resembling millet seed, covering the neck
and chest, sometimes the whole body. Running together
they form blebs, containing a thin offensive scum. The
eruptions are preceded by debility, depression of spirits,
restlessness, cough, tightness of the chest. In a few days the
sour perspiration is manifested, which points out the trouble.
If it is a mild type, the fever will subside soon after the
eruption ; but if severe, it may continue, and develope
vomiting, delirium, and coma ; these are fatal symptoms.
The disease is happily a rare one in the colonies, but it may
occur, so we shall give the treatment recommended by one of
experience in this trouble. Begin with a powder composed
of—

Geranin .... Ten grains
Eupatorium Perp. .... Ten grains.
Compound Powder of Leptandrum ...... Ten grains.

Divide into 21 powders ; give one twice or three times a day.
If these things cannot be had, give a dose of the diuretic
powder instead three times a day. Give a medicated bath of
yarrow, three ounces, in a gallon of water ; simmer the yarrow
for ten minutes in a part of the water, and use as a medicated
bath as directed (see index).

As a daily drink give infusion of the queen of the meadow, one ounce in a quart of boiling water; sweeten with lump sugar, and drink freely. You cannot take too much of it. In change with above meadow-sweet wine (see index) may be taken during convalescence. A good tonic can be given, such as—

Tincture of Golden Seal .... One ounce.
Tincture of Capsicum.................. One drachm.

Ten to fifteen drops three times a day in a wineglass of water. If the cough is troublesome, use the cough syrup.

PEMPHAGUS.

This is another skin disease, consisting of small or large blebs, or vesicles, filled with water, which dry into yellow points. Patches of them, forming scabs, that fall off, leaving the skin red, which in the chronic case heals, it would seem to prepare for a fresh crop, that follow each other in succession. There are the two common varieties—acute and chronic, the former occurring in young children. This trouble is so closely related to eczema that the treatment given there will suit in this case. It sometimes happens that cases will be met with that resist all treatment. We had such a case a short time ago. The doctors had exhausted their patience; we had failed. We heard that a former medical man had cured him with a medicine containing iron. Truly there are more ways of killing a dog than hanging him. Medicine, in disease, is very erratic sometimes.

LICHEN,

In its simple form, is a skin affection which appears in small pimples, principally on the fore arms, but often on the shoulders and breast. It is sometimes attended with severe itching. The colour of the pimples, which appear in clusters, is dark red or white. There are other forms of the trouble which are generally given other names, but as they are all relatives, arising from similar causes, (extreme heat, derangement of the stomach and bowels, low vitality, impure air, imperfect nutrition, uncleanliness, syphilitic taint, &c.), they are all amenable to the same treatment. We will act on the advice of Dr. Thompson and let the names of all these skin diseases be like to the limbs joined on a tree—" Work on the root and that subdue, then all the limbs will bow to you." Nettlerash, prurigo or pruritis, or any form of skin trouble that rises in pimples, accompanied with itching, can all be treated by the following plan :—A Thompsonian course once a week will do good by opening up the outlets for impurities ; every night or other night the medicated bath of burdock as recommended in eczema ; dry, and rub in the ointment recommended for itch, (see index). Make a medicine such as that given for eczema ; if this does not answer try any of the blood purifiers ; if possible, find out the cause, and remove it if you can ; keep the bowels and the kidneys free, and in all probability you will overcome these troublesome affections.

ULCERS,

Are open sores or excavations of the skin. They are divided by various names, but for our purpose we may make them into the two ordinary divisions, acute and chronic. The first are generally the result of wounds, which in the healthy condition are healed by suppuration. The external treatment of this class is very simple. Keep them clean, wash with the healing soap and tepid water. If there is much pus or matter coming from them, a few slippery elm poultices will clean them, then apply the healing ointment. To assist the repairing power of the blood take the sarsaparilla compound decoction or blood purifier. Some of the other class of ulcers will yield to this simple treatment, but there is one that is very difficult to heal, that is the varicose variety, which is due to an engorgement and weakness of the surface veins of the leg ; usually situated on the lower part or shin bone. When of long standing there is usually a thickening of the surrounding flesh, called infiltration. The treatment must be both local and constitutional. Fomentation of mugwort, rest, with the leg elevated, and if much inflamed, poultice (see index). The slippery elm is the best suited, but one of the others may agree better; try them till you get the right one. If the ulcer is indolent, *i.e.*, not apparently getting better or worse, sprinkle a little blood-root powder over it before you put on the poultice or ointment; use the ointment of sanicle (see index), if that fails try the others. It need only be said that there are many remedies and treatments for this form of trouble; sometimes the one will cure and sometimes the other. We saw a fine cure made of a very bad leg by the following simple remedy:—When you boil your potatoes (without salt), pour the water upon foxglove leaves, at the rate of an ounce to the pint, cover, and let it stand till sufficiently cool, keep the leg straight, the foot resting on something, and the liquor under the sore part; bathe for 15 minutes, wet a cloth, cover well, and renew when dry. An American doctor says he can cure these troublesome ulcers by the following treatment:—Get a piece of fine sponge, cut it the shape of the ulcer, about the thickness of a penny, squeeze it out of carbolic acid,* fit it into the sore, cover it over with strips of adhesive plaster, and bandage the leg from the toes up to the knee; look well to the general health, take one or two of the compound carbon pills after meals, with a Thompsonian course and a combination of alterative herbs. If the sanicle ointment does not benefit, try the healing, or one made of vaseline and extract of stramonium, one ounce of the former with half a drachm of the latter. Patience and perseverance, if all things are equal, will conquer.

BOILS,

Are well known, but poorly appreciated. There is an idea that the cause is richness in the blood. If this were true then poverty of the life element would be preferable. As far as observation goes it seems they come on people with rich blood as well as those with poor. The most reasonable conclusion as

---

* Squeeze the sponge out with a knife, and take out the excess by pressing between a cloth, as it may injure the fingers.

to the cause is obstruction to the cutaneous blood vessels with
some morbid matter in the blood. They generally come in
crops, the first consideration on the appearance of one, which
comes as a harbinger of the rest, is a preventive. There are
two medicines reputed—1st. The sulphate of calcium in
pills, one-eighth of a grain in each ; two of these taken twice
a day is said to stop the development. This cure sometimes
succeeds and sometimes fails. The second, which was given to
us recently, is a small nutmeg grated fine, mixed with a little
water, and swallowed the first thing in the morning : miss the
next morning, take another the third morning : miss the fourth,
take another on the fifth ; the three will be sufficient. We have
tried this cure and it is genuine. When taken along with our
ordinary treatment, which is the slippery elm poultice at
bedtime, the discutient ointment through the day, with the
blood purifiers ; and last, but not least, if you want to be rid of
them soon, a course of medicine.

CARBUNCLES

Resemble boils, but usually are a much severer trouble. When
carefully examined, it will be seen that there are three white
spots in the core, while the boil has but one. The inflamed
base is much larger, and the suppurative process slower, while
the constitutional disturbance is greater. The tumours may
vary in size from a watch to a plate. Its appearance is
generally of a dull livid colour. As it advances, the suppurating
tops appear, break, and discharge a thin mattery fluid,
sometimes tinged with blood. The pain is of a burning,
tingling kind, accompanied, if a severe case, with fever of a
typhoid character. This disease, in its grave forms, seldom
attacks the young, the majority of cases being those who have
lived luxuriously and are of a gouty tendency. Sometimes,
however, it will be found in poor and ill-nourished subjects.
Treatment : Attend to the condition of health, that is see to the
blood, stomach, bowels, and kidneys. A Thompsonian course,
being the greatest cleanser of the system, ought to be taken.
The yeast poultice (see index) should be kept applied till the

core has come away. If it is very tedious, dust it with blood-root powder before putting on the poultice. When the remaining sore looks well cleaned, the healing ointment should be applied. If these do not seem to heal, try this :

Fluid Extract of Ergot .... Two drachms.
Oxide of Zinc........................ Two drachms.
Cold Cream.......................... Two ounces.

Spread on a cloth and cover. To assist returning health take a tonic of—

Tincture of Golden Seal................ One ounce.
Tincture of Ginger .... One ounce.

Mix. Dose: A teaspoonful in a wineglass of water three times a day. There is another disease that is confounded with this one. Its true name is anthrax, or malignant pustule. It is a spreading gangrenous inflammation of the skin, caused by the inoculation of a specific poison from affected animals. This is a rare disease, especially in the colonies. In Europe it has several times assumed the character of a plague. The microscope shows that the poison is due to a bacillus of a distinct kind in the blood. It is very fatal, and shows a mortality of 33 per cent.

The treatment we would recommend is, cauterisation with the caustic potash ; the yeast poultice ; sustain the strength by diet, stimulants, and tonics. Should the disease be found in animals, they ought to be destroyed and their carcases burned, so as to prevent the spread of this deadly affection.

ACNE, PIMPLES ON THE FACE.

This is one of the commonest forms of skin disease that we have to deal with. It is an affection of the sebaceous glands and the tissue surrounding them. It is generally confined to the young of both sexes (when not caused by intemperance), is chronic in form and difficult to cure. The causes generally recognised are dyspepsia, high living, disorders of menstruation, uterine trouble, retention of sebaceous matter, &c. ; in some cases we are unable to find

any cause for this troublesome complaint The cures are
many, but often fail to give satisfaction. To begin
with, we would recommend our old friend the course of
medicine once a week. Wash with the healing soap and warm
water, wipe dry, and at bedtime rub in the celandine ointment ;
look well to the stomach, bowels, and liver, and take the
blood purifier. If this fails trv the preceding treatment for
boils, and the liver tonic.

SCABIES, ITCH.

This troublesome condition is caused by a mite, or
microscopic insect that burrows in the skin If allowed to
exist, it soon plays havoc, not only to the skin, but to the
temper of the unfortunate victim whose incessant scratching
has given rise to one of its vulgar designations—the Scotch
fiddle. It generally begins between the fingers and wrist
joints, but is found on nearly all parts of the body ; first in the
shape of small pimples The scratching often causes
wounds on the skin, which fester, and look anything but
inviting. This trouble is not hard to cure if the right
measures are taken We have cured a whole family of ten
who were afflicted for two months by the following means :—
First, we directed them all to get a vapour bath (see directions,
index), then to be rubbed with the itch ointment. We also,
as the skin was involved and wanted healing, gave the
compound decoction of sarsaparilla The cure was soon
complete. This family, in gratitude, strongly recommended
our medicine to others The *rationale* of the cure is, to
destroy the parasites, clean the skin of their nits and debris.
Follow the above treatment, and peace will reward your labour.

URTICARIA, NETTLERASH, HIVES, OR PRICKLY HEAT,

Is an affection of the skin of rapid development. Blisters
of pinkish colour in patches, with stinging, pricking, itching,
or burning sensation. The direct cause is a disturbance of
the cutaneous nerves brought about by gastric irritation, the

result of eating certain kinds of dried shell fish, crabs, lobsters, pork, porridge, and strawberries; too many eggs, continued toast, &c., have all been found inducing causes. The treatment should begin with a change of diet, a simple farinaceous or milk diet for a few days will sometimes be all that is needful to remove it. Sponging with vinegar and water, equal parts, or vinegar alone, will usually cure. An ordinary warm bath of 30 gallons with about half a pound of borax, may be taken, or one gallon as a medicated sponge bath with two ounces of soda, washing with the prickly heat or strong carbolic acid soap, has been found useful; however, the Thompsonian course will cut short its course sooner than any treatment. For an internal medicine the compound powder of mandrake can scarcely be excelled. The blood purifiers, or rhubarb and magnesia, or stomach bitters, are all good. You can take your choice with confidence of a cure soon.

FLUSHINGS, ERYTHEMA.

Some people are very much troubled with these disagreeable symptoms, also called rose rash, inflammatory blush, &c. They are not to be confounded with that too common condition which is vulgarly but truly called whisky face or brandy nose, induced by drinking alcoholic liquors. The causes of these flushings are, disturbance of the digestion, blood irritation, severe exercise, drinking largely of cold water while in a state of perspiration, &c. Symptoms— slight fever, rose-coloured irritate patches appearing on various parts of the body, particularly on the face after meals, continuing so for an hour or two, and sometimes for days.

The treatment for them all is the same, which may be said to be prevention, by keeping the stomach, bowels, kidneys, and liver in good condition. Use an alkaline local bath at bedtime every night while the trouble lasts. Dissolve a piece of washing soda about the size of a large walnut in a gallon of warm water, wash with it, using the healing soap. If immediate relief is wanted through the day, sponging with vinegar will sometimes afford it. Borax and water are recommended, also glycerine and cucumber juice. As an internal medicine, if the symptoms arise from constipation, the comp leptandrum powder, liver tonic or pills; if arising from the stomach, take the spiced bitter powders; if the blood is at fault, the alterative powder or blood purifier will, if persevered with, be found curative. If the symptoms still exist after trying the above, take a course of medicine every week.

DANDRUFF (PITYRIASIS).

Dandruff is a very common skin affection. Its symptoms are so common that we need not describe them at any length. It simply consists of a scaling of the skin in bran-like flakes. Its causes are, low state of vitality, hereditary transmission, syphilitic taint, use of mercury, &c., but we often meet with it when these symptoms are not present. Treatment—look for the cause and remove it; use the healing soap, and a local bath of burdock, rhubarb leaves, or borax and water, wipe dry, and rub in a mixture of equal parts petroleum or vaseline oil and spirits of wine. If in the head the best remedy we have found is our rosemary tricopherus, which is composed of castor oil, spirits of rosemary, &c. Use night and morning, applying the brush at the same time.

TINEA VERSICOLOR,
(Or as we would term it YELLOW DANDRUFF),

Is a vegetable parasite which appears in front of the chest, of a dark yellow colour. It is supposed to be caused by a low state of nutrition, excesses, and sweating, but being infectious, it is more likely to come in this way. It is not likely to be mistaken, as it itches well, and you can seemingly scrape it off with your nails, but it requires a poison of some kind to destroy it.

DIRECTION.—Wash the parts well with warm water and soap, dry, and paint with the following solution:—Corrosive sublimate, four grains; water, two ounces; shake till dissolved. This is a certain cure; ointments would remove it, but they

.are not so pleasant. If you prefer an ointment, use either the blood-root, tar, or itch (see index).

LEPROSY.

This is one of the oldest and most dreadful of diseases; it is mentioned in Scripture many times, and in the earliest of medical books. Although not so common as in Scriptural times it is found more or less all over the globe; in Norway, Iceland, Spain, Portugal, Italy, and Southern Russia. The disease has disappeared in Eastern Europe; in India and China it is very common. The Chinese take it with them almost wherever they go. Forty years ago the Hawaiians or Sandwich Islanders knew nothing of it; now a tenth part of them are lepers. One island is set apart for them. It is well known from whom they got it; the Chinese have over-run the islands and given them this plague. We do not wish to increase the prejudice that exists against Chinamen, but if they do not adopt our civilised mode of life, they ought to be watched and kept from swamping the colonies, where even now leprosy is among them. While it is figuratively true of us all that in the midst of life we are dying, this saying has its literal rendering in the leper. The outside of the body is decaying piecemeal. It usually takes 10 years from the commencement of the disease till death, which must be welcome to the sufferer, terminating his misery. The disease has two forms, and various manifestations. The first stage is the appearance of blotches in patches, from the size of a finger nail to that of the hand, on the skin. These grow in size, darken in colour, take on a bronze gangrenous tint. The face is generally first invaded, but the whole body, even the palms of the hands and soles of the feet are sometimes covered. It is said to be caused by a parasitic growth (Bacillis). The most melancholy thing about it is its incurability; things innumerable have been tried, but all seem to fail. The old adage, " while there is life there is hope," should prevent the patients or their friends sitting down in despair without trying anything. Those who have lived in infected districts only mention five things as having any beneficial effect upon it. Creosote, in half drop doses, given in pill form three times a day, has been praised by some; salycilate of soda, half to drachm doses, three times a day; Hoang-Nan is the Chinese remedy, but has failed to do any permanent good; Gurjun oil has been highly spoken of, but the Chaulmoogra oil has gained most favour. It is given internally in 5 to 10 drop doses, three times daily, and an ointment of 10 grains to the ounce; apply outwardly. We have seen and handled a dead leper, and from the general appearance we should conclude it a disease of the blood. Attempting to cure is only experimenting. Had we the treating of a case we should try our favourite remedy the Thompsonian course and the best blood purifiers. Some time ago we noticed an alleged cure by a plant found in Mexico, but it, like all other things, has not stood the test of time. It is to be hoped that in the not distant future a remedy will be found for this loathsome and fatal disease, for up to the present all that medicine can do is to mitigate symptoms and prolong life

LUPUS VULGARIS.

This is sometimes called scaly leprosy. The difference between this non-contagious form and the preceding class is very clearly set forth in the Law of Moses (Leviticus xiii and xiv.): "If in the leprosy there be a white tumour of the skin and it has turned the hair white in it, and if there be quick flesh within the tumour, then it is an old leprosy of the skin; but if the leprosy spread abroad in the skin and cover the whole skin of disease from his head even to his feet, the person shall be pronounced clean." The latter is what we understand by scally leprosy as it is met with nowa-days. It is in patches of various sizes covered with white scales on a raised surface, resembling psoriasis, of which it seems to be an aggravated form. The diganosis may be somewhat difficult, but the treatment is the same as that for eczema. Follow out the directions and medicines given there, and good will be sure to follow. As the proverb says, "in all labour there is reward." There is just one other form of lupus that makes the life of some of our race miserable; that is the variety seen on the face, which in its progress often eats away the nose We sometimes see these cases, the sight of which moves our pity. Of all the remedies that have been tried, there is but one we find that is claimed as a cure, that is chromic acid in a solution of six grains to the ounce of water, paint on to the affected parts three times a day. The American doctor who gives this cure reports several successful cases Ointments of crysarobin, 20 grains to the ounce of vaseline; proligalic acid, 20 to 40 grains, to the ounce in ointment; are also recommended. The constitutional treatment is not of much avail, still it ought not to be neglected. A good blood mixture, with attention to the skin and digestive organs, will help nature to throw off this incumbrance

SCURVY (Purpurea),

Is a skin disease generally resulting from a want of vegetable diet and eating salt meat. It is well-known to sailors, especially those who go on long whaling voyages. We have seen it, however, in persons who had a good opportunity of getting a vegetable diet. The commonest form of it is scurvy in the beard, called sycosis. The treatment for general scurvy is avoidance of the cause or causes; a vegetable diet; water cress and cold infusion of clivers, or a tablespoonful of the juice, a course of medicine once a week. If the patient is weak a tonic of golden seal and cayenne, one ounce of the first and half ounce of the second, dose a teaspoonful, or the stomach bitters. As an application we have found the hypo-chloride of sulphur ointment splendid; two drachms to the ounce of lard or vaseline, applied twice daily seldom fails. Make the medicine given for ulcers (page 318), in addition to the infusion of clivers. If you want to save yourself from

SCURVY IN THE BEARD,

Which is another form of the above, don't shave. It is an unnatural custom and is often the cause of infection. If you have this trouble, wash every night in an infusion of celandine herb, dry well and rub in the above ointment; it will soon cure; take the medicine as directed.

SCROFULA

Is another form of blood disease, which affects the glands in some parts of the body, principally under the chin and about the ears. The swellings are usually very slow. When this is the case, rub them night and morning with turpentine and lard, two of the former and one of the latter, as recommended in mumps. If they break, poultice them with slippery elm till they present a clean aspect, and are reduced to near their normal condition; then apply the healing ointment. Make the medicine recommended for ulcers (page 318). Take a wineglassful 4 times a day. and a course of medicine once a week. There are many other forms of skin disease, which we have not space to notice; they may all be treated on the foregoing plan. We will close this division with a rather peculiar one sometimes met with.

ICHTHYOSIS, OR FISH SKIN.

The symptoms are a dry, rough, scaly condition of the skin, chiefly affecting the hands, feet, and limbs; having a disagreeable smell, irritation. itching, and uncomfortable feeling. Treatment—a medicated vapour bath of marsh-mallow, healing soap, and soothing ointment. Begin with one every night, lessen as condition improves, keep the system right, and take a teaspoonful of cod-liver oil in cream four times a day. This is a simple and effective remedy.

INTERNAL INFLAMMATIONS.

INFLAMMATION OF THE BRAIN (Phrenitis).

Beginning from above downward we find the first organ liable to inflammation, is the brain. There are two degrees of this trouble, first, congestion, which means a certain amount of stagnation in the blood-vessels. This condition may either be removed or it will pass into the second stage of acute inflammation If the coverings of the brain only, are the seat of the inflammation, it is called meningitis. The causes are, whatever leads to a determination of blood to the head, or prevents a free circulation in it, &c. The remoter causes are. strong fits of passion, intense application of the mind, violent exercise, injuries to the head, intemperance, exposure to great heat of the sun, and the effect of inflammation in some other part of the body. This is called symptomatic. With a knowledge of the law of circulation we can see at a glance that the blood has partly receded from other parts of the system, and it is by this knowledge we must be guided in our efforts to cure.

TREATMENT.—If we can discern the first condition or congestive stage, which may be known by the fullness, pain, throbbing and heat, give a Thompsonian course every other day if the symptoms continue As a daily medicine make a decoction as follows·—

Rosemary herb .... One ounce.
Skullcap .... One ounce.
Wood Betony .... One ounce.
Catnip .... One ounce.
Boneset .... One ounce.

Simmer in a quart of boiling water for 10 minutes; keep on the cover; when taken off the fire stir in a level teaspoonful of cayenne; let it cool, strain, press through a cloth, and give a wineglassful every hour while the violent symptoms con-

tinue; afterwards it may be given less frequently. A pillow
of hops has been recommended. also cloths laid on the head
wet with vinegar or cold water and vinegar. The bowels must
be kept open either by the compound powder of mandrake or
an injection This treatment will seldom fail to restore the
patient. When the severe symptoms have ceased, give some
of the convalescent medicine (see index). Let the diet of the
patient be principally milk, bread, &c.; nothing of any
irritating nature must be given.

INFLAMMATION OF THE EAR (OTITIS).

This is a very painful affection, on account of the large
number of nerves surrounding the organ. The causes of it
are numerous and not always easily traced; blows, cold winds,
standing in draughts, exposure, &c.

SYMPTOMS.—Great pain noise or ringing in the ear;
sometimes in severe cases delirium; swelling, and redness
may be seen at the opening.

TREATMENT.—That recommended for inflammation of
the brain with local application will cure it. Apply a poultice
of scalded hops, after putting in five drops each of laudanum
and glycerine, renew it as often as cold It will generally
be found on inspection that the throat is affected; if so, use
the herbs for steaming recommended in diphtheria (page 307)
also the quinsy embrocation (see index); for milder forms
there are several drops for easing the pain The juice of
onions and laudanum equal parts. five drops put into the
ear gives instant relief Or take—

EAR DROPS

Oil of Sassafras ....,,.... Half ounce.
Oil of Sweet Almonds ....,,.. Half ounce.
Tincture of Opium....................,,.... Half ounce
Camphor......................,,,..., ..., One drachm.

Dissolve, warm it, soak a pledget of cotton wool, put into the
ear and bind over, if the pain is great an anodyne should
be given. Those who are subject to this complaint ought to
put a little cotton in their ears in cold windy weather and
while sleeping. For chronic inflammation or running at the

ears an application of the drops morning and night, and a
course of blood purifiers, with the weekly course of medicine,
will be the best thing.

INFLAMMATION OF THE EYE.

Having already pointed out the general treatment in
children's diseases, it will be sufficient to give a few extra
recipes and directions The plan of treatment is the same
for all local inflammations : equalise the circulation, and
withdraw the abnormal pressure of blood from the part. There
is an old gentleman living near this city who was very ill.
He went to Sydney for treatment, and an eye doctor there
recommended cold water to the eyes and hot water cloths to
the back of his head. This did him good. He was also
advised to let his hair grow long, which he did. He is now
taken for a Christian Israelite, but he has never had a bad
turn with his eyes since. Doctors differ very much here as in
other treatment, one preferring cold water, another hot. While
attending a New York clinical lecture, an amusing incident
occurred. A very smart young professor was pointing out
the benefits of hot water on the eyes of a young patient who
stood beside him He said, " You see, gentlemen, what a
benefit is derived from the application of hot water. We
ordered this girl to bathe her eyes with hot water, and a great
improvement is the result." The girl looked up and said,
" Sir, it was cold water you told me to use, and I used it."
The professor's face shone like the head appendage of a
Spanish rooster. In addition to what we have already said
and given as remedies, an excellent eye-wash is composed of
one grain of sulphate of hydrastis to one ounce of distilled or
rain water. We have seen a severe inflammation subdued in
a day with a lotion of one grain corrosive sublimate to four
ounces of water. Old chronic cases are greatly benefited by
causing a fresh or acute inflammation. The eye is painted
with an infusion of jequerity-bean, three to five per cent ; that
is, 100 parts of water, three to five parts of the bruised beans.
One bathing is sufficient to light up an inflammation which

will last three or four days, but in subsiding will leave the eyes
in a better condition. Dr. Coffin's plan, 50 years ago, was
similar, but more barbarous, namely, to blow a little cayenne
into them : it did good in the same way as the other. As a
simple astringent wash, the sulphate of zinc, two to four
grains to the ounce, will make a very good one. As the eye
is subject to various diseases, it is next to impossible to deal
with them all in a work like ours.

INFLAMMATION OF THE THROAT (Quinsy).

This is a complaint to which some young people are
subject. The causes are colds brought on by damp feet or
exposure of some kind. The symptoms are manifest ; pain,
swelling of the throat, which appears congested. It usually
leads to suppuration and breaks, discharging a quantity of
matter. When the trouble is detected, or symptoms point to
it, no time should be lost in taking a course of medicine.
After the course put on the

Quinsy Embrocation.

Carbonate of Ammonia .... Quarter ounce.
Potato water .... One ounce.
Sugar of Lead .... One ounce.
Camphor .... Quarter ounce.
Saffron .... Thirty grains.
Spirits of Wine .... One ounce.

Dissolve the camphor in the spirits.

Mix the others, warm a little, dip a piece of flannel in it, and
put it in front of the throat ; cover it, and renew when dry.
Use the anti-febrile and inflammatory gargle (page 211), and
drink a decoction of bitters.

PUTRID SORE THROAT (Cynanche Maligna).

Putrid sore throat comes on with cold, shivering, nausea,
vomiting, restlessness, thirst, debility, fever, oppression of the
chest, flushed flace, red eyes, hoarseness of the voice, hurried
breathing, soreness of the throat, swelling of the tonsils, &c.
The treatment of this affection is similar to that recommended

for diphtheria (see page 306). The regular treatment in the
New York Ear and Throat Clinic is, tincture of iron 20 drops
three times a day in water. Here is a better mixture:

Tincture of Iron .... One ounce.
Glycerine.......... .... One ounce.
Tincture of Quassia .... One ounce.
Water .... Two ounces.

A teaspoonful three or four times a day. Dr. Coffin's
treatment is a strong decoction of horehound, barley bark,
ground ivy, agrimony, raspberry leaves; half ounce of each to
the pint; to which a teaspoonful of cayenne pepper is added.
Half wineglassful every two hours, a hot brick in the vinegar
cloth to the feet, and an opening pill, composed of rhubarb,
valerian, gum myrrh, and cayenne, equal parts, two for a dose.
If the disease advances he recommends an emetic followed
by an injection; the throat to be well steamed by inhaling
the steam of yarrow in infusion, and rubbed with the
stimulating liniment, composed of cayenne pepper and
common salt, of each a teaspoonful, and vinegar half a pint.

INFLAMMATION OF THE LINING OF THE CHEST
(PLEURISY).

This is a somewhat common ailment. The pleura is a
transparent membrane which lines the inner walls of the
chest and covers the lungs. In health this membrane secretes
a liquid which lubricates the surface, allowing the lungs to
play freely. This membrane is easily inflamed, and takes on
what is called a white heat inflammation. The causes of
pleurisy are similar to general inflammation: colds, sudden
stoppage of perspiration, wet clothes, exposure, and injuries
to the chest. Treatment: Our old song, some will say—give
a course of medicine; yes, and there is nothing better to
begin with. After the patient is in bed put on a poultice, the
compound mustard (page 234); apply as directed. Make a
medicine as follows:—

Pleurisy Root, in powder .... One ounce.
Lobelia............................. One drachm.
Composition .... One ounce.

Infuse in a quart ot boiling water, stir well, let it stand covered, by the fire, half an hour , pour off the clear, sweeten, keep warm and covered, and give a wineglassful every hour. Keep the hot brick and vinegar cloth to the feet, and relieve the bowels with the compound mandrake or leptandrum powders, or an injection   After the poultice has been on an hour or so, take it off and heat it over steam   If the pain is very great rub the chest with the compound anodyne or soothing liniment, then replace the poultice.   When the severe symptoms have passed give patient a convalescent medicine, No. 6, or if a tonic is needed make a decoction of—

Horehound .... One ounce
Vervain............................ One ounce.
Mullen .... One ounce.
Comfrey Root...................... One ounce.
Water .... One quart

Simmer the comfrey root 15 minutes, put in the others and simmer five minutes longer, cool, strain, and if preferred sweeten ; give a wineglassful three times a day.   After recovery it would be well to wear a chest protector, one that covers the back also   There is not much difference in the various forms of inflammatory chest diseases, so that the treatment above will do for all, at least in the acute form.   For any that may have passed into the chronic state, the various cough mixtures and medicines found in the formula and in our descriptions of the properties of the herbs—the expectorant class especially—can be tried.   As we promised some information as to the sounds in the chest in health and disease, we will now try and make the reader understand them.

SOUNDING THE CHEST.

To understand the different sounds of the chest the first thing is to get the healthy sounds well in the mind. Get a person in good health to practise upon. Let him be stripped to the waist : look at the chest—is it barrel-shaped or pigeon-breasted ? This condition is found in asthmatical people Look if both sides of the chest expand with the inspiration ; put a tape round in a line with the paps when the chest is empty take the measure when expanded with the deepest inspiration again measure—the average difference being 1½ inches—if 2 inches it is good, if only one the lungs are weak : if much less some trouble may be expected. This part of examination is called inspection, the next is palpation, feeling Not much can be learned by it in chest complaints. Still. if both palms are put on the chest, and the patient or person be asked to count 1, 2, 3, you will find the sound conveyed to the hand, this is called vocal fremitus In congestion of the lungs and pneumonia the sound will be very distinct, or as it is termed exaggerated The next proceeding is auscultation The ear or stethescope is placed on the chest between the ribs, and the healthy sound on the right side will be a breezy one, as if you were blowing gently into a handful of fine wire, on the left you will hear the heart's beat, which you will perceive is double, a sound somewhat similar to one produced by striking the heel of your hand first, then the point of the middle finger on the table The lower half of left side of chest is occupied in front by the heart, the upper part by lung tissues. In bronchitis there will be a wheezing, whistling sound on inspiration, and a blowing one on expiration ; this, accompanied with the cough, will generally determine it to a practised ear In pleurisy, if unaccompanied with any other disease, there will be the friction or dry rubbing sound, with feeble breathing sounds, from the inflamed condition of the pleura, and diminished motion of the chest. If adhesion of the pleura takes place, which it frequently does, these sounds will not be heard. In pneumonia, when advanced, the lung becomes like the liver, almost solid, so that little or no sounds come from the inflamed part. The bronchial breathing will be more manifest. In advanced consumption there will often be heard hollow sounds, between blowing and whistling, over certain parts; this denotes a cavity. If the patient whispers while the ear is over the place, the voice can be heard in it; when the disease is situated in the lower lobes, the sounds can be heard better at the sides and back. Percussion is the third method of diagnosing the chest complaints. To do it the forefinger of the left hand is laid on the chest, between the ribs, and tapped upon by the fore and middle finger of the right hand. In a state of health, the sound produced will be semi-hollow, or as the Scotch would say, boss. Tapping down the right side, when you come to the edge of the last rib, the sound will change to dull solid; this is over the liver. On the left side dulness will be found over the region of the heart; these sounds agree with those heard by auscultation, and are generally taken as confirmatory. In pleurisy it often happens that there is a secretion of water in the chest. Careful percussion will enable the height to be ascertained to which it has risen. This condition is called in simple language, dropsy of the chest. We might make this plainer if our space permitted us, but it is only practice that can enable any one to note with certainty the difference between the healthy and abnormal conditions of the chest.

INFLAMMATION OF THE LARYNX (LARYNGITIS).

This is not a very common trouble, but we have seen several fatal cases of it, that is, where it became eventually chronic and ended the life of the patient. It is known as consumption of the throat. When it is of a tubercular order and hereditary there is not much hope of a cure, alleviation, under these circumstances, is about all that can be expected.

CAUSES are such as are common to all inflammations with generally a few predisposing ones : mercurial druggings, tartar emetic, and some kinds of employment where there is much irritating dust.

SYMPTOMS.—The same as generally precede inflammation are present here. An uneasy feeling may be felt for one or two days followed with some fever, alternate fits of heat and cold. It is important to know these warning symptoms, as we need not wait to see where the inflammation is going to settle before we attempt to drive it out of the system. Our first step in meeting the intruder is the course as applied by Thompson. Very often there is no more of a trouble after this treatment has been adopted; if, however, acute laryngitis has been established, its symptoms are sufficiently plain. There is hoarseness, difficulty of swallowing, roughness and dryness of the throat, pain at the projection called Adam's apple, and more or less of troublesome cough. An examination will show the redness and swelling which are also present in the higher parts of the air passages. These symptoms may increase in severity even to a fatal termination. Presuming that the course of medicine has been taken and the patient in bed with the hot brick to the feet and the usual vinegar cloth, a poultice of slippery elm three parts, mustard one part, should be applied over the throat and renewed or warmed up when cool. Keep up the perspiration for three or four hours by giving an infusion of angelica herb, dry, one ounce to one pint of boiling water, with 10 grains of cayenne pepper; let it infuse 20 minutes by the fire, strain, sweeten with treacle, give every 15 minutes till it is all taken: after this let the underclothing and bed-clothes, if wet with perspiration, be changed; dry and warm those to be put on; see that this is done without exposing to cold.

CHRONIC LARYNGITIS.

It so happens that the most of the cases we meet with are of a chronic form, owing their existence principally to the neglect or maltreatment of acute throat troubles—cutting out the tonsils and the uvula, leeching, blistering, mercurial and other poisonous drugs. The symptoms are, more or less of an irritating cough, hoarseness, loss of voice, expectoration of tough mucus, at times tinged with blood; breath generally offensive, with a soreness in the part affected ; but this is not always felt.

TREATMENT : In this case we must do all in our power to assist nature to repair the injuries done to this delicate part of our body. Everything then of the remotest cause must be avoided. If caused by public speaking, this should be given up, especially if the speaker is in the habit of speaking in a high tone ; working at unhealthy occupations where mineral or even wood dust is inhaled, &c. If accustomed to shave, stop the practice ; let your beard grow sufficiently to cover the neck, which should be kept warm. Look to the condition of the digestive and other organs. If the constitution is not too low we would certainly recommend a course of medicine once a week. Use as a gargle—one part of tincture of bloodroot in seven of distilled or rain water. As it is not always possible to reach the part with a gargle, a bent camel's hair brush, made for the purpose, should be applied with the liquid to the place. A slippery elm poultice at bed-time, kept on all night, and kept warm, and an ointment rubbed in in the morning, prepared in this way—

Bloodroot, in fine powder .... Quarter ounce.
Vaseline........................ One ounce.
Lanoline........................ One ounce.
Lobelia .... Quarter ounce.
Powdered marigolds.............. Quarter ounce.

Rub well together on a slab, and rub in for five minutes gently, then cover the throat with a piece of flannel If the throat is irritable dissolve a piece of gum arabic in the mouth, or chew a bit of slippery elm bark or sassafras bark ; try them all ; keep the feet warm and dry.

MUMPS (PAROTITIS).

This trouble is usually a juvenile affection, consisting of a swelling of the glands surrounding or above the throat. It generally lasts about seven or eight days, then subsides In this case there is not much medication needed. Bathe the swellings in an infusion of bitter herbs ; feverfew is good.

Keep a hot flannel on the throat; give a dose of the compound mandrake if the bowels are not too open. It will be well to keep indoors, and if there are other children, keep them apart, as it is very infectious. It sometimes happens that the swelling will subside in the glands of the neck and appear in the breast or the testicles; in this case, it is affirmed by an American doctor of experience, that a mustard poultice put on the neck will bring it back to the neck if desirable. This, however, may be doubted; but it seldom happens, and when it does, judgment must be used as to what should be done. If the swelling should remain take the medicine used for scrofula (see index), and rub in an ointment composed of two parts of lard and one part of turpentine; rub together, apply by gentle rubbing to the swelling twice or three times a day, and attend to the general health.

INFLAMMATION OF THE HEART

May be either that of the pericardium, or sack in which the heart is inclosed, or the heart itself. The trouble is not a common one   When it does exist, it is generally the result of acute gonorrhœa or rheumatism. It may be induced by severe pain, such as results from burns. &c.

The symptoms are, severe darting pain, violent palpitation, feeling of oppression, faintness, difficult breathing, hiccough. If the disease advances, the symptoms become insupportable; breathing is difficult, a cold perspiration breaks over the body, and the patient sinks exhausted. The treatment must be prompt. See to the ventilation of the room, get the patient in the easiest position, so that he can breathe freely, keep the room quiet, and allow no unnecessary intrusion, quietness being indispensable; put a hot brick to the feet, and the compound mustard poultice over seat of pain. As a medicine prepare an infusion of—

Antispasmodic Powder .... Half ounce.
Motherwort......................... One ounce.
Sweet Bugle (Lycopœus Virginicus) .... One ounce.

Infuse in a quart of boiling water ; strain, sweeten with lump sugar, and give a tablespoonful every hour with one drop of tincture of veratrum. Attend to the bowels by giving a dose of compound powder of leptandrum. Let the food be light and nourishing. The digestive food is always of this class. There are other diseases of the heart which we will deal with further on.

INFLAMMATION OF THE STOMACH (GASTRITIS).

Any of the organs of digestion may become inflamed, and since the whole body is dependent for nourishment on the healthy performance of digestion, it need not be emphasised that the danger is great, and the utmost care in the treatment of inflammatory conditions of these organs of digestion should be exercised. First, and also the most important organ, the stomach claims our attention. Being an internal organ, it is not so much subject to dangers arising from exposure to colds, &c. ; therefore, it is not often the seat of inflammation, and if it had a fair and rational treatment at the mouth of its possessor, it is doubtful if it would be inflamed at all ; therefore the first cause may be put down as errors in eating, and especially drinking. Some poisons destroy life through causing the stomach to inflame. Like other inflammation, there are different degrees of it, from a slight attack to one that may prove fatal in 24 hours. Symptoms : Pain or uneasiness is first felt, which may increase to a burning severe pain, with constant nausea and vomiting ; it will increase by pressure. A strong desire for cold drinks, a deep inspiration by filling the chest and producing pressure will cause pain. The tongue is usually red, with sometimes a whitish fur in the middle. The bowels are constipated, unless some part of them (the mucous coat) is inflamed, which may cause a diarrhœa. The pulse is rapid with wiry feeling, skin hot and dry, breathing hurried, and the urine high coloured. The most comfortable position is the back, on which the patient lies with the legs drawn up. The depression of spirits and anxiety is great. If the treatment has not been prompt and

successful the disease advances the tongue becomes dry
and pale, the pulse feeble and threadlike, the body becomes
much emaciated. Delirium, hiccough, vomiting dark matter,
coldness of the feet and hands, may be regarded as fatal
symptoms; or a sudden cessation of pain, which has often
given false hopes to the patient's friends and an unskilful
doctor, is the sign that inflammation has had its most dreaded
termination—gangrene or mortification. Treatment : If it
has been caused by, or as it may follow the taking of poisons
(see antidotes), if the stomach is loaded with indigestible
food and any of the symptoms above felt, it should be relieved
at once by a good emetic, a teaspoonful of fluid extract of
lobelia or emetic powder; this followed by a cupful of
slippery elm gruel will prevent its progress and from becoming
chronic. A case happened some time ago of a young man in
Southland who died suddenly before medical aid reached him.
He had been out rabbiting, and coming to his hut hungry he
prepared one for supper, but did not cook it properly ; next
day he was found dead, and a post-mortem showed his
stomach was distended, inflamed, and mortifying. When the
stomach is not loaded and yet inflamed, nothing of an irritating
nature must be given either in medicine or food. Slippery
elm tea or a decoction of marshmallow root, with a little milk
and sugar to make it palatable, may be freely given. If the
patient can sit up give a vapour bath, put to bed and give an
injection as follows :

Slippery Elm powder .... A teaspoonful.
Coarse Brown Sugar................ Two ounces.
Mugwort Herb, dry .... Half ounce.

Infuse the herb in a pint of boiling water, let it stand till
blood-warm ; strain ; rub up the sugar and the elm powder
together, add a little of the infusion at a time so as to blend them
together into a smooth liquor ; inject gently into the bowels.
This is an important item in the treatment ; it soothes and
sustains. If the first portion is thrown out, give the rest ; put
on hot fomentations of the above herb with a teaspoonful of

cayenne to each pint ; keep the flannels hot by renewing with the hot infusion. If these do not lessen the pain apply the compound mustard poultice over the stomach or seat of pain. If the tongue is inflamed do not give an emetic, but the injection every six hours. To allay the vomiting, if it should continue, make an infusion of spearmint, half an ounce in a pint of boiling water, to which add a teaspoonful of bicarbonate of potash. Give a teaspoonful or two occasionally while the vomiting continues. For a daily medicine make a decoction of—

Slippery Elm Bark	One ounce.
Marshmallow Root...................	One ounce.
Sweet Flag Root	One ounce.
Raspberry Leaves	One ounce.
Dandelion Root	One ounce.

Simmer in three pints of water 15 minutes, strain, and give a wineglassful every two hours ; keep up the heat at the lower extremities and on the surface, and nature will do the curing. If the pain should be great, it would give the patient ease by giving a teaspoonful of the following mixture not oftener than every hour: Muriate of Morphia four grains and infusion of slippery elm four ounces. If the pulse is very quick, put in a drachm of the tincture of veratrum viride, or if not to be had four drachms of tincture of gelsemine. Let the food be of the lightest nature—barley water, whey, toasted bread dissolved in water, and milk, digestive food, chicken broth, &c., given about blood-warm.

CHRONIC INFLAMMATION

of the stomach must be treated more by diet than medicine ; light farinaceous food taken in moderate quantity. The digestive food, with plenty of milk, is one of the most soothing. If there is acidity take a tablespoonful of lime-water in half a cupful of milk three times a day ; this may be alternated with stomach bitters powder or stomach powder for indigestion ; or ten grains of golden seal ; take after meals ; look after the general health, and take three to four courses of medicine. To put a compound galbanum plaster over the stomach is recommended by men of experience ; it cannot do harm but will soothe and protect, at least in some measure.

INFLAMMATION OF THE LIVER (HEPATITIS)

It is generally supposed that the liver is more subject to disease than the other organs. Some medical men are in the habit of putting down to the liver any derangement which they cannot fully understand. In Coffin's Botanic Guide to Health he gives an illustration of this in the parting charge of an old doctor to one of his pupils who was starting out in practice. You will meet with many cases, said he, that will perplex you, on account of their obscurity. You can call them liver complaint, and prescribe mercury ; and in treating children the same doubtful cases will trouble you. You can call their ailment worms, and give them mercury. So it happens that hundreds die of supposed liver complaint ; yet when post-mortem examinations are held, the liver is found to be the most healthy organ in the body. Formerly the true cause of most of these supposed liver complaints was the mercurial drugging so largely practised. Still, like every part and organ, it may become inflamed from the usual causes—cold, intemperance, blows over the region, intense heat, high living, &c. Symptoms : It commences with a chill, followed by more or less of a fever, a pricking pain on right side, which may extend up the back to the right shoulder. When very severe there will be difficulty of breathing and pain on coughing, as the diaphragm presses on the liver. Sometimes the whites of the eyes are tinged with yellow, there is a bitter taste in the mouth, the tongue is coated brown or yellow, loss of appetite, urine high coloured, depression, &c.

Treatment : When the tongue is heavily coated, give the vapour bath and an emetic, one drachm fluid extract of lobelia in a half pint of decoction of dandelion. If the bowels have been costive, it will be well to relieve them with an injection of warm water, into a pint of which put a teaspoonful of tincture

of lobelia. Put the compound mustard plaster over the seat
of pain, and make a decoction of the following :—

Leptandrum or Black Root.............. One ounce.
Dandelion .... Two ounces.
Liverwort .... One ounce.
Juniper Berries...................... One ounce.
Capiscums.......................... One drachm.

Bruise the roots and simmer in three pints half an hour; then put
in the other, let them stay five minutes longer, strain off, cool,
and give a wineglassful every two hours till the bowels move
two or three times a day ; then regulate the dose accordingly.
The above mixture may be changed for the hepatic powder,
and, if needed, the liver pills When the severer symptoms
are subdued, a light nourishing diet, the dandelion coffee, pure,
will be much better as a diet drink than tea or the ordinary
coffee.

INFLAMMATION OF THE BOWELS (ENTERITIS).

This, like that of the stomach, is a very dangerous and even
more painful form. To understand it aright it is necessary to
briefly consider the anatomy of the intestines The smaller,
which is the longest portion of the alimentary canal, is a
tube about an inch in diameter, composed of three coats It
is coiled up in the abdomen When it is in a high state of
inflammation the walls swell to such an extent that the tube
is closed, and as post-mortem examinations prove, it may
become in some of its parts more like a tumour than intestine.
This fact will prove the fallacy of the usual treatment,
which nearly always results in death to the patient
in from one to four days. Symptoms: It is usually
ushered in by a chill which lasts some time, followed
by severe pain in the abdomen ; shooting and cutting
round the region of the navel, obstinate costiveness, the
bowels being closed up, urine high coloured, pulse rapid
and contracted, and an intense desire to move the bowels.
The patient usually cries for this, and herein is the cause of
the irrational and often fatal treatment of giving purgatives.

We heard a lecture on this subject from Professor Whitford of Chicago Eclectic Medical College, in which he gave his experience of many cases he witnessed treated and killed by this purging process, especially when calomel (a preparation of mercury), was the agent used. One case was a young man who had two old doctors. The first one gave ten grains of this poison which had no effect on him, unless to cause more irritation; this was doubled in a short time. The other doctor called to consult approved of the treatment; another dose was given, they being determined to get a passage; they succeeded in getting one, but it was just under the ribs, causing speedy death. Another case, Whitford was called to consult on with a young man fresh from one of the leading allopathic colleges. When he saw the patient and learned the fact that he had given him an irritant cathartic, he took him into the next room and told him he had killed the patient, which time soon proved true. He also informed us of another doctor who had four cases, all of which died, and in every one case the purging treatment had been used. The professor had been called too late to prevent this, and did not think it then prudent to tell the doctor, as he was coming to graduate at the Eclectic College. After hearing the above lecture he followed the old professor to his room and said, " Professor, why did you not tell me I had murdered those four men ?" Another interesting case mentioned was that of two lawyers, leading men in the city, who lived near each other, were friends, and strange to say were both taken about the same time with inflammation of the intestines. The first one had two of the leading allopathics, who treated him by trying to get his bowels to move. The other sent for Professor Whitford who found him suffering intense pain and calling for something to move his bowels. It took him, he said, half an hour to convince him that it was almost certain death to give him a cathartic. He told him that if he would follow his instructions faithfully he had no doubt but that he would be able to be at the funeral of his friend, whom the doctors were physicking and would surely kill. His patient consented to his treatment, and although not able to attend the funeral or the other, yet he saw the mournful procession from the window of his house. The causes of enteritis are exposure of the abdomen to colds, stricture of the bowels, violent blows, eating unripe fruit, wounds, chronic constipation, and irritating, purging agents. Treatment : Put a hot brick, rolled in a vinegar cloth, to the feet, rub over the abdomen with a mixture of turpentine and oil equal parts, then apply a hot poultice of linseed meal or slippery elm, or both combined (or hot herbal poultice as recommended in diphtheria, page 307), mixed with an infusion of poppy leaves or capsules. Do not give any opening medicine until the inflammation has susided, which will be in from two to four days, when they will usually relax themselves. To relieve the intense pain and fever symptoms the professor abovementioned recommends two drops of tincture of aconite with the 18th of a grain of morphia in half a wineglass infusion of peach-tree bark every hour, till pain and vomiting are subdued. As morphia and aconite are dangerous drugs, the utmost care must be taken in their administration. The mixture should be prepared thus :—Get the peach bark, infuse one ounce in a pint of boiling water, when cool, strain, and add a teaspoonful of the following to every tablespoonful dose of the infusion of the peach :—

Tincture of Aconite................ One drachm.
Muriate of Morphia................ Three grains.
Water .... Four ounces.

Mix. Dose, a teaspoonful every one, two, or four hours in the infusion. When the inflammatory symptoms are gone, use the digestive food, brown bread, milk, and other light food. (See convalescent foods and drinks, index.)

PERITONITIS.

This inflammation differs little from the former ; it is sometimes present with it. The peritoneum is the inner lining of the abdomen ; also the covering of nearly all the internal organs. It is a very delicate membrane, and is subject to intense inflammation. The symptoms are very similar ; treat in the same manner. If the poultice does not give the desired relief, make a strong infusion of cayenne, and foment for half an hour : then bind a cloth saturated with it over the part. If objection is made to the morphia and aconite mixture, make a decoction same as in inflammation of the stomach. Give the diaphoretic powder, and, if needed, a slippery elm injection with a half teaspoonful of laudanum in it.

INFLAMMATION OF THE SPLEEN

Resembles that of the liver, but the pain is on the left side. Treat in the same way outwardly. If it is chronic, a medicine may be prepared of the following :—

Spleenwort	Two ounces.
Liverwort	One ounce.
Dandelion	One ounce.
Bog-bean	One ounce.

Simmer ten minutes in a quart of boiling water, take a wine-glassful three times a day : the liver pills when required. A porous plaster may be put over the left side, well towards the back. In the acute stage, if the compound mustard plaster does not take effect, use pure mustard.

INFLAMMATION OF THE KIDNEYS (NEPHRITIS).

The kidneys are probably more subject to inflammation than any of the other organs. It is known by the following symptoms :—Pain in the back above the hip bones, shooting down towards the bladder, urine high coloured, diminished in quantity. There is usually a numbness of the thighs and surrounding parts. This inflammation, if neglected or improperly treated, is apt to leave a chronic affection behind, which will sap the foundations of life, causing dropsy, Bright's disease, &c. Its causes are, hard drinking of malt or spirituous liquors, sudden chills while in a state of perspiration, falls on the back, riding, jumping, retention of urine, gravel, gouty, and rheumatic tendency, taking cantharides, turpentine, &c., &c.

It generally begins with alternate fits of heat and cold, fever, hot dry skin, fainting, weakness. If it is not met and successfully treated, bloody urine may be passed, and even pus, when some portions of the kidneys suppurate (the usual division, acute and chronic). The object of our treatment is to subdue the inflammation and prevent the suppurative process. First, we must try and find out the cause and remove it. That done, we must look to the nursing, and the ventilation of the room. The reader will remember our advice against the common practice of giving strong diuretics while the acute symptoms last. The kidneys must have rest. If the patient is strong enough the course of medicine will be safe. If, however, the symptoms are too far advanced, give a medicated bath, prepared thus :—Infuse three and a half ounces of marshmallow leaves in a gallon of boiling water ; cover, let it stand till cold enough, then let the patient stand in it while he is sponged all over for five minutes ; rub dry, and inject into the bowels the slippery elm injection, let it be retained as long as possible. This done, put on the compound slippery elm poultice, and give a drink of the elm gruel, a teaspoonful of the powder to the half pint. Keep the hot brick to the feet ; give a wineglassful of the infusion of jaborandi leaves every hour, or sufficient to keep up perspiration. As a diet, the digestive food should be given freely. As the inflammatory symptoms subside, lessen the dose of the jaborandi, and prepare a decoction of the following :—

Dandelion Roots	Two ounces.
Tansy	One ounce.
Kidneywort	One ounce.
Marshmallow Roots	One ounce.

Bruise and simmer the roots in three pints of water 20 minutes, then add the herbs, simmer five minutes more, strain hot on two ounces of gum arabic, give a wineglassful from four to six times a day. If vomiting (which is sometimes present) should occur, give the mint tea with a teaspoonful of the bicarbonate of potash to the half pint, a tablespoonful every hour while required. If the trouble should become chronic, the decoction must be continued, the back rubbed with the tincture of cayenne or the anodyne liniment, or a compound cayenne plaster put over it. As a change with the decoction, see diuretics; try them and persevere.

INFLAMMATION OF THE BLADDER

Is known by burning pains felt in the lower part of the abdomen, and around the region of the bladder. There is a great difficulty in voiding the urine, although there is at the same time a constant desire, accompanied generally with a desire to go to stool The water is of a thick red colour, and comes away in drops, with intense pain, at times tinged with blood. When the disease is neglected or improperly treated, it often leads to very serious results. We have known it produce ulceration, stranguary, and chronic inflammation of the parts. In treating it, much will depend upon the strength of the patient and the stage of the disease It has been removed in the early stage by simply applying flannels as hot as they can be borne, wrung out of a strong decoction of marshmallows, and the same given internally with buchu and composition freely, until perspiration began. Keep up this treatment till the pain is relieved. If it persists, give an injection of slippery elm and the same decoction as in the former case—the digestive food and a light and nourishing diet The ulmaria wine may be taken during convalescence. As an aperient medicine the dandelion pills will answer.

FEVERS

May be said to be a diffused inflammatory process over the system. Of the many theories which have been put forward to account for the fever condition, the most reasonable and concise is that it is an effort of nature to throw off poisons from the body. Our space being very limited we have no room for theorising further upon this diseased condition. There are certain symptoms that are common to all fevers: lassitude, weakness of the muscles, with an expression of inward distress, aversion to action either of mind or body, chilliness. These may be called induction signs of fevers in general, which are usually succeeded by alternate chills and heat, restlessness, a sensation of soreness, flushing of the face, dryness of the skin, which is hot to the touch; the pulse is quickened, with headaches and wandering of the mind. These symptoms clearly indicate that fever is present and should be attended to at once, as in most fevers nature needs assistance to throw them off. Causes of fevers are divided into three; first, the remote, which may be said to include every departure from the laws of health; which predisposes the system to disease; the intermittent extremes of heat and cold, marsh damp, vegetable and animal effluvia. Intermediate causes: A morbid condition of the stomach and bowels, and obstruction to the circulation of the fluids. The proximate or exciting causes are, violent exercise, infection, poisonous matter in the blood, that excites the heart to an unnatural speed, which, unless checked, would soon exhaust the system. The indication for treatment in all fevers is to open the pores of the skin, clear the intestines, cleanse the stomach and the kidneys. Our readers, we think, know by this time how to do this. The Thompsonian course cannot be excelled for this purpose; if taken in time, it often, so to speak, sends the fever about its business; but while this is applicable to all fevers, there are special features in each variety of fever that may need peculiar treatment. Again we would ask our readers who can spare the time to read up the herbs and you will find several of them good for fevers which may be used if any of those now prescribed do not seem to be meeting the case.

SIMPLE FEVER

Is a condition which is sometimes found without any other symptoms. There is a quickened pulse, with a slightly raised temperature, especially at night. This may be regarded as a warning which, if neglected, may develop into something worse. Our treatment for this is simply a course of medicine and a few doses of fever powder, with the stomach bitters through the day and the liver or dandelion pills, if needful, is all that is likely to be required.

INTERMITTENT FEVER OR AGUE.

This fever is prevalent in low marshy districts during wet weather. It is called intermittent because of its regularly leaving and returning at stated times, sometimes every day, or every second, third, or fourth day. The paroxysms consist of three stages—first, a hot fit, then a cold shaking fit, and lastly a sweating fit. Treatment: If the system is strong we would recommend a Thompsonian course of medicine twice a week, or in its absence the hot brick and vinegar cloth and the fever powder. As a daily medicine make up a decoction of the following :—

Peruvian Bark...................... One ounce.
Virginia Snakeroot................. Half ounce.
Pennyroyal .... One ounce.

Simmer the roots in one quart of water for 15 minutes; take off the fire, put in the herb with one ounce diuretic powder ; stir, let cool, strain, and take a wineglassful four to six times a day, according to severity of case. Before the cold stage is expected a cupful of composition tea ought to be taken. While we are confident that the above treatment will cure, we know also that other mixtures do it. They may be preferred and possibly suit better in some cases. The following two are from a standard author. Take—

Salicin.......................... Twenty grains.
Hydrastis .... Twenty grains.
Cayenne........................ Ten grains.

Mix and divide into twenty powders, and give one three times a day. This rarely fails to meet the severer cases ; or take—

Quinine .... Twenty grains.
Eupatorium .... Twenty grains.
Cayenne .... Ten grains.

Divide and take same as former.

BILIOUS OR REMITTENT FEVER.

Bilious fever is found to prevail in most low marshy districts during the latter end of summer after heavy rains. The symptoms are, pains in the back, slight cough, restlessnes, sallow countenance, eyes yellow, mouth dry and parched, with bitter taste. In this case it seems the liver is at fault, as there is often felt oppression in the region of it ; and the bile in the blood, indicated by the colour of the patient, shows the principal seat of the trouble to be located in that organ. The symptoms by which it is ushered in are like those of the preceding. The chief points of difference are in the appearance of the skin and the continuance of the fever state, which while it remits in its severity at some time in the day, does not leave the patient free at any time during its continuance. It commences with langour, drowsiness, yellow tinge in the skin, bitter taste in the mouth, headache, fever, thirst, sometimes vomiting of bile. As a rule there is constipation, the tongue is often coated with a light brown colour, there is also oppression of the breath, and in severe cases delirium, the stools are very unnatural in colour and offensive. The cause of this fever, in addition to the climatic, are, bilious temperament, weakness of the stomach, which cannot digest fats, intemperance, in both eating and drinking.

TREATMENT.—Samuel Thompson never failed to cure this fever by his course of medicine. If you look up his poetical directions you will see a specific for it. It is generally thought that it must run a certain course in spite of any treatment. We are positive this is not true. We can produce living testimony to prove our statement that it can be cured in three days. Here is a case in point. A Mr. Glass sent for us to see him. We found him with the well-marked symptoms of this fever; gave him a vapour bath, and left him the lobelia emetic to take. We called on the following evening, and were surprised when the person himself opened the door to us. We asked him what became of the fever? He replied that it went away with the emetic. We need not give any other treatment. After the course of medicine the stomach bitters will complete the cure; but should the patient or his friends not like this treatment, thinking it too severe, then begin with a purge of the compound mandrake powder; put the hot stone to the feet, and an hour or so after the physic has been taken begin with the fever powder. When the fever is at its height, sponge the body over with an alkaline bath. It can be done in bed if the patient is too weak. The assistant nurse can hold up the blankets while the sponge is being applied to one side of the the body and then to the other. Make a medicine thus—

Bogbean .... One ounce.
Agrimony............................ One ounce.
Clivers .... One ounce.
Raspberry Leaves .... One ounce.

Infuse in a quart of boiling water; strain, and give a wineglass-ful every two hours. If the bowels are costive, give the antibilious powder in sufficient doses to keep them open ; as a cooling drink, an infusion of balm in a decoction of slippery elm bark, boil an ounce in three pints of water 30 minutes. When you take it off the fire, put in an ounce of balm ; strain, sweeten with white sugar, and give as much as the patient desires. The balm wine, the hepatic or curative powder may be given in change. When convalescent give light food. If desired the quinine mixture—given for intermittent fever—might be taken instead of or in alternation with the infusion.

YELLOW FEVER

Is but an aggravated form of bilious fever. Treatment and medicine the same.

SLOW OR NERVOUS FEVER.

This kind generally attacks people of a relaxed and debilitated constitution, and has its origin in the digestive organs, which fail to nourish the system. It is ushered in by indisposition for a day or two, generally after some great excitement, but it sometimes comes on so slowly that its immediate cause cannot be traced. There is depression of spirits, want of appetite, weariness, chills, flushings, heat in the hands and soles of the feet, and coldness in other parts of the body. As night advances the symptoms increase till the fever is well marked. As this is a condition generally accompanied by weakness, our treatment must be to strengthen the patient and allay the nervous irritation. The first thing to be done is to allay the fever; for this purpose put patient to bed in a warm, well ventilated room with a hot bottle or stone to the feet. Make the following infusion :—

      Skullcap .... One ounce.
      Valerian, in coarse powder .... One ounce.
      Fever Powder .... One ounce.

Steep in a quart of boiling water thirty minutes, strain sweeten, and give a wineglassful every hour during the height of the fever till the pores open and the temperature falls. As a daily medicine the spiced bitters will be found an excellent tonic. Should the fever be persistent, and if the foregoing treatment fails after a week's trial, give the quinine and the hydrastis as in intermittent; look well to the stomach and bowels, also the kidneys, and use suitable medicine to remove obstructions. Perhaps some reader will ask us, Where is the course of medicine, is it not indicated in this form of fevers ? Not if the sufferer is in a feeble state of health; if there is ordinary strength it will be beneficial. The fever powder and the hot stone will answer the purpose. If the tongue is coated, the lobelia emetic is indicated, and may be taken

through the lobelia pills, where it is not desirable to excite
the system too much. If our thoughtful readers have followed
us (as we would like them to so far in our work), they will see
that we are not tied down to a few things So to speak, the
whole list of herbalism is before us, and if that is not
enough the regular medicine list is at hand Use your
judgment till a suitable medicine to meet all ordinary
indications is found. Nervines, tonics, and sudorifics are
the medicines required in fevers of a nervous kind.

TYPHUS FEVER

May be classed under the heads of putrid, malignant, or
spotted, &c. It commences with loss of appetite, restlessness,
giddiness in the head, depression of spirits, heats and chills,
with frequent vomiting; bowels generally confined, although
diarrhœa sometimes accompanies it. There is often a cough,
red and watery eyes, with bleeding at the nose, and difficulty
of swallowing. As the disease advances, red spots appear on
the abdomen, with loss of blood from the mouth and bowels:
the memory becomes imperfect, delirium sets in, followed by
great prostration, a black crust covers the lips, teeth, and
tongue; the stools become watery and oppressive; the fatal
symptoms are when the patient becomes lost in a dull stupor;
a twitching of the lips, eyelids, jaws, and hands, may be
noticed, followed by low murmurings, hiccough, catching at,
imaginary objects, and finally death. From the above symptoms it will be seen how grave a form of fever this it. The
causes of it are bad sanitation, keeping on wet clothes, lying
in damp beds, wet feet, blood poisoning, &c. As before
stated, we should not wait to see a full development of the
disease. It is a blessing that we have got in the course of
medicine a means of preventing the development of this and
other fevers of the most dangerous kinds. Steam, it may be said, is
the greatest physical power in the world, and in curing disease,
especially fever, its power is hardly known; it is superior to
warm baths, as it seems to persuade the pores of the skin to
open and let out the poisonous matters, which is one of the

exciting causes in fevers. Therefore, we say begin with a course of medicine. Let the room be well ventilated with a current of air in it, so as it does not come in immediate contact with the patient. If the weather is cold, let a fire be kindled, as this will help the ventilation ; a hot stone or brick to the feet, and small doses of fever powder, to keep up the perspiration for four to six hours ; the digestive food to be given at intervals as the stomach can bear it. As a medicine to give in alternation with the fever powders (which ought to be discontinued when the fever abates), take—

Wild Indigo Root .... One ounce.
Peruvian Bark .... One ounce.
Wood Betony .... One ounce.
Vervain............................ One ounce.
Rasp Leaves....................... One ounce.

Simmer the root and bark in three pints of water for 30 minutes ; stir in the herbs and leaves; let it stand covered till cold ; strain, and give a wineglassful three times a day, and a dose of the fever powder three times a day; every two hours give the one or the other; to relieve the bowels give an injection of—

Slippery Elm .... One teaspoonful.
Gum Myrrh .... Half a teaspooful.
Raspberry Leaf Tea .... Half a pint.
Brown Sugar..................... Two teaspoonfuls.

Blend the elm and the sugar together with the powdered myrrh, add a little at a time till it is smooth and blood-warm ; inject it into the bowels gently and keep it in as long as possible. Let the patient drink freely of raspberry leaf and slippery elm tea, or if not, cold water. Change the sheets, and clothing daily ; see that they are warm and dry when put on. Let the passages of the bowels be removed at once. Keep young children out of the room. It is well to get a practical nurse, if not, an elderly person who has been accustomed to the care of the sick. If there is a black crust on the teeth and tongue, wash with an infusion of gum myrrh and raspberry leaves made hot with a little cayenne, or weak solution of Condy's fluid. Support the strength of the patient while the medicine and treatment are driving out the disease ; and in nearly every case when the directions above are carried out, a cure will be the reward.

There is a simple remedy for fever of a putrid form like the above in its severest type, that is yeast. Dr. Fox in his admirable book " The Working Man's Model Botanic Guide to Health," quotes out this remedy at length, which, on account of its importance, we present to our readers.

" During my residence at Brampton, near Chesterfield," writes Dr. Cartwright, " a putrid fever broke out amongst us. Finding by far the greater number of my parishioners too poor to afford themselves medical assistance, I undertook, by the help of such books on the subject of medicine as were in my possession, to prescribe for them. I attended a boy about fourteen years of age, who was attacked by the fever. He had not been ill many days before the symptoms were unequivocally putrid. I then administered bark, wine, and such other medicines as my books directed. My exertions were, however, of no avail ; his disorder grew every day more and more untractable and malignant, so that I was in hourly expectation of his dissolution. Being under the necessity of taking a journey, before I set off I went to see him, as I thought for the last time ; and I prepared his parents for the event of his death, which I considered as inevitable, and reconciled them in the best manner I could to a loss which I knew they would feel severely. While I was in conversation on this distressing subject with his mother, I observed, in the corner of a room, a small tub of wort working. The sight brought to my recollection an experiment I had somewhere met with, of a piece of putrid meat being made sweet by being suspended over a tub of wort in the act of fermentation. The idea flashed into my mind that the *yeast* might correct the putrid nature of the disease, and I instantly gave him two large spoonfuls. I then told the mother, if she found her son

better, to repeat the dose every two hours. I then
set out on my journey. Upon my return, after a few days,
I anxiously inquired after the boy, and was informed that he
was recovered. I could not repress my curiosity, and though
greatly fatigued with my journey, and night was come on, I went
directly to his residence, which was three miles off, in a
wild part of the moors, and to my great surprise, the boy
himself opened the door, looking well, and he told me he had
felt better from the time he took the yeast.

"After I left Brampton, I lived in Leicestershire. My
parishioners there being few and opulent, I dropped the
medical character entirely, and would not prescribe even for
my own family. One of my domestics falling ill, the apothecary was sent for. Having great reliance on the apothecary's
skill and judgment, the man was left entirely to his management. His disorder, however, kept gaining ground, and the
apothecary, finding himself baffled in every attempt to be of
service to him, told me he considered it to be a lost case,
and in his opinion the man could not live twenty-four hours.
On this I determined to try the effects of yeast. I gave him
two large spoonfuls, and in fifteen minutes from taking the
yeast, his pulse, though still feeble, began to get composed
and to fall. In thirty-two minutes from his taking it he was
able to get up from his bed. The expression that he made
use of to describe the effect of his own feelings was, that he
felt 'quite lightsome.' At the expiration of the second hour
I gave him sago, ginger, &c., and in another hour repeated
the yeast. An hour afterwards I gave the bark, as before ; at
the next hour he had food, and an hour after that another
dose of yeast. He continued to recover, and was soon able
to go about his work as usual.

"About a year after this, as I was riding past a detached
farm house at the outskirts of the village, I observed the
farmer's daughter standing at the door, apparently in great
affliction. On inquiring into the cause of her distress, she
told me her father was dying. I went into the house and

found him in the last stage of putrid fever. His tongue was black, his pulse was scarcely perceptible, and he lay stretched out like a corpse, in a state of drowsy insensibility. I immediately procured some yeast, which I diluted with water and poured down his throat. I then left him with little hope of his recovery. I returned to him in about two hours, and found him sensible and able to converse. I then gave him a dose of bark. He afterwards took, at proper intervals, some refreshment. I stayed with him till he repeated the yeast, and then left him with directions how to proceed. I called upon him the next morning at nine o'clock, and found him apparently recovered. He was an old man, upwards of seventy." (See also our New Zealand Remedy, page 52.)

TYPHOID FEVER.

There are not many outside the ranks of the profession that can tell the difference between this form of fever and the former. Putting it in as few words as possible we may first point out their similarity. They are both continuing fevers, both dangerous. Typhus is characterised by great prostration and a general dusky mottled rash without a definite affection of the bowels. Typhoid is characterised by the appearance of rose-coloured spots, chiefly on the abdomen, with a specific lesion or ulceration of the bowels ; the one may run into the other. They are both caused by distinct animal or vegetable poisons, or both combined. Typhoid is more common to the young than the advanced in life, also more prevalent in autumn, or as the Americans say, the fall. As this form of fever is the most common and the most to be dreaded in the colonies, our readers will excuse us for dwelling upon it at some length. Some writers speak of a predisposing cause resulting from an earlier affection of the mesenteric glands ; but while that may be so, it is evident that many are attacked who have passed through life without any ailment of the kind. There can be no doubt that the exciting cause is the poisonous effluvia of decaying animal and vegetable matter. Dr. Murchison in his book, "The Continued Fever of Great

Britain," cites the following cases: (1st.) 20 out of 22 boys at
a certain school were seized with fever, accompanied by
gastro-intestinal irritation. Two of the fatal cases were
examined, and the usual lesion of Peyers' glands—(these glands
of the intestines were first discovered by an anatomist named
Peyers)—was discovered. The cause was attributed to the
opening two days before of a drain at the back of a house
which had been choked up for many years, and the
distribution of its offensive contents over a garden adjoining
the play-ground of the boys. (2nd.) In 1835 an epidemic of
enteric (typhoid) fever desolated the district of Auvergne,
nearly half of the inhabitants were affected and about one
third died. The cause was traced to a stagnant pool which
was a receptacle for dead animals and the sewerage of the
district. Three times did the pestilence return, and each time
the wind was blowing over the affected water   (3rd.) All the
residents in a farm-house in Peebles, 15 in number, were
seized with a fever accompanied with so much gastro-intestinal trouble that suspicions of poisoning were entertained
Three of them died   The only explanation of the outbreak
was that all the drains in the vicinity of the house were
choked up and obstructed with the accumulation of filth from
privies and the farm-yard   In these cases we have a clear
evidence of the origin of the disease It is a matter of
dispute as to its being infectious from person to person, the
opinion is, however, almost unanimous now that it is   Some
affirm that it is caused by alvine discharges of typhoid
patients. About five years ago a terrible visitation swept
away thousands in and around Plymouth (America) The
cause was traced to an infected person whose secretions
found their way into the small river which supplies the district.
It is well to know these things, as we see how to prevent those
terrible visitations. The symptoms of typhoid fever are not
so plain at the commencement as to make it certain even to
the experienced, the incubation stage of most fevers being
much alike ; we may be guided by the fact of its prevalence
(where it is so). Look well to the sanitary conditions present

give a treatment suitable to the symptoms, and wait. Hooper, a great authority on pathology, that is, describing diseases, says : "Great muscular prostration and early head symptoms. with depression of the senses and mental faculties, mark the onset of typhus, whilst symptoms more or less obscure of gastro-intestinal disturbance indicate the presence of enteric-typhoid fever ; but sickness and diarrhœa may be absent. Even head symptoms may be present from the first of the disease. Although the diagnosis may be difficult at first, yet it is no longer so when the disease has advanced. Tender-ness about the navel and lower right side. with a thickly coated aphthous tongue may inform us that the disease is typhoid and not typhus. The stools are light ochre-coloured, and the eruption appearing on the abdomen make it pretty certain. As the disease advances the tongue and lips crack and are more or less covered with little ulcers. If the fever is protracted these spread over the mucous membrane of the throat, but the virulence of the disease spends its force upon those glands of the intestines called Peyer's patches, situated on the lower portion of the ilium These inflame and ulcerate : all post-mortems demonstrate this It may be interesting to give the average ages of liability. The mean age of 1772 cases admitted into the Fever Hospital. London, during ten years was as follows One half were between 15 and 25 : one fifth under 15, less than one seventh were above 30, and less than one sixtieth exceeded 50 The mortality, which is not given, sometimes is very great, the approximation is one third. There is one peculiar fact, that typhoid is more prevalent among the rich and fortunate than the poor in proportion to their numbers Carrying the distinction of these two forms of fever to a fatal end we find that in typhus it is generally preceded by deep sleep. torpor, or coma, about the fourteenth day, while typhoid, by extreme debility about the fourth week, This is the rule, the exceptions are many.

TREATMENT —On account of the want of success in treating this disease in the past, some doctors have affirmed that there is no treatment for it; yet these same gentlemen have prescribed their drugs, made their visits, and got their fees. The students in colleges were told that as there is no recognised treatment, everyone must treat it according to his liking. This advice may be very good for experienced practitioners, but to give it to young students is to carry out the figure of a Dr. Amblert, who likened the doctor going into the sick-room blindfolded, armed with a club. He meant to strike the disease, but too often struck and killed the patient. Mineral drugs are no use here, but we are thankful that the Botanic Materia Medica contains many agents that have been proved efficacious.

What are the indications for treatment? Remove the poison through the outlets, the skin, stomach, bowels, kidneys, and lungs. Some of our medical critics may say, What has the stomach got to do with it? We reply, it is the centre of sympathies, and in treating it we treat all the system. See that hygienic measures are carried out; good fresh air to breathe, as well as cleanliness, is absolutely needful. Begin with, if the symptoms are not too far advanced, a course of medicine, if too weak, the medicated foot bath. (See index.) Give an injection of digestive food every day. As a drink give freely of raspberry leaf and slippery elm tea. Make a medicine as follows :—

Cranesbill Root	One ounce.
Stillingia Root	One ounce.
Black Root	Half ounce.
Wild Indigo Root	Half ounce.
Ginger	Half ounce.

Simmer in three pints of water half an hour; strain, and give a wineglassful four times a day. If the bowels are not sufficiently relaxed, give the compound leptandrum powder. A light slippery elm poultice may be put on the abdomen. Prepare the emetic after the bath thus—

Bayberry, in powder .... One drachm.
Ginger. in powder .... 20 grains.
Lobelia Herb and Seed, in powder,
    mixed .... Half a drachm.

It will be well to weigh them. Infuse in a pint of boiling water; stir, let it cool, sweeten with lump sugar, and give in wineglassfuul doses every ten minutes Vomiting may commence before it is all taken. Persevere, however, give the rest, it will do good. Careful nursing, with the above treatment, and a light fever diet (see index) food for the sick. This with the blessing of God. will cure or lessen the mortality that has hitherto prevailed in typhoid fever. If the skin is dry and hot, give the fever powder in sufficient doses to correct it.

DISEASES OF DIGESTION, &c.
INDIGESTION OR DYSPEPSIA

Is one of the most common troubles of civilised life. There are few people who have reached maturity but have felt at least some of the symptoms of it. Why is it so common ? The answer is simply, we do not live according to nature. If we did so, we should not be troubled with dyspepsia. The causes of indigestion are many. Hereditary transmission—this is a law of nature which is more or less demonstrated everywhere. Parents with weak stomachs have children similarly affected, or at least disposed to be so; but personal indulgence is by far the most common cause. Eating unwholesome food, or too much even of wholesome, late suppers, want of exercise, drinking spirits and liquors otherwise than to quench the natural thirst, too much indulgence in tea, and especially smoking narcotic tobacco, and last, but not least, mineral drugging. These are the principal causes of this trouble. The symptoms are many : Want of appetite, uneasy feeling in the region of the stomach, belchings of wind, eructations of food, sallowness of skin, heart-burn, headache, constipation, &c. Treatment: First, self-denial—that is abandon every habit that you think or suspect is a cause. If you are living on too rich a diet, simplify it; use brown bread, not much animal food, the less the better ; be regular in your habits, attend to the laws of health, and it is more than likely that nature will do the rest. But it is right to help her in her work of restoration, especially if the trouble is of long-standing, or, in other words, has become chronic. The medicines that we would recommend are all of them harmless, being the simple remedies of nature. For the milder forms of indigestion, the stomach bitters are the simplest and probably the best remedy. Take them as recommended, or in smaller doses to begin, and you will have the stomach restored to its natural condition soon. If you prefer a more pleasant medicine, make a decoction of the following :—

Agrimony	One ounce.
Centuary	One ounce.
Golden Seal	Half ounce
Ginger	Half ounce.

Bruise the roots, and simmer in a quart of water 20 minutes ; strain, and, if there is acidity of the stomach, sweeten with glycerine. If the disease has become chronic, it will be necessary to take a course of medicine once or twice a week. Dr. Fox has a mixture which has proved itself a blessing to many, especially where there was nervous debility. It is—

Peruvian Bark	Half ounce.
Juniper Berries	One ounce.
Gentian	One ounce.
Valerian Root	One ounce.
Quassia Chips	Half ounce.

Add three pints of water, boil down to a quart ; strain, and

take a wineglassful three times a day. Regulate the bowels
if you can by your diet. If you are costive, the bilious
powder, dandelion or liver pills may be taken. As a help to
our readers to determine what is the best diet, we will give the
following table of nutriment and food digestion which was
compiled by Dr. Bermount as a result of his observations
into the stomach of St. Martin, the man that had a fistulous
opening into that organ :—

AMOUNT OF NUTRIMENT CONTAINED IN 1,000 PARTS.

Bones	510	Sole		210
Mutton	290	Brain		200
Chicken	270	Haddock		180
Beef	260	White of Egg		140
Veal	250	Milk		72
Pork	250	Wheat		950
Blood	215	Nuts		930
Cod-fish	210	Peas (dry)		930
Barley	920	Cherries		250
Cereals	890	Peaches		200
Beans (dry)	890	Gooseberries		190
Rice	880	Apples		170
Bread	800	Pears		160
Rye	792	Beetroot		148
Oats	742	Strawberries		120
Almonds	650	Carrots		93
Tamarinds	840	Cabbage		73
Plums	290	Turnips		42
Grapes	270	Melons		30
Apricots	260	Cucumber		25
Potatoes	260			

TIME TAKEN TO DIGEST.

	H.	M.
Rice, boiled soft	1	0
Apples, sweet and ripe	1	30
Sago, boiled	1	45

	H.	M.
Tapioca, barley, stale bread, cabbage (with vinegar) raw, boiled milk and bread and milk cold	2	0
Potatoes roasted, and parsnips boiled ..	2	30
Baked custard	2	45
Apple dumpling	3	0
Bread, corn, baked, and carrots boiled ..	3	15
Potatoes and turnips boiled, butter and cheese	3	30
Tripe and pigs' feet	1	0
Venison	1	30
Oysters undressed, and eggs raw	2	3
Turkey and goose	2	30
Eggs, soft boiled, beef and mutton, roasted or boiled	3	0
Boiled pork, stewed oysters, eggs hard-boiled or fried	3	30
Domestic fowls	4	0
Wild fowls, pork salted, and boiled suet ..	4	30
Veal roasted, pork and salted beef ..	5	30
Beef	3	30
Mutton	3	0

HEADACHE,

Usually a symptom of indigestion, but as it is sometimes the only symptom, we may give it a separate treatment The causes are, intense study, worry, biliousness, indigestion, sluggish liver, sultry weather, exposure to the sun, and often symptomatic of other diseases. Removal of the causes will generally remove the effect. Don't overlook this because it is simple. Medicine: We have generally found the headache pills all that was required. Take them as directed, and for immediate relief use a lotion of anodyne liniment and water, of each a tablespoonful, salt a teaspoonful. Mix and saturate a cloth, lay it on the parts, or a mixture of eau de cologne, ether and chloroform, equal parts ; wet a cloth, and pour on a few drops of the mixture; lay on the seat of pain. This is also good for neuralgia and nervous pains in any part. The latest remedy, and a very successful one, is the anti-pyrin; 5 to 8 grains taken in a little water will soon give relief. A decoction of rosemary, catnip, wood betony, and balm, is also an effective cure. There are other herbs which are good, as a look over the Botanic Materia Medica will show.

HEARTBURN,

Also a symptom of indigestion. Some are troubled very much with it. To cure thoroughly the cause must be removed. The stomach put right, this symptom will disappear, unless it is caused by a peculiarity as in some people who cannot take certain kinds of food without having heart-burn. We have known persons, who were in average good health, who could not take oatmeal without having this disagreeable trouble. Experience will teach one to avoid articles of diet that disagree. As prompt remedies are demanded, we will give one or two that claim to be certain cures. First, there is the bicarbonate of soda a half to a teaspoonful, which, in many cases, acts like a charm, but it is not wise to use much of it, seeing it is likely to injure the stomach. A mixture of rhubarb and magnesia, two of the last and one of the first, a quarter to a half teaspoonful, or a piece of spanish juice, dissolved in the mouth, is a favourite remedy with some. Then there are the

HEART-BURN LOZENGES.

Prepared Chalk	Four ounces.
Gum Arabic	One ounce.
Grated Nutmeg.....................	One drachm.
Powdered Sugar	Six ounces.

Mix into a mass with sufficient water; roll, divide into usual-sized lozenges; take one or two when required. Using glycerine for sweetening is also a preventive. To correct the stomach take a course of stomach bitters. There is a severer form of, or a similar complaint to the above, called

WATER BRASH.

It is known by a burning at the stomach, accompanied with risings of a watery insipid fluid. The attacks usually occur when the stomach is empty, although they may occur at any time. The cause is indigestion. Dr. Beach gives a very good remedy for this symptom. Take—

Alexandria Senna	Two ounces.
Jalap	One ounce.
Fennel Seeds........................	Half ounce.
Brandy or Spirits	One quart.

Steep a week, shaking up. Dose, from a tea- to a tablespoonful one to three times a day as it affects the bowels. A teaspoonful of this tincture with one of tincture of tolu may also be taken with advantage. Dr. Fox gives the following as his remedy :—

Gum Benzoin	Half ounce.
Gum Storax..........................	Half ounce.
Gum Guaiacum	Half ounce.
Gum Myrrh..........................	Half ounce.
Gum Balsam Tolu	Half ounce.

Bruise, put in a bottle, and add—

Oil of Wintergreen....................	Half ounce.
Oil of Hemlock	Half ounce.
Spirits of Wine, pure..................	24 ounces.

Shake up daily for a fortnight. Some of it may be used after standing one day. Dose, two teaspoonfuls in two table-spoonfuls of water, sweetened, three or four times a day. In severe cases the dose may be doubled. Let the food be of the most digestible kind, and seek to remove the cause—indigestion—and this effect will cease.

VOMITING,

While generally symptomatic of other troubles, sometimes occurs as primary ; the stomach will reject all food and medicine. If the cause is known, apply suitable remedies to remove it. The mint mixture recommended for inflammation of the stomach (page 340) should be given. After this has been tried and failed, take a hot foot-bath of mustard and water, and an emetic of lobelia. The liver pills or liver tonic has done wonders in this condition. There is a well-known case in the Timaru district of a young woman who met with an accident, a fall. After a time vomiting began, which continued for over a year, during which time she was under the care of doctors all round, also in the hospital, with no benefit. She had wasted to a shadow. An operation was thought the only chance she had, but its dangerous nature was made known to her parents. They would not consent. It is well they did not, for in all likelihood it would have ended her pilgrimage. As a last resort (and this is often the case) we were applied to. Our manager,   gave her the liver tonic and slippery elm for food. This medicine acted like a charm—her life was saved. A decoction of bitters with eight or ten bitter almonds, bruised fine, and prepared with it may be taken. The stomach bitters, will also cure.

COLIC

Is characterised by cramp-like pains in the bowels, which when pressed are relieved . there is often also retching, nausea, and spasms of the muscles of the abdomen, griping and twisting pains, around the navel. The causes of colic are, accumulation of irritable substances in the bowels, biliousness, worms, metallic lead poisoning, strangulation of the bowels, or obstruction of any kind. There are three varieties— hysteric, bilious, and painters' colic. Treatment: If the bowels are confined, or in any case if the pain is great, give the elm injection, into which put half a teaspoonful of essence of peppermint or half an ounce of the infusion in half a pint of water, with which make the injection. Take the

COLIC POWDER,

which is composed of equal quantities of marshmallow and calamus roots powdered; a teaspoonful in a cup of warm water, sweetened. This will be improved if a half teaspoonful of antispasmodic tincture or 20 of the cholera drops are added, should there be looseness of the bowels. Rub in the anodyne liniment from five to ten minutes , then put on a cloth wrung out of hot water. As a preventive medicine, take a decoction of

Dandelion	One Ounce.
Calamus	One Ounce.
Marshmallow	One Ounce.
Valerian Root	One Ounce.
Mandrake	One Ounce.
Chillies	One Drachm.
Or Cayenne, Half Drachm	

Boil in three pints down to a quart, and take a wineglassful three or four times a day. Take the nerve pills if it is hysterical, the bilious powders if of the bilious and painters' kind, to move the bowels. We feel certain of a blessing if you should have colic and carry out our directions.

FLATULENCY, OR WINDY STOMACH,

Is another symptom of indigestion, which may be treated as its cause. In addition, the carminative drops, which are thus compounded —

CARMINATIVE DROPS.

Oil of Caraway	One ounce.
Oil of Juniper	Half ounce.
Antispasmodic Tincture	One ounce.

Mix, shake well, and give six drops on a little sugar after meals about half an hour, or four times a day. The compound carbon pills should be taken also.

JAUNDICE.

This is a trouble the nature of which cannot be mistaken, as the yellow skin is an unmistakable symptom. It is caused by an obstruction in the gall bladder, usually through cold or catarrh, which produces an inflamed condition of the duct that conveys the bile to the intestines. One of the common inducing causes is a disgusting sight or smell. A person we knew was one day jumping a fence, and landed on the putrid carcass of a cat. This gave him an acute jaundice. The cure of this trouble is not difficult, unless it be the result of liver disease, when it is only cured by treating the liver. (For treatment, see inflammation of liver) Simple jaundice is cured by the following treatment : For half an hour foment over the liver with flannels wrung out of a strong alkaline solution, four ounces of carbonate of soda or soda crystals to a quart of boiling water ; after this put on a poultice of linseed or oatmeal, made with the alkaline solution. Take a decoction of barberry bark or fringe tree bark, one ounce to the pint, a wineglassful four times a day, and keep the bowels lax with the bilious powder or liver pills An American doctor, speaking of the virtues of the fringe tree (or chionanthus virg.), tells of a hotel-keeper who sat outside his place looking more yellow than a Chinaman. The doctor asked him why he did not get his trouble cured He said, "I wish I knew how." He told him to come round to his office. He came and got the medicine The doctor says in two days he began to bleach out splendidly. Lobelia inflata, which, (see index), is another cure Altogether there is a number of remedies. We only wish every other liver trouble was as easily cured as jaundice.

CONSTIPATION.

This habit may be more or less constitutional, or as it is very often symptomatic of other troubles. It is caused directly by a loss of muscular activity of the intestines, which in good health have what is termed a peristaltic action, a worm-like downward motion. The liver also is usually implicated and sluggish. There is no need to speak of symptoms, as there are few who have not experienced the difficulty of evacuating the bowels in consequence of the hard impacted fæces. Treatment: We wish to impress upon the minds of readers, those who suffer, the necessity of studying their diet and endeavouring to remedy the evil by it, instead of the various nostrums sold everywhere in the shape of pills, mixtures, &c., which often increase the difficulty. We have known of persons who could take 12 Holloway's pills at

night, and in order to induce them to start, six more in the
morning. A gentleman came into our shop one evening,
and said, "Well, Mr. Neil, these dandelion pills have had
a wonderful effect on me. Not long since I was so costive
that I could take a whole box of Holloway's pills at one time
with only a motion or two, then I would be as bad as ever.
I have taken one box of your pills; it has lasted me some time,
and now I only need a dose now and then." Very good, but
we are sorry to confess that our pills are not always so
successful; no, it is better to try other means first. As a diet
use the whole meal bread, a plate of porridge in the morning
or at bedtime, the dandelion coffee instead of the ordinary
coffee or tea, stewed fruit, roasted apples, the yolks of two eggs
with milk. Try to get an evacuation regularly every morning. Massage or rubbing over the bowels from left to
right in a circle has been found helpful. If you know of
any cause, such as smoking, want of exercise, &c., it must
be given up; the loss of whatever pleasure may come from
it will be fully and more than fully made up by a return to
health. Medicine: Several of the botanic authors recommend
bullocks' gall made into pills with lobelia, valerian, and cayenne.
Get the fresh ox gall, evaporate to the consistency of tar, put
two parts of lobelia and one of cayenne, make into a proper
consistency, roll into ordinary sized pills, and take two or three
three times a day, as many as will keep open the bowels. The
latest remedy, cascara segrada (see index), is highly commended.
The bilious powder is good and does not bind up after. The
liver tonic and liver pills are effectual with some. Among the
cathartics some suit one, some another. Try again till you
find the right one.

DIARRHŒA OR SUMMER COMPLAINT

Is another common ailment which is not hard to remedy if it
is taken in time. The cholera drops, the recipe for which we
now give, is almost specific.

CHOLERA DROPS.

Tincture of Cayenne .... One ounce.
Tincture of Rhubarb .... One ounce.
Tincture of Catechu .... One ounce.
Essence of Peppermint .... One ounce.
Tincture of Opium .... One ounce.
Spirits of Camphor .... One ounce.
Oil of Pennyroyal................... Quarter ounce.

Shake up, and give for an adult 15 to 30 drops, a quarter to a half teaspoonful, in a little warm water. sweetened, every half, one, or two hours, till relieved. Look up the class of astringents, and you cannot go wrong in using them as directed!

DYSENTERY

Is an aggravated form of the above. In addition to the looseness, there is great straining and often blood present in the discharges. The cholera drops will generally cure this also. If not, take the following remedy :—

Oil of Cinnamon .... Half drachm.
Oil of Peppermint .... Half drachm.
Laudanum......................... Half ounce.
Proof Spirits .... One pint.

Dessert-spoonful given every three to four hours.

Dr. Fox's astringent powder is. we have found by experience, an excellent cure It is compounded thus—

Turkey Rhubarb .... One ounce.
Catechu .... One ounce.
Tormentil.......................... One ounce.
Prepared Chalk .... One ounce.
Gum Myrrh .... One ounce.
Confection Aromatic .... One ounce.
Bayberry .... One ounce.
Cinnamon .... One ounce.
Opium .... Quarter ounce.

All in powder. Pass through a sieve, or mix well. The adult dose is a teaspoonful in a half cup of warm water, sweetened, three

or four times a day ; children, according to age. The digestive
food should be taken, and if the case is a severe one, a slippery
elm injection, with half a teaspoonful of the astringent powder,
should be given   Let the food be of a light and mucilaginous
kind.   The blessings of those who have been ready to perish
have come upon us for our successful treatment of these bowel
complaints.

FALLING OF THE BOWELS.

This condition is often the cause of chronic diarrhœa, and
dysentery. It is caused by a lax condition of the sphinctre
muscle of the anus, and it is cured by a removal of the cause,
and the application of astringents   An American gives this as
a remedy : Return the gut, and select a small round piece of
alum ; melt the angles off it in warm water : push up till it has
passed the sphincter : it will dissolve. Two or three applications
will suffice.   In some old patients it may be needful to get a
truss.

NIGHTMARE (Incubus)

May also be included in diseases of digestion, as it is generally
found in connection with dyspepsia   The sympathy between
the stomach and brain is a recognised fact which may account
for the unnatural dreams which accompany the affection. The
dreamer imagines himself falling down a precipice, about to
be torn by wild beasts, or an impossibility to breathe.   There
is a semi-consciousness with it which makes one try to awaken
and cry out.   The cause, weak stomach, nervousness, great
anxiety, constipation, eating late suppers, eating indigestible
food, &c.   The subject is generally lying on the back   In the
effort to awaken, the sufferer groans and often rolls out on the
floor.   People think lightly of these symptoms, but they are
sometimes fearfully distressing, and we are inclined to the
opinion that nightmare is often the cause of death in those
found dead in their beds. We have often felt that if we had
not wakened when we did, death would have resulted.   To
prevent, avoid all excesses, take a vegetable diet, a cup of
composition at bed-time, small doses of the stomach bitters,

keep the mind as well as the body pure.   The sum up of advice
is, correct digestion and tone up the nerves.

GALL STONES.

These concretions in their passage through the gall duct
cause the most excruciating pain.   The trouble is not always
understood.   We have known of a sufferer under our treatment,
and that of some doctors, without the true cause of his pain
being discovered.   The usual mistake is to suppose the pain
to be colic.   The symptoms are, acute pains of a sharp-cutting
nature, felt about an hour after meals.   When the effort of
nature to send out the gall to carry on the work of digestion
takes place, these pains are most distressing, causing the
patient to double up and even faint away.   The cause is not
easily found out—it is the bile salts that crystalise and form
into stones.   From the fact that oil is the best treatment yet
found, it may be inferred that there is a want of the fatty
element in the blood, or a failure of the liver to secrete it.
Bilious people are most likely to suffer from gall-stones, as
most of them cannot take fats.   To cure—when the pain is felt,
take a dose of hiera picra, as much as will lie on a sixpence.
Follow this with from a quarter to a half pint of salad oil.   If
you cannot take it simple, it may be disguised in milk.   To
ease the pain, make a poultice of equal parts of powdered
lobelia, slippery elm, and belladonna.   Apply over the parts
hot, and give a dose of anodyne tincture if the pain
continues.   Use the liver pills to keep the bowels free.   This
treatment, with a course of medicine every week, will cure and
prevent severe returns of the trouble.

CHOLERA MORBUS (English Cholera).

This complaint usually comes on very suddenly in hot
sultry weather.   The causes are given, as deficient food, putrid
meat, irritating foods, severe purgations, marsh poison,
obstructed circulation, &c.   The symptoms are, severe
griping pains, purging, vomiting, the tongue is furred, the
pulse quick, feeble, and sometimes irregular; there is thirst,

anxiety, cold sweats, a blue appearance of the face, extreme debility; if the disease advances, cramps and hiccough occur. It may terminate fatally in 48 hours or less. In the treatment of this trouble the botanic system is most successful. Thousands have been saved by it. Our want of space forbids us giving many such examples. We will give, (1.) A merchant in his office was taken suddenly ill. The blood seemed to recede from the surface of his body, intolerable pains, and the other symptoms. An herbalist friend happened to call just then. He ran out and procured some of Coffin's anti-cholera powder (see index), put a full teaspoonful in a half pint of hot water; there was no time to wait for it to settle; he drank it. In a short time he gave him another. This removed the trouble that in all likelihood would have sent him to his grave. (2.) A man after returning from his work took ill in a similar way. He went to the closet in the garden. His wife wondered why he stayed so long. She went out and found him apparently dead. She ran to the house, where she fortunately had cayenne pepper. She put about half an ounce in a cup half full of water, sweetened, and got it down his throat. In a few minutes she got him into the house, when he soon recovered. (3.) An old man living by himself was nearly dead; to use his own way of putting it, his inside was purged out. Our country traveller gave him a teaspoonful of the cholera drops, and then sold him the 1/- bottle. In half an hour his bowels were settled; his life saved. These cases will show the power of our simple remedies. The cholera powder will, as a rule, be all that is needed, but if the painful straining is very great, give the remedy for dysentery, also injection; hot cayenne fomentations over the abdomen. and the slippery elm food will complete the cure.

ASIATIC CHOLERA

Is similar to the above, but partakes more of the character of a plague. Its first appearance was in India in 1817. In a few weeks after its outbreak 10,000 people were swept away; the year following 1800 deaths took place in Calcutta in three months from it. Russia and England were visited in 1829, and the number of deaths in England was 101,000. There was another visitation in 1849, and the last in 1885. We remember both of the last, and they were terrible. It is to be hoped that in these colonies we shall never have such an ordeal to pass through. It may be all very well to boast of our better conditions, sanitation, &c., but it is not always possible to avert it. These dispensations of Providence are sent to remind us that we are mortal and win us to righteousness. The cause of cholera is said to be a specific bacillis which poisons the blood, robs the body of heat, &c. The blood-poison acting on the nervous system causing the terrible cramps with spasms and diarrhœa which are the chief symptoms of the deadly disease. The treatment must be very prompt. The patient, as soon as the symptoms are detected, should get a large dose of the cholera powder, then, if able, the steam bath, or get a tubful of hot water, stir in mustard, stand him up to the knees and bathe the body for five or ten minutes ; put to bed with hot bricks to the feet and sides. Keep on with the cholera powder or drops, give the digestive food, and the blessing of saving him who was ready to perish shall be yours. For the experience of an eye witness see page 18 ; and as a preventive when cholera is in the district or county, see charcoal (page 48).

WORMS.

As we have already in our treatment of children's diseases dealt with worms, it will only be needful to treat of one principal kind, not common in juveniles—that is the tape variety. The symptoms caused by this parasite are not very clear, as they often are connected with other troubles : sickness at the stomach, pain sometimes, the appetite is voracious, wasting, and more or less hypochondria, the knowledge of having such an unnatural companion giving rise to it. Its existence is generally known from seeing portions of it in the evacuations. It is white, tape-like, but notched at the sides, and it seems to have a wonderful power of life, as parts or half may come away, yet it lives and grows sometimes to enórmous lengths. Dr. Beach, in his Reformed Practice of Medicine, mentions the case of an American lady who was infested for thirty years, and passed in that time pieces that, if joined, would reach one mile in length. We made a present of one which we had expelled from a person, 33 feet in length, to the Otago University Anatomical Museum. To kill this parasite is sometimes very easy, at other times nót. We have known of persons suffering for years, although they had tried many doctors and remedies. We have generally found the following treatment successful :—First, eat no supper, but before going to bed take one drachm of extract of male fern in two ounces of the mucilage of gum acacia. In the morning take a tablespoonful of honey. In an hour after, before breakfast, take two tablespoonfuls of castor oil on a teaspoonful of bilious powder. When you feel that your bowels are going to move get a chamber half full of hot water, evacuate the bowels, and in all probability you will see the worm. Wash it and see if the head is there ; if not you had better repeat the same process in a fortnight. The object in using the hot water is to keep the worm, which is not dead, warm, for on feeling the cold it will cling to the bowels and only a portion will come away. There are several other remedies which promise much, but we do not think any of them will be superior to this one, however, as we wish to give something to fall back upon, we will give one or two. Cowhage half a teaspoonful in arrowroot jelly, eat garlic and fine salt, take a purge twice a week with the compound mandrake powder. Kamala, a teaspoonful, may be taken instead of the cowhage. Kusso is another remedy. Half an ounce of it is taken in the morning, followed by a brisk purge ; one dose in the week is sufficient of it. The very latest remedy is the cocoanut. Grate the whole of an ordinary-sized nut, take it all, in an hour after take a good purge. Examine the evacuation, and if there is not any part of the tape worm you may feel certain you do not have the trouble at that time. Having giving the treatment for ordinary worms, we will simply give directions for making

WORM SUPPOSITORIES.

Take oil theobrom. or cacao butter. powder in a mortar. Mix two teaspoonfuls of worm powder, a teaspoonful of powdered aloes, one of gum arabic : beat them into a mass, and mould them into round pyramids about the size of a very small thimble. One may be inserted in the anus at bedtime and allowed to dissolve. Suppositories may be used for piles and womb troubles, prepared with suitable medicines.

PILES (HEMORRHOIDS)

These painful tumours are caused by an obstruction to the circulation of the blood in the parts around. The hemorrhoidal veins are engorged, swell, and form the piles. They are caused by constipation, taking purgatives too frequently, patent pill swallowing. sitting on the damp ground, pregnancy, sedentary occupations, unhealthy state of the liver, &c. There are three kinds : the external, the internal, and the bleeding. Symptoms · Pain, principally felt at stool. The external may be seen as small round projections of a livid colour. The internal are recognised by the pain they cause, and are also seen by the speculum. Either of these form the bleeding ones. Treatment : The first thing is to cure the costive habit. For this take a teaspoonful every morning and evening, if necessary, of the electuary of senna. This sometimes will cure of itself. Wash night and morning with a strong decoction of yarrow made warm each time ; after washing, wet with the extract of witch hazel. Another treatment : Take the bilious powder to regulate the bowels, a dose first thing in the morning ; then the pile powedrs three times a day, and apply the pile ointment ; third, take a teaspoonful of the following :—

Fluid extract of Wa-a-hoo Bark .... Half ounce.
Fluid extract of Aloes .... Quarter ounce.
Fluid extract of Stoneroot (Collisonia) Three drachms.
Glycerine .... One ounce.
Water, to make .... Four ounces.

If a teaspoonful is too laxative take smaller doses. It is affirmed after years of trial that this will cure nine out of ten cases. Where there is much pain an ointment may be applied, made thus :—

Vaseline .... One ounce.
Sulphate of Morphia .... Four grains.
Tannic Acid .... One drachm.

Use night and morning or twice a day. When the tumours bleed a suppository of tannic acid or a strong solution of the same should be used. Suppositories are made by mixing the ingredients with a substance that will hold them together. (See treatment for worms). There are various operations for piles, but it requires experience to do them.

URINARY DISEASES.

Besides acute and chronic inflammation of the urinary organs there are a few other complaints that occur in connection with them. Before particularising them we think it needful to give our readers a brief analysis of the urine, which we quote from a reliable source.

BRIEF ANALYSIS OF URINE,

AND ITS SIGNIFICANCE IN DETERMINING DISEASE.

Healthy urine in colour varies from a pale straw to a brown yellow; it is generally a yellow amber. Pale urine, when it indicates disease of an anæmic form ; coloured urines —reddish-yellow to red—indicate febrile conditions ; dark coloured urines—brownish to blackish—contain abnormal pigments, requiring examination The specific gravity of urine is from 1005 to 1030, generally 1015 to 1025 : average daily quantity 40 to 55 oz. ; solid matters, 600 to 1200 grains. The natural reaction is acid ; sometimes after meals, neutral or alkaline. Alkaline urine generally indicates some disease by which (1) some portion of the urine is retained and an alkaline fermentation is set up ; or (2) some increased secretion of mucus. If the litmus paper used to test the alkalinity remains blue after drying, it is alkaline through some fixed alkali, potash, soda, or an alkaline earth. If in drying the paper resumes the red colour, it is made alkaline by a volatile alkali (usually carbonate of ammonium, from the decomposition of urine). The latter is always pathological. The urine may be abnormally acid, tending to form calculi. In chronic and acute diseases the amount of free acid generally diminishes, but it increases in pneumonia and rheumatic fever

1. First class of deposits, uric acid, urates, phosphates, hippuric acid, lime oxalate, mucus, epithelium, and pigments. Uric acid deposits resemble grains of sand of a yellowish, reddish, or brownish colour Uric acid is insoluble in hot water, and soluble in the alkalies—soda, potash, ammonia. Test (muriatic acid) : Add to sediment placed on a glass slide one drop of strong nitric acid ; evaporate and add one drop of ammonia. A beautiful violet colour will indicate the uric acid Clinical significance—meat diet with little exercise, gout, diseases of the liver, chronic diseases of respiratory organs, chronic bronchitis, emphysema of lungs, pneumonia, rheumatic fever, skin diseases, acute inflammation of kidneys. The urates are the most frequent deposit in urine ; they are soluble in hot water, and in the alkalies. When cool, turbid urine is heated to 100 degrees Fahr., if it becomes clear, a urate is present. The muracid test given above is applicable. The acids decompose them, giving free uric acid. Clinical significance—similar to uric acid. Phosphates : The earthy phosphates of lime and magnesium occur as precipitates ; they are soluble in acetic and the stronger acids. A few drops of

any acid will cause them to disappear. Clinical significance —Amorphous lime phosphate occurs when the urine becomes alkaline under vegetable diet, and after nervous exhaustion; the crystalline lime phosphate usually indicates grave disease, as consumption, cancer, diabetes; the ammonia smell almost always comes from the decomposition of urea. Lime oxalate: This deposit is crystalline in form, and is best recognised by the microscope: in excess it is the oxalic acid diathesis. Mucus: It occurs in small quantities in healthy urine. It appears as a light cloud, which slowly sinks to the bottom of the glass. It has the colour of the urine, when filtered it is transparent and glairy; it entangles the other deposits, and they conceal its presence. It is more ropy than pus, but frequently the microscope is required to distinguish between them. When pathological it comes from a chronic inflammation, or an ammoniacal decomposition of the urine in the bladder.

2. In the second class of deposits (those foreign to healthy urine) the chief forms are, pus, blood, oil, and chyle. Pus: It is found in turbid urine, having a whitish deposit of ropy consistency. A few drops of liquor potash, turn it into a semi-solid, ropy. gelatinous mass, well shown when dropped from a test-tube. Pus, in small quantities, especially in females, may have no clinical significance; but when it forms a visible deposit it becomes important. It may come from any part of the genito-urinary tract, or from any abscess opening into it. Blood: When it appears as a sediment, it is usually of a blood red colour, (uric acid is more of a dark brown colour.) It is best detected by finding the blood corpuscles under the microscope. It indicates a hemorrhage in the urinary tract, which may come from a variety of causes. Oil: It is recognised under the microscope, and usually indicates fatty degeneration of the kidneys.

3. The third class of substances in the urine which indicate disease give no deposits. They are, albumen, sugar, and bile. Albumen: Albuminous urine has a low specific gravity—1005 to 1015. In acid urine the albumen is coagulated and thereby

detected by boiling Heat does not coagulate albumen in alkaline urine until it is made acid. A few drops of nitric acid will distinguish the earthy phosphates from the coagulated albumen. The former will be dissolved : the latter will become more opaque When the quantity of albumen is small, proceed as follows —Let nitric acid trickle down the sides of a test-tube containing urine. The acid being heavier will sink to the bottom, and the urine will float above. At the junction, if albumen is present, there will be an opaque layer, which gentle heat will not clear away. Albumen in the urine may be due to fatty degeneration of the kidneys, to temporary conditions in the renal circulation (capillary turgescence, fevers, inflammations), to affections of the mucous membrane in urinary tract, and to the mal-assimilation of albuminous foods.

TEST FOR SUGAR.

The specific gravity is usually high. The following is Haines's test :—

Pure Sulphate of Copper......	Thirty grains.
Pure Glycerine	Two fluid drachms.
Pure Caustic Potash, in sticks ..	One and a half drachms.
Pure Water	Six fluid ounces.

Dissolve the copper and the glycerine in a portion of the water and the caustic potash in the remainder. Mix the two solutions, when a transparent blue liquid should result, which should be bottled and laid aside for use. Take about one drachm of the above test solution and boil gently. It should give no deposit. Add 10 or 15 drops of urine. If sugar is present there should be an abundant red or yellowish red precipitate. A white flocculent deposit would indicate phosphates and not sugar. Bile : Put a little urine in a white plate, and add a few drops of nitric acid. A play of colours from violet to green will show the presence of bile.

SUPPRESSION OF URINE.

This is caused by a partial or complete failure of the kidneys to secrete the urine from the blood. It may be due

to inflammation, gravel, wasting as in Bright's disease.
Symptoms—Besides the suppression there is usually a smell
of urine in the prespiration, with feverishness, drowsiness,
and in bad cases delirium and convulsions The first thing
to do is try and find the cause, which will indicate as to the
treatment to be pursued. If the system points to inflammation, follow out directions there given The vapour bath
should be given at once. Keep up the perspiration with hot
bricks in the vinegar cloths to both sides and feet. Make a
medicine of—

Jaborandi...........................	One ounce.
Dandelion	One ounce.
Peletory of the Wall	One ounce.
Tansy	One ounce.
Valerian	One ounce.

Put in three pints of water, simmer 15 minutes, strain, and
give a wineglassful every two hours till symptoms abate. If
the suppression is obstinate a teaspoonful of sweet nitre may
be taken between the decoction. Keep the bowels open and
give a light and nourishing diet. In retention of urine, the
bladder, prostrate gland (situated at the neck), may be
inflamed, or it may be gravel. (See symptoms of inflammation
of bladder and carry out instructions). If symptoms point to
gravel (see index and treat for it), but by far the most common
cause is stricture of the urethra. (See index and treat for it).
Should no cause be found, or the symptoms be obscure, use
a catheter to draw off the water. A decoction of the
following will assist in preventing a return of the retention :—

Marshmallow Root......	One ounce.
Buchu Leaves	One ounce.
Tansy	One ounce.
Slippery Elm	Two ounces.

Simmer in three pints of water 10 minutes, strain, and give a
wineglassful four times a day. If thirsty drink freely of a weak
decoction of slippery elm, sweetened. Add lemon to taste.

INVOLUNTARY FLOW OF URINE.

If this is not, as it often is, the result of other complaints, it can be cured with a decoction of astringents, such as :—

Uva Ursa..........................	One ounce.
Bistort	One ounce.
Beth Root	One ounce.
Sumach Berries	One ounce.
Unicorn Root	One ounce.
Spanish Juice	One ounce.

Simmer 30 minutes in a 1½ quarts of water, give a wineglassful three times a day A sitz-bath of sea water or sea salt and water well rubbed into the loins will be beneficial. If the decoction causes constipation do not stop it but use an opening medicine. This complaint in children is termed

BED-WETTING

The above medicine in smaller doses will do for them. The practice of making them empty the bladder the last thing in the evening should be enforced. In an American journal we see a strong recommendation of one drop doses of tincture belladonna three times a day in a teaspoonful of water. Another recommends red wine, a tablespoonful, three times a day ; another three grains of chloral hydrate. We think that our own is the best ; try it, and if it fails try the rest, but we would say have patience, for it is sometimes hard to cure.

DIABETES.

This is one of the gravest troubles that we have to cope with. Its direct cause may be described as a perverted action chiefly of the liver, although anatomists and physiologists usually give the liver all the blame. It is our opinion that all the digestive organs are more or less at fault. This is clearly shown in the great thirst and generally constant constipation. The kidneys also may be said to work at high pressure, as the enormous quantities of urine secreted will prove. The inducing causes are given as hereditary transmission, indulgence in liquor-drinking, and other excesses, which weaken the vital forces ; however, on this point there is a difference of opinion, which indicates the want of knowledge as to the definite cause. The symptoms are plainer : the almost constant desire to make water and the excessive amount voided ; however, this symptom alone is not enough to determine it. The presence of sugar in the urine will prove diabetes. To find out whether there is sugar the chemical test will show. (See the analysis of urine, page 383). Presuming we have a reader who thinks he cannot test it chemically, and does not care to go to a doctor, and wishes to satisfy himself in a positive way, let him keep all the urine he passes in 24 hours, take a pint of it, evaporate it till there is just a little remaining, put the point of the finger in it, touch the tongue, and if it is sugary the taste will determine the grave nature of the disease, which, like consumption and a few other troubles, has baffled doctors of every school. Treatment : If the disease is detected before the body is wasted, begin with the Thompsonian course once or twice a week. Make a mixture of—

Barberis Aqua Folia	One ounce.
Sweet Bugle......................	One ounce.
Chilies	One drachm.
Cherry Bark	One ounce.
Prickly Ash Berries	One ounce.
Bistort Root	Two ounces.

Simmer in three pints of water down to a quart. strain, press, and give a wineglassful four times a day. By our latest Medical Journal we learn that a Doctor Valentine has discovered that creosote stops the secretion of sugar by the kidneys. He used from four to ten drops a day in two cases, when the sugar disappeared promptly and did not return. Put one or two drops in each dose of the decoction ; begin with one. Dr. Monkten of Hokitika says he has given sulpho-carbolate of soda, from 5 to 30 grains, even in the last stage of diabetes with great benefit. This is a compound of sulphur, carbolic acid, and carbonate of soda. The diet must be as much a meat one as possible, with brown bread and milk, buttermilk preferred. No sugar, but glycerine or saccharine may be used. Keep the skin and bowels clear. The liver pills will answer well here.

GRAVEL AND STONE.

This disease is caused by impurities left in the blood. Small sand-like particles are formed in the kidneys which cause pain in their passage through the ureters or tubes that lead to the bladder and from the bladder when voiding its contents. In severe cases the symptoms are not unlike inflammation of the kidneys, but an examination of urine will show that gravel is the trouble. Treatment: A strong decoction of the diuretics must be given :—

Queen of Meadow Root.............. One ounce.
Wild Carrot Seed .... One ounce
Peletory of the Wall .... One ounce.
Parsley Pert........................ One ounce.

Put in three pints of water, simmer down to a quart, strain, press, and take a wineglassful every two hours till symptoms abate Should the pain be very great, a warm sitz-bath, into which put an ounce of laudanum or a decoction of four ounces of poppy heads, and take a teaspoonful of diuretic drops, prepared thus :—

DIURETIC DROPS.

Sweet Nitre .... Two ounces.
Tincture of Opium .... Half ounce.

A teaspoonful in a cupful of slippery elm gruel every hour till the pain subsides. To prevent the formation be careful with your diet. Take the digestive food once a day and a course of medicine once a week.

Stone is a concretion that when any size forms in the bladder the same treatment will do for it with as much slippery elm as you can take. (See index). Lithontryptics— try them all till you succeed.

ANOTHER URINARY COMPLAINT

Is stricture of the urethra. This exceedingly painful trouble is almost wholly confined to males. It is caused by inflammation and the use of injurious injections. Operations are usually resorted to but are not very satisfactory. The best treatment we can find is tincture of gelsemine, full doses, and warm sitz-baths, with an ounce of laudanum to the quart.

PROSTATITIS,

(Inflammation of the prostate gland) resembles the above. It is usually met with in old men. The same medicine will be suitable, alternating the gelsemine with tincture of staphysagria Rub into the parts the turpentine and lard, given in treatment for scrofula.

BLOODY URINE.

This is sometimes the result of injuries. If so, drink freely of a decoction of comfrey root and elm bark. Rest and nature will repair the injury, if it is not of a very serious nature. If it continues, or when it comes without injuries, take the following mixture :—

Sweet Nitre .... Four ounces.
Tannic Acid .... One ounce
Glycerine .... Two ounces.
Water to fill an eight-ounce bottle.

A teaspoonful four times a day in a wineglassful of the decoction Lessen the dose as the symptoms abate. This we feel certain will cure.

DROPSY

Is seldom if ever an independent disease. but is a result of some other derangement. It is defined as an effusion of serum into the tissue or cavities of the body. Its cause is the antecedent trouble, or a failure on the part of the kidneys to do their secreting work. The varieties are named after the part of the body in which the water is found. In the flesh of

the extremities it is called œdema; when it is diffused, it is
anasarca; in the abdomen, it is ascites; in the chest,
hydrothorax; in the head, hydrocephalus; in the ovaries
it is called ovarian dropsy; and in the scrotum, it is
hydrocele. To cure, our attention must first be directed to the
cause. If this is removed, then the water will be absorbed,
but it is not easy to do this when some of the organs are
diseased, as the liver, kidneys, or ovaries; if we cannot remove
the cause, let us try and get rid of the effect—the water.
Presuming that there is strength enough left in the system,
there is nothing better than the course of medicine. After the
bath and the emetic give eight drops of this mixture—

Podophyllin .... Five grains.
Oil of Juniper .... Half drachm.
Gum Acacia .... One drachm.
Rose Water .... Two and a half drachms.

Rub together till well mixed; put in a half ounce vial; shake
up, and take as above, in an infusion of—

Juniper Berries.............. A wineglassful.

Make a medicine of—

Peletory of the Wall................ One ounce.
Broom .... One ounce.
Diuretic Powder .... One ounce.
Cayenne......................... Half teaspoonful.

In a quart of boiling water.

Let it stand covered one hour; strain, and press through a
cloth, and give a wineglassful four times a day, and as many
of the drops as will keep the bowels free. We have seen fine
cures with the above treatment. If, however, this should fail,
try the diuretics. Dr. Beach gives the following mixture,
which is a very valuable one, but requiring care in its
administration :—

Foxglove Leaves, dry .... One ounce.
Spearmint Herb, dry .... Two ounces.

Infuse in a full quart of boiling water in a covered vessel 12
hours , strain, express, and add half a pint of Holland's gin.

Bottle, and give half a tablespoonful four times a day, gradually increasing to one tablespoonful. He affirms that this medicine will in 24 hours cause a flow of water, drain the cavities of the body, and in cases where there is no organic disease, cure the patient. The diuretic powder and pills alone have cured some. (See also diuretics, page 70).

Dr. Fox's mixture is worth inserting. It is—

Loaf Sugar...................... Two ounces.
Foxglove Leaves, dry .... Quarter ounce.
Pellitory of Wall .... One ounce.
Saltpetre....................... Half ounce.

Put the whole in three cupfuls of water ; simmer 20 minutes ; when cool, strain, clear, and add one ounce of sweet nitre. For those over 20 years give two tablespoonfuls twice a day ; children, according to age. He claims for it what Dr. Beach does for his. He also recommends two cayenne pills to be taken after meals.

NERVOUS DISEASES.

RHEUMATISM.

This painful affection is not generally classed with nervous diseases, but there can be no question that the pain is caused by nerve irritation. While this may be said of all pain, it is especially true of rheumatism. The acute form assumes the character of and is called

RHEUMATIC FEVER.

Causes—Predisposition, exposure to cold, wet clothing, a morbid condition of the blood, caused by the retention of waste products, mercurial drugs, &c. Symptoms : Pain and swelling of the joints, fever, pulse full and bounding. There is pain in the back, stiffness, the least movement, only of the bed-clothes, gives intense pain, causing even strong men to cry out; the tongue is covered with a white thin coating, the thirst is great, the appetite almost gone, the bowels constipated, the urine high coloured. The symptoms are generally increased in the night and remit in the morning, when the patient gets a little sleep. While it is not usually dangerous in itself, it often attacks the heart and either proves fatal or injures the organ, to a greater or less degree. It may also cause an enlargement or distortion of joints, especially of the fingers. In the treatment of this disease the proverbial differing of doctors is apparent. Everyone seems to treat it according to his fancy. There is, no doubt, some excuse for this, as the disease is very erratic, particularly the chronic form. The old and barbarous custom of bleeding has passed away for ever. It is hard to find a reason why it ever had an existence, for, as Dr. Coffin once said, you can never improve the quality of blood by depletion, any more than you might expect to improve the contents of a barrel of beer by drawing off some of it. Our botanic doctors are more unanimous in their treatment of rheumatism. As soon as the premonitory signs are felt, an opening medicine should be given. Half a teaspoonful of fluid extract of cascara segrada, and continued three times a day, then a vapour bath, or hot bricks and vinegar cloths. Keep up the perspiration for six hours by drinking freely of yarrow and composition tea, or, if the pains are severe, take the diaphoretic powder. As a liniment to apply to the painful parts, Dr. Beach recommends—

Oil of Hemlock .... One ounce
Laudanum .... One ounce.
Camphor.......................... Half ounce.
Spirits............................ One pint.

Dissolve; warm by putting the bottle in hot water, paint over with a soft brush, or lay on soft cloths saturated with this liniment, the anodyne, or Rheumatic Pain Cure will generally afford relief. A poultice of bran, scalded with vinegar, has afforded more relief sometimes than liniments. As a medicine take with the cascara segrada a decoction of—

Wood Sage......................... One ounce.
Angelica Root, coarse powder ...... One ounce.
Wintergreen Leaves .... One ounce.
Burdock Seeds, bruised............. One ounce.
Chilies .... One drachm.
Prickly Ash Bark .... One ounce.

Bruise and simmer the roots in two quarts of water half an hour; put in the herbs and seeds, let remain on the fire 10 minutes longer; strain, press, sweeten with sugar, and give a wineglassful every two to four hours. This is the treatment we would recommend first. If it should fail the iodide of potash may be substituted—one ounce in a quart of water. Dose—A tablespoonful 4 times a day. One of our American doctors says he uses in the first stage 20 grain doses of salicine four times a day. If the pain is unbearable, a subcutaneous injection of morphia may be given; but this would not be safe for an inexperienced person to give. However, there are tabloids now with the accurate quantity which are dissolved in a teaspoonful of water, and so many drops injected, by putting the point of the syringe under the skin and pressing the piston; doctors carry them in their pocket-cases. If the pain should locate in the head, it should be bathed with a strong tincture of stramonium. The cascara will keep the bowels free. Keep on with it as an opening medicine, no matter what other things you may use. Give a light milk diet, digestive food. When convalescent, use one of the diet drinks. (See index.)

CHRONIC RHEUMATISM.

The object in treating it is to rid the blood of its unhealthy matter. Give a course of medicine once a week. Take a decoction of—

Liqourice Root .... One ounce.
Sarsaparilla .... One ounce.
Burdock Root .... One ounce.
Prickly Ash Bark .... One ounce.
Sassafras Bark...................... One ounce.
Wintergreen .... One ounce.
Wood Sage .... One ounce.

In two quarts of water. Bruise the barks and roots, simmer half an hour, add the rest, simmer a little longer, strain, and if desired, sweeten, and take a wineglassful four times a day. The rheumatic pills and rheumatic powder may be changed with the above. Just a word or two about the most common kind, which those subject to it describe as a touch of rheumatism. It is not enough simply to rub in a liniment and get rid of the present pain. The germs of the disease are in the system ; try and cast them out. Take the treatment just given for the chronic form, and you will not likely have a touch, or at least not so many of them.

SCIATICA

Is an inflammatory condition of the greatest nerve in the body. It is a most painful affection and one which is not readily cured, as the nerve is imbedded in the muscles of the thigh, it is not easy getting at it with liniments. A hot fomentation of herbs is more effective. Take :—

Tansy .... One ounce.
Marshmallow .... One ounce.
Southernwood...................... One ounce.
Mugwort .... One ounce.
Wormwood .... One ounce.
Chamomiles........................ One ounce.

Boil in a gallon of water, and when hot enough not to scald put in a bucket, support the leg over it, put a flannel round the thigh two or three times and pour on the hot liquor for a quarter to half an hour. To keep it up in heat put a small hot stone or two into it. Warm and repeat twice daily. Wipe dry, cover with a dry flannel and take this mixture :—

Tincture of Gelsemine.............. Two ounces.
Tincture of Peruvian Bark .... One ounce.
Tincture of Black Cohosh .... One ounce.

Mix. Take a teaspoonful in a wineglassful of the compound decoction of sarsaparilla three times a day. As liniments are sometimes beneficial, and have the advantage of being easier handled than the fomentations, use the one in the following treatment for neuralgia. Keep the bowels open and the skin clean. A vapour bath once a week will be beneficial.

NEURALGIA, OR FACEACHE,

Is another of the same class of nerve affections. When it does not arise from an aching tooth, we have found it yield readily to our treatment. Our mixture is—

Concentrated tincture of Gelsemine.... Four drachms.
Bromide of Ammonia................ Two drachms.
Infusion Peruvian Bark up to .... Four ounces.

Take a teaspoonful three times a day of this mixture, or the tincture of gelsemine in one drachm doses, or the quinine and hydrastin (page 352). As a liniment we have found the one given by Doctor Chase, and called the

MAGIC LINIMENT,

a really good one. It is compounded thus :—

Morphia .... Ten grains.
Chloral Hydrate .... Half ounce.
Gum Camphor .... Half ounce.
Chloroform .... One ounce.
Amyl Nitrate .... Two drachms.
Oil of Cloves .... Quarter ounce.
Oil Cinnamon .... Quarter ounce.
Alcohol, to fill a four ounce bottle.

Directions :—Dissolve the morphia in a little of the spirit, rub the camphor and the chloral hydrate together till they become a liquid ; mix all together except the amyl nitrate, which, being very volatile, must be put in the bottle before corking ; shake, and add four to six drops of sulphuric acidor vitriol, to keep the morphia dissolved. Rub gently over the seat of pain. We have tried this ourselves and found it did what was claimed for it. The objection to it is its high price. We sell it at one shilling an ounce, but it is not often that our own pain-killer fails. We have had people come into our shop almost mad with pain, and after a good rubbing with it go out rejoicing. Neuralgic patients ought to take care of their general health; keep the bowels open, and if the teeth ache get them extracted or stopped. The liniment may be applied to the teeth also.

LUMBAGO (Pain in the Back),

Belongs to this class when it does not proceed from inflammation of the kidneys. The symptoms are, dull pain in the small of the back, stiffness, the urine is generally high coloured, which shows that the kidneys are implicated. The causes are cold, exposure, violent exercise, falls, &c. It is not as a rule hard to cure. First, give a vapour bath, rub the back well with the tincture of cayenne and prickly ash berries, or anodyne liniment, or Rheumatic Pain Killer. Prepare a decoction of diuretics thus :—

Dandelion	Two ounces.
Uva Ursi	One ounce.
Parsley Pert	One ounce.
Buchu	One ounce.
Chilies	Half drachm.

Simmer the roots in three pints of water half an hour, then add the herbs, let cool, strain, and take a wineglassful four times a day. If the bowels are confined take a dose of the golden pills or dandelion at bedtime.

APOPLEXY.

Without doubt this is one of the most sudden and dangerous affections that the body is subject to. Its immediate causes are (1) congestion of the blood-vessels of the brain, (2) rupture of some of these vessels, (3) an effusion and pressure of serum or water in the cavities of the brain. Predisposing causes are, luxurious living, corpulence, continual drinking, or the habit of nipping indulged in by travellers who do business with public-houses, samplers in wholesale stores, want of exercise, &c., &c It may be paradoxical, but we might say that the way to cure apoplexy is to prevent it first by living in accordance with nature's laws. There are certain premonitory symptoms, which, if heeded and the proper remedies taken, would either prevent the attack or greatly lessen its violence. These symptoms are so numerous that we do not think it needful to give them all. The principal are, dull heavy feeling in the head, giddiness if attempting to stoop, an unusual tendency to sleep, engorgement of the veins of the forehead, and loss of memory. These symptoms being marked in stout plethoric people advanced in life, should induce measures to be taken to ward off a possible and near attack. The first object is to equalise the circulation, exercise in the open air, but not too fatiguing, hot foot-baths, cold applications to the head, keep the bowels free with the compound mandrake or leptandrin powder, dandelion or liver pills, become as nearly as possible a vegetarian, use the digestive food, drink meadowsweet tea or ulmaric wine, or a cup of composition at bed-time. These measures will in all likelihood ward off the threatened blow, but should it come, as it often does, without these warning symptoms being given or heeded, the patient falling down insensible, showing by the livid countenance, stertorous breathing, swelling of the veins, bloodshot eyes, and frothing at the mouth, that it is apoplexy we have to deal with, open the collar or neck-wear, vest, &c., get a hot foot-bath with mustard nearly up to the knees, apply cold water to the front and top of the head, rub the back of the head with tincture of cayenne or pain-killer. Keep up this treatment for 20 minutes, if the patient does not come round before this, give an injection of the slippery elm, into which put a teaspoonful of the antispasmodic tincture and a tablespoonful of olive oil, put to bed with a hot brick in a vinegar cloth to the feet, prop up in a reclining posture to favour the return of blood from the head. When the patient can swallow give half a teaspoonful of the antispasmodic tincture, repeating it every hour till the symptoms have abated. When convalescent carry out the directions for prevention. Take a course of the blood purifying medicine. Keep the skin, bowels, and kidneys free with suitable remedies.

SUN STROKE

Is very similar in its manifestations to apoplexy. Treat it in the same way: cold water to the front and top of the head, hot to the back and neck; the hot foot-bath, &c.

EPILEPSY,

Called falling sickness, now commonly known as fits, is a sudden deprivation of the senses, with more or less convulsions. The trouble is most common to young people, who may be otherwise in good health, The fit may have premonitory symptoms, or come on at once, and after continuing from a few minutes to an hour, will pass away, leaving the patient usually as it found him. The causes of these dangerous visitations are, injuries to the head, water on the brain, deformity in the skull, tumours, affection of the spine, violent affections of the nervous system, sudden fright, fits of passion, emotion of the mind, worms in children, hereditary predisposition, and retention of menses, &c. Often it is impossible to assign any cause. The symptoms are well known, especially after one or two have taken place. It is likely, however, to be mistaken for apoplexy by the inexperienced. There are two or three points of difference which will distinguish them. In apoplexy the pupils are dilated, in epilepsy contracted. In the former convulsions are not frequent; in epilepsy they are present, the teeth firmly set, and the tongue often badly bitten. These and the oft-recurrence of epilepsy will show the difference between the two forms of fits.

TREATMENT.—When the patient feels the symptoms of a coming attack, which are various—headache, giddiness, specks floating in the sight, tremour, cold numbness of the limbs—let full doses of the antispasmodic tincture be given every hour. If the stomach is loaded, let an emetic be given, and an injection, unless the bowels are free. This will often ward off or lessen the severity of an attack. A piece of wood, in the form of a gag, should be carried or at hand. When it does happen, open waistcoat and neck surroundings, put the wood in the mouth to prevent the tongue from being chewed; then as gently as possible give in sips the antispasmodic tincture, half a teaspoonful in half a cup of water, sweetened. When recovered, a regular medicine should be taken. Make a decoction of—

Wood Betony .... One ounce.
Vervain............................ One ounce.
Catnip .... One ounce.
Fit Root .... One ounce.

Simmer in three pints of water ten minutes ; strain, and add one ounce of antispasmodic tincture. Take a wineglassful three or four times a day.   Rub the spine from the neck down with the stramonium ointment; keep the bowels free with the compound rhubarb pills. If the patient is of a robust constitution, a course of medicine once a week would be advisable, (if caused by painful menstruation or suppression.) (See index.) There are other remedies which have been found good. The simplest of all is fine salt, a teaspoonful in water twice a day; extract stramonium, two to three grains, in pill form night and morning. Dr. Chase gives oxide of zinc in powder, commencing at half a grain up to three grains three times a day with the stramonium ointment to the spine. There is another—the velerinate of zinc, same doses, and the bromide of ammonia, in a half to drachm doses, three or four times a day. This is combined with the potass salts. Caution.— People subject to fits should not follow dangerous occupations, as serious consequences may happen. Avoid fat meats, excesses of all kinds, live on plain food, never load the stomach, but rise from the table with the appetite unappeased.

PALSY (PARALYSIS),

Is a loss of power, partial or complete, in a part or parts of the body ; it very often affects only one side.   This is due to

the fact that the brain is divided into two halves, each
half sending its nerves and stimulus to the opposite side of
the body. When only one side of the body is affected it is
called hemiplegia; when the upper or lower portion, para-
plegia; if only a limb, it is paralysis. Causes: Obstruction,
pressure on the nerves by tumours, effusions, dislocations,
injuries especially to the head or spine, atrophy of the brain,
lead poisoning. It often follows an attack of apoplexy; in
short, anything that enervates the system may be an inducing
cause. Treatment: Should the attack come on suddenly,
as it often does, with excitment and twitching of the muscles,
a strong nerve sedative must be given. The following is
good :—

Gelseminum .... Half ounce.
Spirits of Camphor .... Half ounce.
Ether............................ Quarter ounce.
Laudanum........................ Quarter ounce.

Mix, and give a teaspoonful in a cupful of the infusion of
hops, valerian, or skullcap. Give this every half hour till the
spasms relax. If the patient is in good health the course of
medicine once or twice a week will do good; if too weak for
this, use the milder means to restore the natural circulation
of the blood. If the lower part of the body is paralysed and
the bowels lose power of action, an enema of elm and antispasmodic powder or tincture will be required. Local steamings
to the parts affected, and stimulating liniments should be used.
Keep the bowels open with the Comp Leptandrum Powder.
Make a mixture of the nervines :—

Prickly Ash Bark...................... One ounce.
Valerian .... One ounce.
Skullcap .... One ounce.
Wild Cherry......................... One ounce.
Poplar Bark......................... One ounce.

In three pints of water. Boil down to two, strain, add two
ounces tincture of cayenne. Take a wineglassful three times

a day, and a teaspoonful of tincture avena sativa in warm water, sweetened if preferred.

HYSTERIA, OR HYSTERICS,

Is a nervous trouble, supposed at one time to be due to uterine derangement, but it is found to happen when, to all appearance, the womb is in its normal condition. The causes are, sudden emotion of the mind, irregular menstruation, indigestion, constipation, worms, &c. Treatment: Give antispasmodic tincture, put the feet in hot water and mustard, put cold water on the face and head. Prevention: Correct the digestion, treat the symptoms as directed under respective heads, calm the mind, take out-door exercise, weather permitting, seek cheerful company, live in hope—the hope of eternal life and happiness, which is within the reach of all. (See New Testament.) Some of our readers may scoff at this advice. We give it, however, in the conviction that it is the very best that can be given, not only for the life to come, but also for the present.

ST. VITUS DANCE (CHOREA).

This disease consists of a partial loss of control over the voluntary muscles. Nervous derangement is the direct cause. It is often confined to one side of the body or only a part of it, and may be induced by anything that throws the system out of harmony. Treatment: Nervine medicine. Take the nervine pills and a mixture of—

Skullcap	One ounce.
Burdock Seed, crushed	One ounce.
Wood Betony	One ounce.
St. John's Wort	One ounce.

Steep in a quart of boiling water, when cold strain, and if preferred sweeten and take a wineglassful three times a day; children according to age. Rub the spine with a strong

SOOTHING OINTMENT.

Vaseline	One ounce.
Extract of Stramonium	One drachm.
Extract of Cannabis Indica	Half drachm.

Rub in night and morning, attend to the general health, and we feel certain a cure will result.

LOCKJAW (TETANUS),

Is usually a fatal nerve affection. When treated by the profession we think we are justified in saying all the cases that have occurred in Dunedin have been lost, and why? Simply because the doctors refused to try the means which have saved hundreds. The last case that happened was one in point. A builder trod on an upturned nail, which penetrated the sole of his foot. In a short time symptoms of lockjaw appeared, which advanced till they were firmly set. Two of the leading lights in the profession were in attendance trying many things. A friend of the patient came to us and asked if we could cure it. We replied that we thought so, in fact we were confident. He hastened to inform the friends and ask them if we might come and treat him. He was told that they had the best medical advice, and preferred to leave the case in their hands, but the case soon slipped out of their hands into the grave. The causes of this much-to-be-dreaded condition are severe injuries, especially to the palms of the hands and soles of the feet. Treading on rusty nails is the most frequent cause. When the accident happens wash in warm water, apply pledgets of lint soaked in tincture of gum myrrh over the wound for an hour; keep them soaked; then put on a poultice of slippery elm and lobelia, renew when cold. This may prevent the spasm, if not, give the vapour bath and the antispasmodic tincture; rub the neck and jaws with it, put to bed, hot brick to feet, and if relaxation has not taken place continue the tincture every half hour till it takes effect, then in smaller doses with doses of nerve powder. Dr. Coffin's treatment was a teaspoonful of cayenne and the vapour bath. In cases where you cannot get the patient to swallow give an injection of slippery elm with a teaspoonful of the antipasmodic tincture in it, or a teaspoonful of the antispasmodic powder. Persevere with the medicine and give one, two, or three vapour-baths till they take effect, about six hours apart. It may be a hard fight for life, but we have never heard of failure when similar means have been used.

GENERAL DISEASES.

HYDROPHOBIA (Rabies).

It is a blessing that this distressing and dangerous disease is unknown in the colonies : it is generally communicated by the bite of a rabid animal—mostly the dog. The poison is absorbed into the circulation in a shorter or longer time. The symptoms of the disease—inflammation and pain—take place at the wound. Spasms of the muscles, a dread of liquids, especially water, are manifest. These give the disease its name. In severe cases the wretched sufferer will try to bite even his own friends, because he is now mad. His saliva, coming in contact with a wound, would communicate the poison. It sometimes happens that a number of persons will be bitten by a mad dog, and only one or two will develop the disease ; this is no doubt on account of the saliva being wiped off in the passage of the teeth through the cloth when bitten. The wound should be washed by syringing out with warm water, then a solution of caustic potash ; then apply the yeast and elm poultice, and give a course of medicine as soon as possible, and one every day till danger is past. Give a strong decoction of the bark of the roots of the ash tree and skullcap ; drink freely of it, a quart a day. A French doctor was cured himself, and he cured 80 others by the vapour-bath alone. If the dread of water should prevent the administration of medicine, give by the rectum, the antispasmodic tincture or the fever powder. A teaspoonful of either may be injected. Pasteur's method has not been so successful as the above simple means in curing this dreadful disease. A German remedy is to wash the wound in vinegar and water, and pour on it hydrochloric acid, which neutralises the poison.

SNAKE BITES.

In some parts of the colonies snakes are common, and colonists are often bitten. The first thing to be done is to put a ligature tightly around the limb. a short distance above the bite ; the wound must be sucked vigorously, even if the patient cannot do it himself. There is no danger, as you can swallow the poison, it kills only through contact with the blood. Next put on a poultice. Mashed onions and salt are recommended, or slippery elm yeast with charcoal, and lobelia. Before undoing the ligature. which should be kept on for fifteen to thirty minutes, let out the blood gathered in the superficial veins ; then dose the patient with whiskey and ammonia— ammonia one part. whiskey nine. Give it till intoxication, and keep it up till danger is past. It is wonderful how much can be taken while this poison is in the blood. Produce a free sweating by means of hot bricks and vinegar, and after 1½ hours give the ash and skullcap infusion as in the last It is affirmed that this is a perfect antidote by one who has seen severe cases treated by it and cured.

COLD AND CATARRH.

The causes of cold are too numerous to mention, nor is it necessary, since every one knows when they have taken one. neither age, sex, nor constitution is exempt from cold, for all are liable to it. We shall simply say that a cold is the first ta ge of fever or inflammation occasioned by obstruction in the circulation of the blood or closing up the pores of the skin, which are the natural outlets for the exhausted or waste material brought to the surface of the body, and discharged through the million little outlets prepared by nature for this purpose. This wasted material is the refuse of the blood, and can be no more suffered to remain without doing injury than can the refuse of the food taken into the stomach and bowels after the nutrition has been extracted. We all know the danger of confined or obstructed bowels, but overlook the danger of obstructed perspiration.

The symptoms are, tightness of the chest, running at the nose, stiffness, and soreness of the eyes, sneezing, listlessness pains in the head, cough, shivering, &c. If the cold is very severe it is called influenza, and is sometimes epidemic. Some time ago it was very common in Melbourne. An amusing story is told which illustrates the power of faith as a factor in the healing process. A young man, clerk in a shipping office, was coughing and sneezing at a great rate, when one of his companions asked him if he had heard of the new remedy. He replied, "No; but I wish I could get something that would cure me; what is the new remedy?" The other said, "It is two pills, they are called the genuine Mozambique Pills, one shilling each; but you do not want any other medicine, as a cure is certain." "Well, I'll try them, will you get me two, here is the two shillings? The other replied that he would when he went to lunch. After dinner he rolled up two pills out of bread crumbs, called at a chemist's, got a small pink pill-box and a dust of magnesia, and took them to the influenza man with directions to take them on going to bed. In the morning, when asked how he felt, he replied that he was very much better, and he believed that the pills had done him a deal of good. It took the joker all his time to keep from bursting. However, it leaked out during the day how he had been sold. He hit upon a plan to make it even with his funny companion, so he put in a small advertisement, intimating that this cure for influenza— the real Mozambique pills—could only be obtained at (giving the joker's address), who, when he had set himself for a quiet evening at home, was called to the door to see someone who wanted Mozambique pills. We did not learn how he got out of the difficulty, but it is affirmed that there was knock after knock at the door for these pills that night. Practical joking is generally paid back with interest, as it was in this case.

The causes of colds are as well known as the symptoms, and yet most people act as though they did not know them, they are so careless in exposing themselves. In addition to the one already mentioned—neglect of the skin—there is no greater one than that of cold and damp feet. What may be called the two cold-producing areas of the body are the feet and neck. In civilised life the feet are encased in boots, which hinder the free perspiration, causing a dampness, which is re-absorbed. This is one way colds are induced; keeping on damp clothes is another; a damp cold atmosphere, and sudden changes from heat to cold, standing in draughts, &c., are all known causes, which, acting on a system not in the best of health, cause the condition so well known. We need not point out the folly of neglect, for although colds may come and go without treatment, it is not always so; sometimes they come and stay, or in going leave something worse behind. Let no one then neglect to shake them off as soon as possible by a proper treatment: take the stitch in time. Now, our readers may anticipate our advice—the course of medicine, or a modified form of it, the composition powder, the vapour bath, and the lobelia emetic, will cut it short; or the yarrow treatment (page 79). There are few simple colds that will withstand these, but if they have get a hold on the system a continuance of the above or stronger measures must be adopted. The Balm of Gilead (see index) will cure both coughs and colds. If it is severe, as in

BRONCHITIS,

Treat as directed for inflammation of the chest, using the balm, hot bricks, &c. The cough powder is also good. There are numberless remedies for colds and coughs, two or three of which we will give besides the above, which are first in point of merit.

No. 1.

Horehound........................	One ounce.
Hyssop	One ounce.
Yarrow	One ounce.
Ground Ivy.......................	One ounce.
Chilies.......	One drachm.
Linseed	Two drachms.
Or Slippery Elm	Four drachms.

Simmer in three pints of water; cool, strain, add half a pound
of lump sugar; warm; dissolve, and add two ounces of
tincture of lobelia. This is equal to half an ounce of the herb,
which may be simmered with the herbs instead. Take from a
half to a wineglassful four to six times a day.

No. 2.

For a hacking cough take—

Syrup Ipecac.....................	One ounce.
Syrup Tolu	One ounce.
Tincture Wild Cherry	One ounce.
Balsam Peru	Half ounce.
Essence Peppermint	Twenty drops.

One or two teaspoonfuls four to six times a day.

No. 3.

Take of—

Saltpetre........................	Quarter ounce.
Oxymel (Honey) of Squills	Half ounce.
Ipecacuanha Wine.................	Quarter ounce.
Spirits of Sweet Nitre	Two ounces.
Tincture Digitalis................	One drachm.

Add water to six ounces, one to two teaspoonfuls, four times a
day. This one is good when there is pain in the back. These
will suffice; if not, look up diaphoretics and stimulants, and
try them. When there is cold or catarrh in the head, take the
headache pills, and inhale the vapour of menthol or essence of
eucalyptus in this way: get a cup half full of hot water, put in a

pinch of menthol, or a half teaspoonful of the eucalyptus, and draw in the steam. The menthol is the best. It is also good for running at the nose.

CHRONIC CATARRH.

This condition, the result of neglected colds, is very stubborn, and, in some cases, incurable when it is connected with a syphilitic taint. Whatever kind of medicine is taken, the course of medicine once a week is invaluable, and should not be neglected. Use the compound decoction of sarsaparilla or the mixture (see p. 393), the inhalation of menthol or yarrow ; and as the throat is generally implicated, use the gargle as in chronic laryngitis, with a syringeful up the nostrils. There are several kinds of snuffs prescribed, which may be tried as helps to remove it :—

> Morphia .... Four grains.
> Cinnamon, in powder................ Two drachms.
> Trisnitrate of Bismuth .... Four drachms.
> Snuff up occasionally.

Another :—
> Golden Seal, in fine powder.......... Half ounce.
> Morphia .... Five grains.
> Gum Arabic....................... Half ounce,

Or pinus canadensis instead of the golden seal ; an infusion of the pinus or hemlock bark, one ounce coarse powder to a pint of boiling water, with four ounces of the white extract of witch hazel. Mix, and use as a gargle, and syringe up the nostrils. Keep the bowels and the kidneys clear, and great benefit, or a perfect cure, will be the reward.

BLEEDINGS.

External are usually the result of cuts or wounds. If a clean cut, and not severing any of the arteries or large veins, the simplest treatment for them is to draw the edges together and keep them in position by a strip of adhesive plaster. If it is only a small cut a rag with a little wound salve or Friar's balsam will be sufficient. If an artery is cut it will be needful to put on a ligature above the cut, holding the finger, thumb, or hand over the wound while this is being done. As a blood stauncher Dr. Chase gives a mixture, claiming that it will stop bleeding from any, even large blood-vessels. Mix:

Whisky	Two ounces.
Castille Soap.......................	Two drachms.
Carbonate of Potash...............	One drachm.

Scrape the soap fine, dissolve in the spirit, and add the potash; keep corked. Warm it and soak pledgets of lint and apply them. They will need to be repeated if the wounds are deep or limbs torn off. A strong solution of alum is also good, or tannic acid.

INTERNAL BLEEDINGS

From the nose, if caused by falls or blows, are as a rule easier stopped than those which are spontaneous. Simple bathing in cold water with alum or vinegar added, if not severe, will be sufficient. A cup of composition to equalise the circulation will be beneficial. If the bleeding continues after simple means have failed, prepare a strong decoction of—

Bistort Root.......................	One ounce,
Comfrey Root......................	One ounce,

To a quart of water; take a cup three parts full of it and fill up with tincture of marigolds; inject some up the nostrils with a syringe; put a teaspoonful of cayenne pepper and sugar in the rest of the decoction, and take a wineglassful every hour till bleeding stops. If it does not stop when this is done, try some of the first styptic mixture; dilute it with an equal part of water, and sniff it or use the syringe If all these fail, which we hardly think they will, try Doctor Coffin's cure, namely: a teaspoonful of cayenne pepper in a cupful of sweetened water. This cured a man whose nose had bled for eight days. In desperate cases try and find out the cause and work for its removal. A hot brick to the feet will draw down the blood from the head, to which cold may be applied.

BLEEDING FROM THE MOUTH, TEETH, AND GUMS.

Strong astringents, washes, or gargles must be used. Look up astringents, (page 28). If a tooth has been extracted and bleeds, the dentist ought to have put in a proper styptic. We have never found any trouble in stopping bleeding with a piece of cotton-wool soaked in chloroform put in the cavity. Blood sometimes comes from the stomach It may be distinguished from that which comes from the lungs by its colour, being dark. The astringent decoction of comfrey and bistort without the cayenne should be taken , with the digestive food and a light diet.

BLEEDING FROM THE LUNGS

At one time this was thought to be a fatal symptom, but there are many cases, some of which we have known, where bleeding occasionally occurred without any great disturbance to the health ; however, it is usually dangerous, and no time should be lost in trying to remedy it. No matter what the causes are, the system cannot afford to lose the blood, especially the pure oxydized as it comes from the lungs. Its bright scarlet colour will determine that it is from them, also the fact that it is raised by coughing. Treatment : Put the feet in hot water and mustard. If there is any ice procurable swallow a few pieces. Put half an ounce of tannic acid into a bottle, fill with hot water, and suck down the steam. Make a medicine of the astringents, thus—

Bistort Root .... One ounce.
Tormentil .... One ounce.
Comfrey Root, crushed .... One ounce.

Simmer in three pints of water for 20 minutes; take off the fire and put in one ounce of sweet bugle herb; give a wineglassful every half hour if the bleeding is much; four times a day if only spitting it occasionally. From an American author we see a simple remedy given—table salt. Dr. Rush cured a patient with two teaspoonfuls when all other means failed; three to six teaspoonfuls daily while it continues. (See page 32 for another remedy).

Bleeding from the bowels is generally caused by piles. However, it may come from other parts of the intestines. If the means used for bleeding piles do not take effect, take the above medicine. All internal bleedings will be amenable to this treatment.

HEART AFFECTIONS.

Palpitation of the heart is usually a symptom of indigestion which, when cured, it disappears. This is the rule; but there are exceptions If the means for the cure of indigestion have failed, take an infusion of tansy and skullcap, one ounce each in a quart of boiling water; half a teacupful three times a day, with two compound motherwort pills night and morning. If the trouble comes from heart disease, take tincture of lily of the valley, a teaspoonful three times a day. The new remedy—tincture strophanthus—two to ten drops three times a day, or cactus grandiflora, twenty drops three times a day

These are given as remedies, and may be tried in turn if the others fail.

HYPERTROPHY OF THE HEART.

This is a condition which results from acute inflammation degenerating to the chronic. The enlargement seems to be in some cases a provision of nature to make up for what is termed valvular insufficiency; that is, some of the blood returns to the heart, because on account of the valves not sufficiently covering the openings. Those experienced in sounding the chest well are able to detect the unhealthy sounds called regurgitation murmurs, besides the greater space the enlarged heart occupies in the chest. The symptoms of this disease are, shortness of breath, especially going up hills or stairs, pain or uneasy feeling over the region, sometimes affecting the arms, palpitation, &c. Treatment: Avoid violent exercise, such as running, jumping, heavy work, excitement of any kind. Attend to the laws of health; that is, keep the organs in good order, and take the following :—

Sweet Bugle .... One ounce.
Motherwort .... One ounce.
Lily of the Valley, in coarse powder .. One ounce.
Digitalis .... Quarter ounce.

Infuse in three pints of boiling water; take a wineglassful three times a day; in summer time only make half mixtures, as they will not keep. Sweetening with glycerine will preserve the herb mixtures. Put a compound gallanum plaster (heart-shaped) on, and take a light and nourishing diet.

OSSIFICATION

Is a condition spoken of, but is never fully developed, as it would be impossible to live with a physical hard heart. We might do without one of the duplicated organs, but we have only one heart, which, when it ceases to beat, we cease to live. Notwithstanding this, there is a disease which consists of a partial ossification of the valves. A chalk-like substance appears on the edges, which gives rise to the trouble. The

general opinion is that this is a result of rheumatic affections.
This deposit is similar to that found in the joints of some
chronic rheumatic patients. The symptoms are similar to the
former, with, in advanced cases, dropsy. It is generally
thought that nothing can be done for such cases of heart
affection, but we think otherwise. The treatment for chronic
rheumatism, in combination with diuretics and heart tonics,
will, at least, benefit and ward off the end. However,
perseverance will be indispensable. We would recommend
the following as a heart tonic :—

> Fluid Extract of Lily of the Valley .... One ounce
> Tincture of Strophanthus .... Half ounce.
> Water .... Eight ounces

A teaspoonful three times a day in the mixture for chronic
rheumatism If dropsy is present, take it in the decoction
recommended for it.

FATTY DEGENERATION

Is another affection to which the heart is liable. It is seldom
found, except in the aged, and is most likely to occur in the
corpulent The same class of symptoms, and a similar
treatment to the above adopted, with the antifat mixture
(See Obesity, index)

ANGINA PECTORIS, OR BREAST PANG,

Is one of the most painful and alarming affections of the
heart. Symptoms : A sudden pain is felt at the lower part of
the breast-bone, which spreads over the region of the heart,
and, in fact, over the chest and arms, there is a loss of
breath, a sense of suffocation, the countenance becomes
deadly pale, there is great anxiety, and a cold perspiration
breaks over the skin When the trouble first commences, it does
not usually last long ; perfect stillness and rest seem to soothe
it away But in time, unless the disease is checked, the
attacks may be so violent that the strongest anodynes must be
given to ease the dreadful pain. The paroxysms, as a rule,
leave as suddenly as they come. The cause is certainly

a spasm, which some high in profession say is neuralgaic Others deny this and affirm it to be rheumatic. It matters little, as they are both of the same class. The cure is the thing to know, and we are happy to say that in the antispasmodic tincture we have a reliable remedy, from a half to a teaspoonful in a like amount of cold or warm water. Taken at the beginning of the spasm, it relaxes at once, and it also acts as a preventive. Look after the general health, take the digestive food, compound leptandrum pd. for regulating the bowels; don't use stimulants, nor engage in violent exercise, for this is usually the inducing cause. The treatment of the faculty is now the inhalation of nitrate of amyl, which is encased in globules, one of them is broken and inhaled. It is well to have something at hand, as it is very sudden. Before leaving these heart troubles, let us give a few symptoms which will enable the reader to determine the four principal heart conditions.

Atrophy or wasting of the heart may be concluded from the general debility of the patient, giddiness, fainting, feeble and irregular pulse, painful and oppressive breathing, cold extremities, puffy countenance, extreme prostration.

Hypertrophy, by the enlargement and increased force of the action, percussion; and inspecting the chest, will also confirm the diagnosis.

Dilatation may be known by the tremulous, fluttering, irregularity of the pulse, fullness of the veins, in some of which a pulsation may be felt, difficulty of breathing, drowsiness, and general debility.

Valvular disease may be determined by the stout, puffy appearance of the patient, difficult breathing. It is generally associated with degeneration of the liver or other internal organs. What Solomon wrote in his book of Proverbs regarding the affections, called the heart—" Keep thy heart with all diligence, for out of it are the issues of life "—we would transpose somewhat and say, Look after your health with all diligence, and your heart will look after itself, as it works on independently of our will power.

CHEST AFFECTIONS.

ASTHMA

Is a spasmodic affection of the nerves of the lungs. Its symptoms are too well known to need pointing out. The causes are hereditary, or frequently the result of chest affections, unhealthy occupations, malformation of the chest, pregnancy, liver and heart affections, neglected colds, &c. Treatment : Attend to whatever complications may exist. When a fit comes on immerse the feet in warm water and mustard. Take composition to equalise the circulation. Burn half a teaspoonful of the asthma powder, and inhale the smoke. This will nearly always relieve the attack, which is all that can be done in most cases, especially when the patient is up in years. Still we can help by judicious medication to lessen the frequencey and force of the spasms. The virtues of lobelia inflata we have pointed out in our description (see page 33). Try this, see its effects ; if it does not cure, make this mixture :—

Comfrey Root	Two ounces.
Skunk Cabbage....................	One ounce.
Solomon Seal	One ounce.

Crush, and simmer these roots in two quarts of water, 15 or 20 minutes, then put in—

Lobelia	Half ounce.
Stramonium	Quarter ounce.
Hyssop	One ounce.
Vervain	One ounce.
Chilies..........................	One drachm.

Let them remain on the fire five minutes more, strain, and add one pound of crude glycerine ; take a tablespoonful three or four times a day. The cough powder may be taken in change with this, or the expectorant, or cough syrup. If the trouble should be complicated with heart or kidney disease, take this mixture :—

Extract of Buchu	One ounce.
Sweet Nitre.......................	Three ounces.

Mix, and take a teaspoonful in an infusion of euphorbia pilefuria (p. 144). There are a host of remedies for asthma, but our space will not allow of more than another in the form of a powder for burning. Take—

Grindelia Robusta	One ounce.
Jaborandi Leaves	One ounce.
Blue Gum Leaves	Half ounce.
Foxglove Leaves.................	Half ounce.
Stramonium.....................	Two ounces.
Cubebs.........................	Half ounce.
Saltpetre	One and a half ozs.
Cascarilla Bark	One ounce.

All ground and mixed. Burn from a quarter to a teaspoonful at a time, and inhale the smoke. Do not smoke tobacco, but a mixture of coltsfoot and stramonium leaves, with a few aniseeds, or the herbal tobacco instead.

CONSUMPTION (Phthisis).

We have no space for the usual long introduction and sympathetic moralisings common to medical writers when introducing this subject. Much of its terribleness belongs to the unfortunate circumstances of the poor in the densely-peopled parts of the older lands ; still it is far too prevalent in the colonies, not so much among the native born as those who have either had it when they came, or were sent out with the hope of a cure. The causes are, hereditary taint, unhealthy occupations, neglected colds, want of attention to the laws of health, dancing in a heated room, going out into the cold, damp atmosphere, self-abuse : in fact anything that militates against the health. The symptoms of consumption are, a higher temperature than normal, a quickened pulse, a short cough, a gradual softening of the muscles and shortening of the breath. These may be considered the premonitory symptoms. They should not be neglected, as in almost every case they grow in intensity. We have noticed persons with hese clearly marked signs who for a long time have resisted the dreaded conviction that their lungs were going, and blamed the liver, which certainly was more or less affected, in sympathy. It is no use shutting the eyes to unwelcome truths, as by so doing the means of remedy are often neglected. The question often asked is, Can consumption be cured ? At one time, after reading some herbal books we did not hesitate to answer, yes ; but experience has taught us to be more careful, and now compels us to say, yes, and no ; having treated a number of cases, some of whom recovered, and some are now covered up in the bosom of mother earth. If the reader turns to page 335 he will see the way in which by sounding the chest we may be more certain in identifying the disease. These, with what we have already given, and the expectoration of matter or pus (which may be known from its yellow colour and density, it usually sinking in water) will determine the grave nature of the disease. It will be asked, How can we know when it is curable or not ? We cannot always tell. However, there are indications which will help us to make a prognosis or conclusion. First, What is the family history ? Is there consumption on both sides ? Is the chest narrow, and are there well-marked hollows on the top of the shoulders ? Can you hear the patient whisper through them ? Is the body much wasted and the expectoration great ? Are there the night-sweats, with hectic fever and diarrhœa ? There is not much hope for such cases ; all that can be done is to alleviate the symptoms as best we can. The more hopeful cases are when the patient has come of a sound family, and the disease has not advanced far ; but human wisdom is very faulty, and hopeful cases are lost, and the hopeless ones saved.

The treatment will greatly depend upon the indications present in each case. Age, strength, and stage of disease, must be considered and treatment adopted. In the first stages many have been cured by Thompson's plan : the full course once a week, with the stomach bitters, and sufficient lobelia in the spirit tincture to keep up a free expectoration. Even in what appeared to be the most hopeless cases, when doctors had given the patient up, this treatment has saved.

Dr Coffin did not enforce the vapour bath or the emetic, but gave the following mixture :—

Raspberry Leaves.................. Half ounce.
Agrimony .... Half ounce.
Clivers .... Half ounce.
Barbary Bark .... Half ounce.
Horehound .... Half ounce.
Ground Ivy .... Half ounce.
Centuary .... Half ounce.

Simmered in a quart of water 15 minutes; strain, and add half a teaspoonful of cayenne pepper and a quarter of an ounce of spanish juice, a wineglassful four times a day. Half a teaspoonful of the acid tincture of lobelia, and a cupful of the stomach bitters, three times a day, is all his treatment, which has been instrumental in rescuing many from an early grave. Dr. Fox's treatment has also cured many. It is as follows: omitting the vapour bath, he prescribed the emetic of lobelia once or twice a week, a poultice of barley meal, one inch in thickness, on the chest during the day, and the following mixture :—

Liquorice Root .... Two ounces.
Cherry Bark .... Two ounces.
Horehound .... Two ounces.
Vervain .... Two ounces.
Centuary........................ One ounce.
Bone Set........................ One ounce.

Add two quarts, boil down to three pints; strain, and add half a teaspoonful of cayenne, and two ounces of

RASPBERRY TINCTURE OF LOBELIA,

made as follows :—

Take half a pound of honey and a cupful of water; let these boil, take off the scum, pour boiling hot upon half an ounce of lobelia herb and half an ounce of cloves; mix well, then strain and add a gill of raspberry vinegar. Take from a teaspoonful to a dessertspoonful four times a day. The above medicine is taken 10 to 14 days, then change for the following :—

Wild Cherry Bark..................	Two ounces.
Comfrey Root	Two ounces.
Mouse Ear.......................	Two ounces.
Columba.........................	One ounce.
Ground Ivy	One ounce.
Peruvian Bark	One ounce.

Boil these in the same manner, and add the cayenne and raspberry tincture. Take also the cough pills made as follows :—

COUGH PILLS.

Gum ammoniacum	One ounce.
Lobelia...........................	Half ounce.
Ipecacuanha	Half ounce.
Black Hellebore	Half ounce.
Extract of Balm of Gilead	Half ounce.
Cayenne	Half ounce.
Gum Arabic Powder	Half ounce.
Oil of Spearmint..................	Twenty drops.

Bruise the gum ammoniacum, add a tablespoonful of water to it, simmer in the oven in a jar a few minutes, and when dissolved add syrup of squills, sufficient to form into pills. Take one with each dose of the decoction. This treatment must be persevered in to the very letter; for the patient may depend upon it no half measure will effect a cure; and the reason that many fail is because they expect to be cured by magic. They take one or two doses, and it is either nauseous or some kind friend tells them it will kill them. They then abandon the treatment, and the botanic system is blamed for not having cured cases where the failure is altogether attributable to the patient.

The emetics are of the utmost importance, as they cleanse the whole system, removing the tough and ropy phlegm, and breaking up the ulcers; the medicines are healing, and while they correct the circulating fluids they also improve the general health. The diet must be light and nourishing—beef tea, mutton chops, sago, tapioca, marmalade instead of butter (see Diet), and exercise in the open air; but damp atmosphere must be avoided. Removing northwards in winter would be advantageous. Intoxicating drinks may not be taken, as they inflame the lungs and aggravate the symptoms. When the patient feels languid, a dose of composition, strained and sweetened, would have a good effect.

The two treatments are about the average of all the botanical doctors we have read from time to time. There are new remedies and modes of treatment announced, with more or less confidence on the part of the discoverers, some of whom are only advertising medicine men who can either manufacture testimonials, or get others to do it. There is hardly a year that does not see some new cure, but the one that sees them in as often sees them out.

What we would recommend ourselves is a course of medicine once a week; the balm of gilead, or Coffin's mixture, in a wineglassful of strong infusion of mullen plant, one ounce to the pint, strained, and sweetened with brown sugar. As a strengthening food and medicine, take a teaspoonful of a mixture of powdered comfrey root and elm, boiled in a half pint of milk; blend the powder with a teaspoonful of sugar and a little milk; add the rest gradually; let it come to the boil. We think this is superior to cod liver oil, still if the stomach is able to digest it, some of the oil may be taken with this, a teaspoonful, stirred up with it will form a partial emulsion. If the stomach is weak, a dose of pepsin may be added to the cupful of elm and comfrey food. We imagine some of our readers say, Who on earth could take all that medicine—balm of gilead, mullen, comfrey, slippery, cod liver oil, pepsin? Yes, and a cup of composition tea to boot. Don't be alarmed. When you may know that it is as much a food as it is medicine. Were it drugs, you might stand aghast, but the simples will not injure. We have met with doctors in America who believed strongly in whisky for consumption. They could not give a clear reason for its curative effect, but affirmed that it hindered the progress of decay in the lungs, they having noted it in their own practice. As we **cannot** afford to despise any remedy which others have found beneficial, we would suggest that a tincture, in which the whisky will be combined with other healing herbs, may be tried. The spirit will extract more of their virtue than water. Take—

Marigold Flowers with the green part
    attached .... One ounce.
Yerba Santa........................ One ounce.
Whisky .... One quart.

Steep together one week, and take a tablespoonful in water three times a day. The inhalation of oil of peppermint, ten drops in a cup of hot water, is also said to cure ; if not, it will do good. Some speak hopefully of creosote, which is now on trial. (See index.) The latest alleged remedy is a high temperature. It is affirmed that the kind of bacillis that infests the lungs cannot exist in a high temperature. Several trials have been made, and it is affirmed that there were indications of cure. This is only on trial, yet it may also do good. Breathe in air as hot as you can three times a day (see index). In the first development of the trouble many have been cured by going to sea, or changing to a higher district and drier climate. All these things are useful to know, although it is not always possible to act out our knowledge. (See food for consumptives.)

To correct the night-sweats, sponge the body over every morning with this mixture :

Vinegar .... One cupful.
Cayenne .... One teaspoonful.
Salt .... One handful.
Water .... One pint.

Take a cupful of sage tea at bed-time. After the hot sweats, rub dry with a warm towel before there is time for the cold stage to come on ; a cupful of composition will be good. Just a word or two on the

FEAR OF DEATH,

which is common to all creatures. This is a natural instinct for self-preservation, and notwithstanding the popular belief which some sincerely entertain, of being in heaven the moment the breath leaves, there is still a clinging to life. The best of men are in no hurry to die, unless their bodies are racked with unendurable pain. Our own belief, which we have as a result of studying the Word of God, is that in death there is no life; that the dead are sleeping in the dust till the trump of God shall awaken them. The righteous will be raised with an immortal pain-proof, glorious body, animated with spirit instead of blood as this one. How about the other class? The Scripture declares they shall perish! Thank God this does not mean they shall live for ever in hell or torment. But excuse us for this digression. Some will say, What has this got to do with medicine? Just this, that a calm and hopeful view of death is conducive to recovery. To our readers who may be consumptive and look, with a certain amount of horror, at the near approach of death, we wish to correct this state of mind. To the believer in Christ, who has done the will of God, there is the glad prospect of an eternal life of happiness, which will be increased with the realisation of this truth, that sin, suffering and death will be no more.

ALCOHOLISM OR DRUNKENNESS,

Although self-induced, it is still a diseased condition of the stomach. The difficulty about cure lies in the fact that the victim is a slave to or a worshipper of the drink, which is his mortal enemy. What power can help a man when he is bent on his own destruction? That Power which he does not seek, nor will till he sees his own helplessness and sin. Some of this sort even try to excuse their folly. Here is an example: A friend of ours was holding forth on the Melbourne wharf one Sunday. In his discourse he mentioned that the religion of Christ was the only one that commanded a man to love his enemies. Later on he turned on drink and denounced it as an enemy of man. After his discourse, one of his hearers, we suppose a drinker, saw a point and said, "Mister, did you not say that we were to love our enemies?" "Yes," replied our friend. "And you also told us that drink was our enemy, then according to your own argument we ought to love drink; that is just what I do." The lecturer, who was a sharp-witted little man, scratched his head, and replied thus: "Yes, I told you to love your enemies, but recollect I never told you to swallow them." This is wherein the evil lies. Still there are many victims who wish to be cured of the love of drink. This being so, we rejoice in the fact that there is an abundance of remedies. 1st. Commence with small doses of stomach bitters, keep on for three months and victory is certain. 2nd:—

Red Peruvian Bark .... Two ounces.
Cinnamon .... Two ounces.
Cayenne Pepper .... Half ounce.
Rectified Spirit .... One pint.

Infuse one week.

Dose: A tablespoonful in water three to six times a day. 3rd. A Russian doctor gives it as a certain cure. (Get a doctor to do this):—A subcutaneous injection of strychnine one grain, in 200 grains of water. Inject five drops once a day for eight or ten days, and the cure is complete, the subject will then have a perfect loathing for spirits.

ACCIDENTS.

BURNS AND SCALDS.

The treatment of these painful sores is very important. In the first place our object is to ease the pain; in the second, to heal the parts in such a manner as that no scar or as little as

possible will be left. There is no pain so intense as that of
burning, and it is from this that the danger to life is great. It
has been proved that if but one third of the surface of the
body is burned or scalded death will certainly result from the
great pain, which the heart and nervous system are unable to
stand. This fact gives the lie to that horrible dogma which
some men teach and are foolish enough to think that it is
taught in the Bible, that the damned shall be forever burning
and never die. The second death is death and not life in
hell-fire, which place is also to be burned up. We cannot
think or write on this subject without feeling contempt and
indignation at such a God-dishonouring doctrine. But to
return, what shall we do in cases of burns or scalds? Nature,
we might say, teaches us. Apply cold water, wet soft cloths,
lay on the parts, renew when the pain returns, or keep them
immersed in the water. It will depend upon the extent
of the injury how long it will take to remove the pain. When
it is nearly gone, prick the blisters, cover with the healing
ointment spread on the surface of an elm poultice
made with cold milk. If the pain is great give a teaspoonful
of the anodyne tincture and composition tea. Do not
disturb the dressing for two days. When you dress it let
out any new blisters. Put on the ointment and poultice again
and renew once a day till the sore is clean, then dress with
the ointment till well. If the burn has been very severe, care
must be taken to prevent as much as possible the formation of
an unsightly scar. Apply a poultice of marigold flowers pounded
with a little castor oil or olive oil. There are a number
of remedies, as the linseed oil, lime water, and soda and water,
covering with flour, painting with varnish, &c., but in simple
burns we think none will surpass what we have given. If the
mouth should be scalded, gargle with borax and cold water,
drink slippery elm gruel with a little oil. In case of the clothes
catching fire, roll in blankets or carpets, get into water as soon
as possible, keep the whole body in with just enough out to
breathe with. If the face is burnt, wet cloths should be laid on
and renewed to keep down the pain; give the composition

powder and the anodyne tincture.   We have not seen or known of it being given, but a subcutaneous injection of morphia to deaden the feelings would keep away the fearful pain which is the chief cause of death in our opinion.   If what is termed proud flesh occurs it may be touched with the caustic potash or a little burnt alum sprinkled over before renewing the poultice.   Dr. Skelton gives as the best poultice, equal parts of slippery elm and white pound lily root powder mixed with sweet oil.   Dr Fox recommends a pint of linseed oil poured on cotton rags, set fire to, and the oil that drops from them to be used as a dressing.

Following the above we might now deal with other accidents of a like nature.

DROWNING

Is one of too frequent occurrence.   If the person has not been so long in the water as to preclude the hope of restoration, he should be, if a child, laid across the knees and moved gently to get the water out of the lungs and stomach.   If a grown person, lay him over a barrel or chair.   When this is done strip and wipe dry, put in warm blankets with hot bricks to fee and sides.   If the weather is warm and the sun shining, lay him in it.   The whole body should be rubbed well.   While this is being done one should hold the nostrils and blow into the mouth ; a bellows may be used, or the warm breath to inflate the lungs   Then make pressure on the chest to expel the breath.   Repeat this for some time.   Occasionally turn the patient over in such a way as to let any water out of his mouth. A stimulating enema may be given and the antispasmodic tincture in usual doses.   Another way the one recommended by the National Life Boat Society, is to raise the arms above the head as far as possible and lowering them alternately, make pressure on the chest to assist in its contraction and expansion.   The pressure should be made when the arms are lowered.   Persevere.   It takes sometimes two hours to revive one.   As an encouragement to perseverance it is affirmed that persons have been under the water for hours and restored by the above means. We have not seen it recommended, but the galvanic battery might be of use in the work of restoration. Try it if the above fails.

FREEZING.

In restoring animation in cases of apparent death or the stupor which precedes it, remove to a cold room, and if there is snow at hand rub the body with it till a natural redness appears. Give for a warm drink a teaspoonful of cayenne tincture in water, sweetened, every 15 minutes. Use the means to restore breathing as above, take into a warmer room, very gradually restore outside temperature, for the thawing process must, to be safe, begin from within. If any of the parts are frost-bitten the same care must be taken not to apply heat outwardly; if ulcers result (see page 318), treat for them. Do not be in a hurry to get dead parts amputated as nature often does more in restoring them than we think. A line of demarcation will form as in mortification. Some may say freezing is not likely to happen here, but it has happened. We know a young man who lost both lower limbs and is now walking on artificials.

CHILBLAINS

Are the mildest form of frost-bites. There are a great number of people who suffer from them, especially the young. To prevent them we would recommend a free use of composition tea; wear warm gloves, thick stockings and roomy boots. If not broken rub them with the external pain-killer or chilblain liniment, or a solution of washing soda (strong), iodine, creosote and oil of cade are also given as remedies. If broken use the chilblain or healing ointment.

FALL OR BLOW.

If the injury has been to the head, give antispas. tinc. and the treatment for apoplexy, (page 395); if to the body or limbs, see that no bones are broken; if they are, a medical man will be required, but it is not always easy to get them, so it will be in place to give a few hints on

BONE-SETTING.

When a bone is broken there results a greater or less degree of inflammation, which may be said to be the first process in repair. If the bone can be set before this has had time to develop, so much the better. Supposing we have a simple fracture, all that can be done is to put the limb in its natural position in splints with the comfrey poultice. (See page 68.) If there is swelling and deforming, caused by the muscles drawing the broken edges past each other, then put flannel round, and pour water as hot as can be borne, which will cause the muscles to relax, the bones now drawn into position must be secured by the splints and bandages.

DISLOCATIONS

Are reduced in a similar way. We are sorry space forbids us to go further into this.

STARVATION.

This may happen. A person found nearly dead must be very gently treated. The sensation of hunger is caused, figuratively speaking, by the stomach eating itself when it has nothing else to eat. As starvation of a serious kind will have caused injury to it, it will be better to give an injection of warm milk into the rectum; add slippery elm after a little, then give the digestive food by the mouth, with a little wine or tincture of marigold, in warm water and sugar. Gradually give the solid food as the stomach recovers, which it does soon under this treatment.

LIGHTNING STROKE,

Although it is of rare occurrence, so much so that medical writers seldom mention it, still it has and may happen at any time. The treatment is to dash cold water on the face and head; let it run down over the body. If this does not revive the sufferer in five minutes, strip off the clothes, dig a hole, bury up in a sitting position to the neck. The object is to abstract the electricity out of the body. As soon as the eyes open, shade them.

Take him out, move into a cool place, and wash with cold water. A hot drink of composition will finish the cure, if the injury is not beyond recovery.

NOXIOUS VAPOURS, GASES, &c.

Expose the patient to the open air, dash cold water on the face ; use the means for respiration in drowning.

ACCIDENTS WITH POISONS,
(See page 177.)

HANGING OR CHOKING.

In hanging, after cutting down loosen the rope and any clothing about the neck and chest ; place the patient in an easy position, give a dose of antispasmodic tincture ; if you cannot get it down the throat, give it by injection ; put a hot brick to the feet and sides. This treatment may restore, providing the neck is not broken. Choking by food sticking in the air passage generally happens with children. The custom of clapping them on the back will be first adopted. Examine or feel if you can remove the morsel with your fingers. A small pair of bent forceps, if at hand, may reach it. If the patient is getting black in the face, and an almost certainty of death, there is no time to run for a doctor, cut into the wind-pipe in this manner : Midway between the projection called Adam's apple and the top of the breast-bone, where you may feel the wind-pipe, make a perpendicular cut, about half an inch ; put on some of the blood stauncher, (page 408), if you have it ; if not, cut down till you come to the wind-pipe, pierce that carefully, then slip in a hollow, small tube, an open quill or pen-holder, or anything that will keep the wound open and let in and out the breath. Some of the faculty may blame us for giving such advice, but the proverb comes to our rescue—A drowning man will catch at a straw. If it is the only chance, why not use it ? Get medical help if you can.

FAINTING

Is a condition usually caused by a shock to the system, either mental or physical, although it often occurs from extreme debility. The direct cause is a partial stoppage of the heart's action. This is a wise provision of nature, which is sometimes the means of saving life. For instance, a person gets a limb torn off, or a lesser accident, in which some of the arteries are cut or torn. Were the heart to continue at its usual pace, the life current would escape, and, in all probability, the sufferer would bleed to death; but the blood pressure being lessened, the arteries and veins have time to contract, and the patient recovers, except in extreme cases.

TREATMENT.—Having already treated upon some accidents that cause fainting, we will only remind the reader that the causes should receive attention, and point out what is to be done. First, suppose it happens in a meeting. Remove to the open air, or into an airy room, lay on the back, wet the temples, rub the hands, apply the smelling salts to the nose. If the patient is not revived soon, give some antispasmodic tincture—tincture of cayenne or ginger. If any of the blood-vessels have been wounded, now is the time to bind them up. Where fainting results from sheer weakness, find out the cause and work for its removal; tonics and nervines are indicated here.

DEATH.

To determine when it has taken place, if breathing and circulation have ceased, life is gone. By holding the polished blade of a razor or knife to the mouth or close to the nostrils, if there is no moisture on it then there is no breath. Darken the room, hold a candle behind the fingers, if dead the red semi-transparence will be wanting. Place your ear over the left side of the chest, and if there is no heart-beat, circulation has ceased. These, with the coldness, the glazed eyes and deadly pallor proclaim too unmistakably that another soul is dead.

GENERAL DISEASES.

CANCER.

There are few troubles that are so much dreaded as this one. Some people are made miserable by anticipating it when there is any kind of lump or swelling about them. This is foolish, as it will not help us even if we are going to become victims. Those who are labouring under it and have the sentence of death upon them (which we all have), it requires strong faith to keep up their spirits. Some time ago we attended a lady who was dying of the disease. Her faith was bright, she told us that those gracious words of the apostle gave her comfort, "'All things work together for good to them that love God.' (Rom. viii.) Even this cancer is working for my eternal good." True, in the case of every believer in Jesus, although all cannot realise it as she did. But cancer is a serious thing nevertheless. A short description will suffice to point out the principal forms of it.

SCIRRHUS (Carcinoma),

Is a hard tumour which is generally developed in the glands. The mammary ones are the most liable to be affected. The size may be so small and the growth so slow that its existence may not be noticed for a long time. During this forming stage it has been checked and absorbed by pressure. A bandage must be made that, like a truss, will keep up a constant pressure, kept on from one to three months, when it will often disappear. This is far better than cutting out, which seldom effects a cure.

SARCOMA

Is another form of cancer. They appear first on the skin as rounded pea or bean-shaped nodules or pimples. The colour is bluish-black, brownish, or iron-gray. They gradually increase and run into each other, when they form various shaped flattened masses. Later on they grow into mushroom forms and then ulcerate. Another form is

EPITHELIOMA.

It begins on the skin, as one or more pale-red or yellow-ish-white and hard waxy nodules (small lumps), which ultimately degenerate into ulcers. There is a form of this called

RODENT ULCER,

Which is most frequently seen on the upper part of the face, having a tendency to eat into the flesh. Of course there is a certain amount of obscurity as to the causes of this dreaded malady. Heredity has not been well established, as it develops for the first time in families which, as far as it is possible to know, never knew it. Then again the victims of it have had children, grand and great-grand, who never developed cancer.

An American doctor, writing in one of the leading Medical Journals, says that one of its chief causes is mercurial drugging. He recalls the history of several families to prove this, showing that after a course of such physicking cancer made its appearance. We are convinced that he was right. It has often been known to result from blows, wounds, &c. One of the worst we ever saw was caused by a jag from a whin. What may be called the pathological cause is the abnormal multiplication of cells at the cancer spot. It has not been decided amongst scientists that these cells are different from the ordinary ones of the body, but they multiply so fast as to crowd out the vessels which supply nutriment, and, as a result, the tumour dies and corrupts away.

The first form, Scirrhus, is the most common, so much so that it is the only one that many of the writers mention. As we remarked before, that the knife so commonly used is the only treatment that the average medical doctor considers worth thinking about, the proverb that experience teaches a certain class does not seem to fit here, for it has been proved over and over again that excision does not cure but rather increases the mischief. Dr. Monro, of Edinburgh and Aberdeen, says that of 60 cases of operation for cancer only four were free of the disease in two years. Is it possible to cure it at all, some may ask ? Our reply is, that it has been cured, when taken in time, by the pressure referred to. Even when turned to ulceration there have been cures accomplished by means of the treatment we shall now give. Supposing that either the pressure has failed or has not been tried, and that the tumour is growing, then it will be best to treat it as follows :—Make a paste of equal parts of blood-root, in powder, chloride of zinc and flour, with aromatic sulphuric acid. This is spread on small strips of cloth-cotton. Make incisions into the tumour, half an inch apart, into which insert the bits of cloth with the paste. *Cover up, bandage, and in about two weeks the dead mass will come away, leaving a healthy sore, which may be healed with the healing ointment. The following pill to be taken.—Blood-root ½ oz. and mandrake ½oz, mixed into a mass with extract of dandelion, and one or two pills taken three times a day. If the paste gives too much pain, the sulphuric acid may be substituted by water. Another paste is made with the white of eggs and salt : rub together in a mortar, as much salt as can be taken up. The American doctor, who gives this last mixture, says it will draw the man out of his boots. Dr. Beach gives as his treatment a discutient ointment, made of bittersweet, bark of root, stramonium, hemlock, and belladonna leaves, dock and poke roots, equal parts of each ; bruised, and covered with spirits. Simmer over a very slow fire, then cover with fresh butter ; simmer till the leaves feel crisp ; strain into an earthenware pot, and rub in for half an hour before the fire, or heat enough to melt it. After the rubbing, a plaster of the extract of hemlock is put over ; keep on 12 hours ; take off, repeat the rubbing with the ointment and the plaster ; a good blood mixture to be given at the same time.

The dock-root alone is said to have cured several bad cases. It consists of a poultice of the bruised roots applied. The directions recommended are to get the narrow-leaved

---

* It will require an experienced person to do this operation properly.

dock roots, wash them well, boil them till soft, pour off the water, wash with it as hot as can be borne ; fill the cavities, let it remain there two minutes, then peel the skin off the roots ; mash, then lay them on fine gauze ; dip a linen cloth in the decoction, and lay on the gauze ; repeat this every eight hours, night and day ; drink also a wineglassful of the decoction, with quarter a wineglass of wine, sweetened with honey, three times a day. Another remedy is to wash three times a day in a solution of borax (as much as the water will take up), then dust in bismuth powder ; take internally wineglass doses of decoction of blue-flag root. Another :—Chromic acid, from a six to a ten per cent. solution, painted on three times daily. Dr. Fox applies the tincture of blood-root, blue flag, and sweet clover ; lay on saturated cloths, renewing often every two or three hours. If the system is low, he recommends a blood tonic mixture, thus :

Quassia and Dock Root, each .... One ounce.
Cinque Foil .... One ounce.
Bittersweet .... One ounce.
Agrimony .... One ounce.

Put in two quarts ; boil down to three pints, then add a tea-spoonful of cayenne and two ounces of decoction of red Jamaica sarsaparilla. Take a wineglassful three times a day and a poultice of spotted hemlock leaves on the cancer. If it is smelling badly, a poultice of yeast, elm, and charcoal, or elm, blood-root, and lobelia, in powder. Now some of our readers, who are the victims or their friends, may say, Which shall we try first ? We reply, If needful, try them all, the simplest first. If the cancer is in the stomach, take the dock tea, a wineglassful, and the three tinctures, in half teaspoonful doses ; if in the womb, inject the dock decoction and, if possible, the blood-root, and zinc, paste, or paint with the chromic acid. Where life is involved, do not mind the trouble.

WHITE SWELLING.

This is an affection usually of the knee joints. In its mildest form it is called housemaid's knee, the result of much kneeling and scrubbing on the knees. To prevent this, girls should have something soft under them when kneeling at work. When symptoms of it appear the cause must be abandoned at once, even if a situation must be given up. If continued it may lead to the most serious consequences. The first thing in the way of treatment is a course of medicine, this will throw off the waste material; then take a decoction of the following :—

Blue Flag........................... One ounce.
Poke Root .... Half ounce.
Burdock Root .... One ounce.
Bittersweet Bark................... One ounce.

Bruise, and boil these in two quarts of water half an hour, then add—

Clivers .... One ounce.
Wood Sanicle .... One ounce.
Chilies .... One drachm.

Take off the fire, stir, let cool, sweeten, and take a wineglassful three times a day. Keep the bowels free with dandelion pills. Steam the knee over bitter herbs, such as wormwood, mugwort, and tansy. Hold the knee over the vessel, cover with a blanket or flannel to keep in the steam. Put a hot stone in to raise up steam when it is not sufficient. After the steaming wipe dry and rub in the following liniment :—

Tincture of Bistort .... Two ounces.
Compound Soap Liniment .... Two ounces.
Laudanum .... One ounce.
Oil of Hemlock .... One ounce.

Mix. Keep a cloth saturated with it on all the time, except during the steaming, which ought to be done three times a day. Rest in the horizontal position is needful, that is, keep the leg resting and straight out while you are sitting. Don't stand or walk any more than you can help. If the disease is in the hip-joint it must be treated in a similar manner, and perseverance alone will cure. When it has become chronic, operations are often resorted to but seldom effect any good. It is only through the blood and good local remedies that we can hope for a cure.

GOUT (PODAGRA).

It is commonly supposed that the rich, or those who live on the fat of the land, are the only subjects of this malady. While this is the rule, there are exceptions which we have met with, although they are few. The cause is usually high living, wine-drinking, and want of exercise, which produce the exciting cause, namely, a retention of waste products in the blood, which deposit about the joints, excite the nerves, and cause the excruciating pain, so common a symptom. This, with swelling, stiffness, and loss of power in the joints, are the symptoms of the disease. Treatment: We think the advice of the celebrated Dr. Abernethy to the rich old gourmand who consulted him for this disease would cure the most of sufferers with gout, viz.: earn a shilling a day and live on it. Our first advice, though not in the same words, is much the same. Abandon luxuries, take exercise in the open air, attend to the laws of health, take a course of medicine once or twice a week, and the following medicine :—

Queen of the Meadow Root .... One ounce.
Burdock Root .... One ounce.
Bittersweet Root................... One ounce.

Bruise, and simmer in two quarts of water half an hour, then stir in—

Senna .... One ounce.
Clivers .... One ounce.
Wild Pansy .... One ounce.

Take off the fire, let cool, strain, and take a wineglassful four times a day; apply the anodyne or liniment cum opii (page 213.) At bedtime make a strong decoction of mugwort and poppyheads, bathe the parts while it is hot, then mix up an elm poultice, put and keep on all night. There are many reputed cures. Cold water immersion repeatedly through the day has a good record. Try it when the pain is great. Dr. Fox tells of a man who had it for a number of years and was cured with

Turpentine .... Fifteen drops,

once a day; and cloths saturated and applied to the soles of the feet completed the cure soon, although the treatment was very severe on him for the first week.

WHITLOW AND FELON.

The former of these painful troubles is a small inflamma tion, generally at the root of the nail; the latter, the felon, is at the covering of the bone. This is sometimes called periostitis. Both are exceedingly painful, and are amenable to the same treatment. If taken in time they may be aborted by keeping the finger soaked in hot water, as hot as can be borne, for at least an hour three times a day. One or two days will be sufficient. This may save a month or two of trouble; or, as a medical man advises, the ointment of nitrate of mercury, applied thickly on a cloth, and kept on three or four days. But if it has gone too far for abortion, then apply the following:—Salt, a teaspoonful, roast it on a shovel till the gas and moisture are out; mix this with Venice turpentine, about the same quantity; put it on, and in two days you will find a hole down to the bone. This is rather a painful application. A poultice of spotted hemlock is more soothing, and also a good cure. Drink freely of the composition powder to equalise the circulation, and the alternative pills to increase the renewing power of the blood.

BRIGHT'S DISEASE (ALBUMINARIA.)

Besides acute inflammation, the kidneys, like the lungs, or in fact nearly all the internal organs, are subject to wasting disease. In 1827 Richard Bright wrote a book in which he set forth the peculiarities of kidney disease, and the evidence of their existence in the albumem present in the urine. This is the reason why chronic kidney diseases are called by his name. At one time it was believed that the presence of albumen in the urine was a sure symptom of this disease, which is generally looked upon as incurable. Even to this day some doctors, after examining a person's urine and finding it, will tell him that his case is hopeless. Of course if it is present in great quantity it is a very bad omen. But facts are to hand that albumen has been found in the urine of people in good health, who never had disease of the kidneys, and some have died of the disease, whose urine had hardly a trace of it. We are reminded here of the old proverb on exception to rules; but we give these facts to show that this alone is not sufficient to determine consumption of the kidneys. The presence of tube casts, seen by the microscope, is more certain, but even with these combined, showing the disease, it is wrong to pronounce a case hopeless. While there is life there is hope, even in Bright's disease. The symptoms are, pain in region of kidneys, fulness under the eyes, caused by slight dropsy, gradual loss of strength, swelling at the ankles, poor appetite, constipation, dusky skin. The urine is pale, of a low specific gravity, and shows the presence of the albumen, by the tests given for it on page 382. The causes are, the result of acute inflammation, excessive use of malt liquors, irritative medicines, gouty condition, gravel in the kidneys, obstruction to the circulation, through colds, &c. Treatment :—As in other serious diseases we generally give the botanic first, as it has proved itself a saving one. Begin with a partial course of medicine, thus—

Bone-set Herb.................... One ounce.
Lobelia Herb and Seed .... One drachm.
Cayenne .... Ten grains.
Mandrake, in powder .... Half drachm.

Infuse in a pint of boiling water; stand before the fire one hour, during which time the body should be bathed all over with a decoction of hemp agrimony. After this put to bed, with hot brick to the feet in vinegar cloth; strain the infusion, sweeten with treacle, and give in wineglassful doses every ten minutes till it is taken. Vomiting will commence generally before it is all taken. Continue it. Keep the perspiration up for six hours, and give the slippery elm gruel. As a daily medicine prescribe—

Mandrake Root	One ounce.
Sarsaparilla Root	Two ounces.
Liquorice Root	One ounce.
Guaiacum Chips	One ounce.
Marshmallow Root	One ounce.
Mezereon Root	One ounce.
Chilies	One drachm.

Bruise the roots, cover them with two quarts of water, simmer down to one, strain, and add a quarter ounce of the extract of sarsaparilla; take a wineglassful four times a day. A fomentation of bitter herbs, as southernwood, wormwood, and marshmallow leaves boiled in two quarts of water 15 minutes. A flannel is dipped in this decoction, squeezed out, and laid across the kidneys as hot as can be borne; cover up, and renew in a few minutes, keeping the decoction hot all the time. This must be done for one hour twice a day. Let the food be free from fats. Skim milk, lean meat, no sugar nor starchy foods. Slippery elm we know to be good, and may be taken in the digestive food prepared with the skim milk alone. Keep the bowels free with the liver pills. The above is the substance of the treatment by two of the leading botanic doctors in England who have treated and cured it many times. The eclectic treatment, of which we have just received an example from a well-known and successful American doctor, who gives cases with symptoms and cure. We will quote one case in full :—

Mr. H——, aged forty-three, proprietor of an express company, a hard worker, in health weighing 180 pounds, florid complexion, sanguine temperament, of good family, good habits and strictly temperate, consulted me July 1, 1887. He had been gradually failing in health and strength for several months. More recently he had been failing rapidly, had constant aching in the back, with sharp shooting pain in

the back and in the deep muscles of the limbs and body.
His appetite was poor and his bowels constipated ; he was
restless and uneasy. There was œdema under the eyes, and
the countenance had a dingy, jaundiced and pinched
expression. The urinary examination determined that he
passed from twenty-four to thirty ounces in twenty-four hours.
The colour was very dark. The reaction was acid, and there
was a heavy sediment. The specific gravity was between
1010 and 1012 ; urea, urates, uric acid and the phosphates
were all very deficient. Blood was present in large quantities,
and formed the greater part of the sediment. Albumen
precipitated, formed 25 per. cent. of the bulk of the urine.
There were tube casts also in abundance. This case, from
these symptoms, I diagnosed as a case of true Bright's disease
in an early stage of the severe inflammation, with
hæmaturia, induced probably by overwork—by lifting, perhaps.

For treatment, I prescribed the tincture of the chloride of
iron fifteen drops in water four times daily, with dry cups over
the kidneys. There being no change in one week, I ordered
gallic acid, ten grains alternated with the iron, every two hours.
For diet I proscribed all starchy, saccharine and fatty foods,
and ordered lean beef once daily ; skimmed milk drank freely,
and other nitrogenous food. He continued to lose in strength
and weight until about the end of the first month of the
treatment, when the improvement began—very slow at first,
scarcely perceptible, afterwards more rapid and satisfactory in
every particular. Urine lighter in colour and but little
sediment ; specific gravity increasing and the albumen reduced
two-thirds. Gave one-fourth grain extract of nux vomica four
times daily for another month, and then discontinued the
gallic acid, and gave iron and nux alternately. The improvement was gradual and permanent. He assumed his usual
work in September, at which time the albumen had almost
entirely disappeared, and the urine had assumed the amber-
yellow colour of health ; specific gravity about normal ;
quantity increased by three pints. In January, after a three

months' absence, he returned to say that he was strong and felt well except a sharp pain in his kidneys. Urinary examination showed that I had gone to the other extreme in my treatment. Quantity and colour normal; specific gravity 1032; no trace of albumen; urates and urea in great excess; uric acid in large quantities; other normal constitutents about normal in amount and no blood or casts.

" I ordered the medicine stopped and gradually made a complete change in the diet. For medicine I gave a teaspoonful of the effervescing citrate of lithia in a half-glassful of pure water every two hours, which treatment ultimately removed the excess of waste and irritation, and the man has since continued in good health."

In cases where dropsy supervenes the doctor recommends fluid extract of bitter root. We have quoted from others because we have not had much experience with the trouble ourselves, and the cases we know of having been treated by the faculty with the ordinary treatment, all terminated fatally, so that with Bright's disease the prospects of a cure are not very bright to the patient under their treatment. If any of our readers are labouring under it, we strongly recommend them to try the botanic first; if that fails try the other; and if the kidneys and system have not gone beyond the possibility of repair there is hope.

OBESITY.

Of the two extremes, thick and thin, it is difficult to tell which is worse. We imagine that those on both sides think theirs is the least desirable. It is generally thought that fat people have the remedy in their own hands. This is so, to a great extent, but not absolutely, as some persons have dieted themselves almost to starvation without much, if any, reduction. There are three things which, if used properly, will assist in removing the superabundance of fat—diet, water, and exercise. The mind must be made up to lose the gratification derived from pleasant food. Self-denial is indispensable. As an anti-fat diet the following is the scale given by a good authority :—Breakfast (early) : A little toast or brown bread, tea or coffee, if active exercise is going to be had, a little lean meat or egg. Dinner (mid-day) : Brown stale bread, lean meat, vegetables, plain boiled maccaroni or biscuit pudding. This meal ought to be the last, unless hunger is felt ; if so, a cup of tea with biscuit may be taken. Intoxicating liquors must be avoided. Skimmed milk may be taken. Water, in the form of baths, is strongly advised. (See index.) It is also the best thirst quencher in summer, and may be acidulated. The acid fruits may also be taken. Exercise or work is as needful to correct this habit as the former. It should be done in the former part of the day. Digging in the garden, chopping wood, or anything that will cause perspiration. Do not sleep above six hours. Now if these rules are carried out, you will need no anti-fat medicine, which hardly ever justifies its name, for some people seem to fatten on it. However, we know that it does benefit some people, therefore we will give Russell's remedy, called Anti-fat. This London gentleman got a pound for a 12 ounce bottle, which lasted one week. We make it at a good profit for 5/. Take—

Dock Root	One ounce.
Cocoa Leaves	Half ounce.
Fennel Seeds	Half ounce.

Infuse in a pint of water ; strain, and add—

Tincture of Fennel	Two ounces.
Tincture of Orange	Half ounce.
Tincture of Cardamom Co.	Half ounce.
Tincture of Lavender Co.	Half ounce.
Glycerine	Half ounce.
Ground Citric Acid	One ounce.

Mix, and take a tablespoonful four times a day. The juice of the poke-berry, reduced to pill consistency, and two taken three times a day, is spoken highly of in the States. A course of medicine, once or twice a week, would contribute in the reduction. Patience and self-denial will overcome.

Having now treated the ordinary and most of the extraordinary diseases common to both sexes, we will close this division of our work with the diseases peculiar to women.

DISEASES OF WOMEN.

MENSTRUATION.

It is well known to adult females that girls, when they reach the period of their life, called puberty, have a monthly discharge of blood, mingled with waste products, coming from organs of generation. We think it is but right that mothers should inform their daughters of this natural process, as it often terrifies young girls when the change takes place. The age when the flow appears differs very much. In hot countries, animal, like vegetable life, comes to maturity sooner than in cold or temperate ones, where there is still a wide divergence ; we having known of girls changing at 12 and others at 17, and in extreme cases not till 20. The average, however, may be taken at 14 to 15. In good health there is little or no trouble. With some it is hardly noticed, and every 28 or 30 days the regular appearance of the flow is an evidence of good health. With others there is more or less irregularity for a time till they are fully established. There are three phases of trouble that are connected with the menses : (1) Suppression or (amenorrhœa) ; (2) painful menstruation, (dysmenorrhœa) ; and (3) excessive flow, (menorrhagia.). The first condition is a very common one, and, if neglected, may lead to serious consequences. Waste products of any kind cannot remain in the system without danger. The causes of suppression are, cold, close confinement, fright, debility, acute disease, &c.

Besides the stoppage, the symptoms are, pain in the back and loins, lowness of spirits, headache, fits of heat and cold, weakness. Where there is a full habit of body, the face is flushed, the pulse is usually hard and bounding. Of course these symptoms are not always present, nor in the same degree. We might just hint at the natural cause of suppression, which ought not to be forgotten, as we have met with cases where this was ignored, and, so to speak, bucketfuls of medicine taken to no purpose. Presuming, then, that the courses had begun and stopped, we begin at once to remove the obstruction. Treatment: A hot foot-bath of pennyroyal, with a strong tea of the same. (See page 94.) Carry out instructions, and in all likelihood the trouble will soon be removed. This will also answer when there are symptoms indicating with the age of the girl that the time has come for the menses to commence. If the patient is pale, it will be well to take the female corrective pills or Blaud's, which are now largely prescribed by the faculty in dealing with these cases. If the cause can be traced to any disease, means must be adopted to cure it, as it is not likely the effect will cease before. It sometimes requires patience to get the obstruction removed— 3, 6, and even 12 months—so do not give up trying.

PAINFUL MENSTRUATION.

The causes of this trouble are, nervous irritability, cold, constipation, mental emotions, excesses, &c. Where the pain is regular, it may be inferred that there is a flexion of the womb or a partial stricture.

TREATMENT.—We have found by treatment that sitting over the steam of a bitter herb infusion gives the quickest relief. Take—

Wormwood	One ounce.
Southernwood	One ounce.
Tansy	One ounce.
Mugwort	One ounce.
Water	Two quarts.

Put into a chamber or suitable vessel, and sit over for 15 to
20 minutes; have two or three stones to put one in occasionally
to raise the steam. In bed use hot fomentations or the same
over the lower part of the abdomen. If after lying on the
back for some time the pain continues, turn over on the knees
and chest. If the womb is flexed backwards, this may remove
the obstruction. Drink freely of the pennyroyal tea, and take
this mixture :—

Black-haw Bark..................	One ounce.
Unicorn Root	One ounce.
Ground Pine	One ounce.
Ginger	Quarter ounce.
Tansy	One ounce.

Bruise the roots, and simmer in three pints of water one
quarter of an hour, put in the herbs; simmer five minutes
longer; cool, strain, and sweeten, and give a wineglassful
every two hours till the pain subsides. Here is another
mixture we have found good—

Tincture Cannabis Indicus	One ounce.
Water...........................	Four ounces.

Dose : A teaspoonful three to six times a day. A teaspoonful
of the aromatic spirits of ammonia every hour or two till
relieved is recommended by a good authority in America.
Warm water injections three or four times a day have been
found beneficial. Attend to the skin, stomach, bowels, and
general health, and, unless it be caused by an obstinate flexion
of the womb, you will not likely be troubled with it if you carry
out our instructions.

EXCESSIVE MENSTRUATION.

This trouble is very common and very weakening, as the
loss of blood must always be. There are two ways in which
it occurs: First, excessive flow during the usual times, and
second, a moderate amount continued for three or four times,
too long and returning too often. The causes of this loss are
given as plethoric or full habit of the body, want of exercise,
confinement in close heated rooms, sloppy food, constant

indulgence in tea or strong drink, excess of the passion, miscarriages, a determination of blood to the pelvis, or weakness of the blood-vessel. Treatment :—Endeavour to find out the cause, and if you can, remove it ; attend to the general health, and take the restorative powder (page 229). If there is a full habit of the body take a course of medicine once a week. Should the powder not correct it, make a strong decoction of the following :—

Bistort	One ounce.
Cranesbill.........................	One ounce.
Beth Root	Quarter ounce.
Unicorn Root	Quarter ounce.
Ginger	Quarter ounce.

Simmer twenty minutes in three pints of water, strain, if desired sweeten, and take a wineglassful four or more times a day. Injections of oak bark are beneficial, as they tend to astringe the vessels. Astringent suppositories made with tannic acid may be used in severe cases (page 379).

GREEN SICKNESS (CHLOROSIS).

This disease or condition is found in young girls near the change of life. It is generally caused by a low state of health, tight lacing, suppressed menstruation, a deficiency of the red corpuscles in the blood ; and depraved sexual excitement is sometimes a cause. The symptoms are : The pale-greenish colour of the face, bloodlessness of the lips, weakness, palpitation of the heart, pulse feeble, appetite bad, and lowness of spirits. Treatment : See that every cause is avoided, drink freely of composition tea to restore the circulation. If menses are suppressed take the medicine to premote them, and an iron tonic prepared thus :—

Tincture of Gentian Co.	Three ounces.
Tincture of Peruvian Bark	One ounce.
Syrup of Orange	Two ounces.
Hypophosphate of Iron	Two drachms.

Dissolve the iron as much of it as will in two ounces of boiling water, mix all together, shake up, and take from one to two teaspoonfuls three times a day; a course of medicine once a week, if the debility is not too great, will assist in bringing about the desired health.

WHITES (Leucorrhœa).

This consists of a discharge of white, glairy mucus. It originates in a catarrhal condition of the womb, the mucus membrane and glands of which being in a state of sub-acute inflammation, secrete an abnormal amount of mucus. The process is similar to what takes place with catarrh in the head. The causes are: general debility, the result of inflammation of the womb; colds, gonorrheal infection, or anything that weakens the system, predisposing it to disease. Treatment in this trouble: We must treat it locally and generally, find out the cause or causes if possible and remove them. If there are any complications, such as indigestion, constipation, worms, or piles, seek to cure them; keep the skin in a sound condition. The course of medicine once a week will help the cure. In the summer the cold salt-water bath once a day with brisk rubbing of the skin will be valuable. In the winter the chill can be taken off to suit the weather. Injections are of great service. The various astringents are the class indicated, the favourite of which is oak bark. Take four ounces, simmer in three pints of water to a quart, press, strain, and add—

Tincture of Cranesbill .... One ounce.

Use night and morning, inject a syringeful and keep it in contact with the womb from five to ten minutes. Do this after first syringing out with warm water, as warm as can be borne comfortably. Now make a medicine of :—

Witch Hazel Bark .... One ounce.
Cranesbill.......................... One ounce.
Golden Seal........................ One ounce.
Ginger .... Half ounce.

Bruise, and simmer the roots in three pints of water to a quart ; sweeten, and take a wineglassful three or four times a day. Dr. Fox's mixture, which we have found good, is as follows :

White Pond Lily	One ounce.
Comfrey Root	One ounce.
Tansy	One ounce.
Stinking Arach	One ounce.

Simmer in three pints of water down to a quart, take off the fire and stir in half an ounce of grated nutmeg, half a teaspoonful of cayenne, and half a pound of lump sugar. Take a wineglassful four times a day. Nourishing diet and open air exercise are indispensable. Now, the reason why many women suffer so long, and let their health be undermined is because they will not persevere. This being a chronic disease is often very hard to remove. It will take time, energy, and patience combined with good medicine to remove it.

INFLAMMATION OF THE WOMB.

This organ is like the rest, liable to inflammation. The causes are such as give rise to the inflammatory condition of the internal organs, injuries to the womb, through bad confinements, falls, &c. The symptoms are, pain in the region, which is greatly increased by pressure, fever, loss of strength, thirst, vomiting. The pulse is weak, the bowels confined, and the urine high coloured. If after confinement, the local discharge is lessened, if not altogether stopped.

TREATMENT.—As perspiration is stopped, commence with a course of medicine, given in bed, the hot bricks, &c. Foment with the bitter decoction directed for painful menstruation ; squeeze out the flannels, and lay over the bottom of the abdomen as hot as can be borne. Do this for an hour three times a day till the pain is subdued. As a medicine take—

Boneset .... One ounce.
Ginger .... Half ounce.
Catnip............................ One ounce.
Motherwort .... One ounce.
Pennyroyal........................ One ounce.

Infuse in two quarts of boiling water ; strain, sweeten, and give in wineglassful doses every hour till pain and symptoms abate. Dr. Beach, whose experience in treating such cases was great, gives as an unfailing remedy the following :—

Spirits of Spearmint, or the Tincture of
Green Herb with Holland's Gin .... One ounce.
Spirits of Sweet Nitre................ One ounce.

A teaspoonful in sweetened water often while pain lasts. Keep the feet warm with the hot bottle or brick. If the bowels are confined, give the compound mandrake powder, or, if the pain continues, an injection, with a grain of opium in it, will be preferable.

CHRONIC INFLAMMATION OF THE WOMB

Is often the cause of leucorrhœa, but this symptom is not always present. There is generally enlargement, with a feeling of weight and pain at menstruation, &c. For this condition, drink a decoction of marshmallow root. Sit over the steam of the bitters, as in painful menstruation ; also inject some of the infusion, warm, three times a day. Make pills of the following :—

Macrotin .... One drachm.
Pulv. Ipecac...................... Twenty grains.

Make into a mass with extract of dandelion ; divide into 40, and take one night and morning. Keep the bowels open, and take a course of medicine once a week.

INFLAMMATION OF THE OVARIES (Ovaritis).

The ovaries are two small bodies which are attached to the womb by the Fallopian tubes. They lie at the bottom of the abdomen. There are few women that know anything about them. In their case ignorance is bliss, for it is generally through suffering from them that the knowledge is gained. Sudden stoppage of the courses through cold is the cause most likely to lead to it; but may be caused by other inflammations of the pelvic organs. For the acute form, which may be known from pain in one or both groins, increased on pressure, and chilliness, the treatment is the same as for inflammation of the womb. Athough the acute is not a common trouble, chronic inflammation or disease of the ovaries is often met with. We know of several cases in this city now, where the patients have suffered terrible pain for a long time. It is hard to cure this condition, no doubt on account of the delicate and wonderful construction of these bodies. It is in them where the ova or eggs are formed, which, when impregnated, are the starting point of human life. Of late years the operation called ovariotomy, which is the removal of the ovaries, has given relief to thousands of sufferers whose lives were a burden to them. We, like most other men, would not advise an operation of so serious a nature without trying every other means of cure. The symptoms are more or less of a burning pain at one or both sides near the front projection of the pelvic or hip-bone, with swelling and tenderness or pain on pressure. The round body can often be distinctly felt, which could not be done in a natural condition. Indications for treatment: Promote the healing quality of the blood, equalise the circulation, keep open the pores and bowels, and encourage the secretion of the kidneys. A combination for this purpose may be made thus :—

Black Haw Bark.................... One ounce.
Unicorn Root .... One ounce.
Ginger Root .... Half ounce.

Bruise; and boil in three pints of water 15 to 20 minutes; then put in :—

Marigolds .... One ounce.
Clivers .... One ounce.

Stir, take off the fire, let it cool, strain, sweeten, and drink a wineglassful four times a day. The tea of marshmallow root will also be advisable; and for the relief of pain the following remedies have been tried and found good. If the one does not relieve after a fair trial use the others :—

1.

Extract of Belladonna	Half drachm.
Powdered Camphor................	One drachm.
Blue Ointment....................	Three drachms.
Lanoline	One ounce.

Mix, and spread on a cloth, and lay over the seat of pain.

2.

The Magic Liniment.................. Page 394.

3.

The Soothing Liniment .... Page 213.

If these should fail it might be well to try a small fly blister, just sufficient to cover the painful spot. Warm sitz baths, sitting over the steam as in painful menstruation. If everything fails, and the pain is undermining the health of the patient, it will be well to seek advice as to the advisability of getting the operation for removal of the ovaries done. It is well not to let the system run down too far, for the operation requires a certain amount of strength in the patient to stand it. We have seen the operation performed by some of the experts of New York. It may be interesting and instructive to give an account of it, which will show what some of our citizens have had to pay £50 to £100 for to certain medical extortioners, who, like a class in Scripture, devour widows' houses by enforcing their outrageous fees. The doctors, or some of them, want protection; but it is our opinion the public want protection against their extortion.

OVARIOTOMY.

The subject of the operation was a young woman about 24 years of age. She had suffered a long time with an uncontrollable pain. She was put to sleep with ether, the greatest care being taken that everything likely to be required was at hand, and the skin sponged with an antiseptic solution—

bichloride of mercury or corrosive sublimate, one part in
2000 of water: all the instruments, sponges, and the operator's
hands were dipped in it. A line was drawn from one inch
above the pubic bones to within an inch of the navel. The
professor, keeping the two fingers of his left hand at the lower
end, and on either side of the line, made a straight cut
upwards about half an inch in depth. The blood came
freely, but was dried up with the sponges applied by an
assistant. One or two of the larger veins were compressed
with forceps. Another cut was made, the blood wiped up,
and some larger vessels tied with catgut ligatures which
become absorbed. Another cut and the bleeding stopped in
a similar way. The peritoneum was now reached; this was
picked up with the forceps, and a small hole made in it. At
the end of the cut a grooved director was inserted and pushed
under the line of incision, care being taken that no part of
the intestines were included. The director is like a probe with
a groove on it to guide the lance or scalpel in cutting.
The inner lining was now cut through and the abdomen
opened. The professor introduced the first two fingers of the
right hand and felt for the ovary that had been the cause of
suffering. Fortunately it was not tied or glued to the intestines
or abdominal walls, as is often the case. It was brought out
and examined, and in appearance was like a sheep's kidney,
but a little smaller; was larger than natural and presented the
appearance of disease. A catgut ligature was then tied round
the Fallopian tube that connects the ovary to the womb. This
was to prevent bleeding. The ovary was then clipped off and
cut open, when its diseased appearance was manifest. The
other one was taken out, examined, and to all appearance
was healthy. The professor hesitated for a minute, but made
up his mind that it was better to make sure of no further
trouble, so he separated it in like manner. The stumps were
kept outside till all bleeding was stopped, then sponged and
put back. The abdomen was sponged out, closed, and six deep
stitches put in with silver thread, other six superficial ones
taken to bring the edges together. An antiseptic bandage

was put over and secured with a binder. No food was to be given for twelve hours. Being summer, her drink was to be iced milk and water. This patient made a good recovery. The operation took about an hour. Another we saw by an old doctor took two-and-half hours, on account of the ovaries being bound by fleshy bands to the intestines and abdomen. It does not do to cut these attachments. They must be carefully separated with the finger. As in this case the bleeding had been considerable in the abdomen, it was carefully sponged out. The sponge being held by a holder, which is like a forceps. A glass drainage tube was left in to allow of any matter being sucked out with a syringe every day. It usually takes from twenty to thirty days to recover the wonted health after the operation.

ITCHING (Pruritus Vulva).

This is a trouble that a good many adult females are acquainted with. It consists of itching at the orifice of the vagina. The causes are: disorders of menstruation, the change of life, poverty of the blood, bad digestion, worms, &c. The one symptom is itching. It is possible to confound this with an itching caused by a parasite in the hair, which must be destroyed by the application of an ointment or wash. Strong bloodroot or blue ointment; or fluid extract of staphysagria will destroy these parasites in a day or two. The treatment for the above trouble is, find out the causes if possible, and remove them (see page 317). Carry out directions there given. The following local remedies are recommended in addition:—

(1.)

Carbolic Acid.................... Twenty grains.
Laudanum .... Four drachms.
Hydrocyanic Acid, diluted .... Two drachms.
Glycerine .... Four drachms.

Add water to make four ounces. Apply a soaked pledget of cotton wool to the parts.

(2.)

Cyanide of Potassium .... Four drachms.
Glycerine .... Two drachms.
Simple Ointment .... Two drachms.

Rub together and smear.   Apply on a cloth.

(3.)

Borax Powdered.................... Two grains.
Hot Water .... Half pint.
Corrosive Sublimate .... Ten grains.

Rub till dissolved.   Bathe the parts frequently.   Great care must be taken with these remedies, as they contain poison. The tar and rosewater recommended in eczema may also be used.

ITCHING OF THE ANUS

May be treated in the same way, except when it is internal, then suppositories made as directed on page 379, should be used, containing—

Morphia........................... Half grain.
Carbolic Acid .... Two grains.

Omitting the worm powders if you are certain that worms are not one of the causes.

PUERPERAL, OR CHILD-BED FEVER.

This disease is one which has desolated many homes, depriving children of that most sacred and precious treasure— a mother's love, and the father—of his helpmate. It is now fully established that the disease is contagious, but at the same time it often arises where it is impossible to trace infection. It is often communicated from one to another by mid-wives and doctors. Dr. Young, Professor of Midwifery in the Edinburgh University, gives it as his opinion that in every instance it is communicated. He says that for many years the disease was unknown in the lying-in ward of the Royal Infirmary, but after it was introduced into it, almost every woman was attacked after her confinement. He further says it was only eradicated by the ward being emptied, disinfected, newly painted, ventilated, &c. After this there was freedom from it as before. When it originates in the individual, it is generally believed that the cause is absorption of dead matter The blood or lochial discharge being stopped confirms this view. It follows after what are termed bad confinements, especially when instruments and great force have been used. These, with a certain amount of predisposition and bad sanitary surroundings, may be assumed as the causes of this dangerous fever, which resemble typhoid. Prevention : If our readers will turn to page 270, and read Dr. Skelton's rules, to be observed during pregnancy and delivery, we are certain there would not be so many cases of puerperal fever. Dr. Coffin, who was a little too rough on regulars, blames them for most of this trouble. Giving ergot of rye and physic, he condemns as being a cause. His treatment is very simple, and facts prove it to have been most successful. An infusion of—

Centuary	Half ounce.
Barbary Bark	Half ounce.
Ground Ivy	Half ounce.
Agrimony	Half ounce.
Raspberry Leaves	Half ounce.

Steeped in three pints of boiling water ; strain, add

Cayenne	Half teaspoonful.
Powdered Gum Myrrh	Half ounce.

Give a tablespoonful every three hours ; a hot brick to the feet with the usual cloths. A strong tea of raspberry leaves and white lily root powder ; to a cupful of which add—

Cayenne	Half teaspoonful.
Valerian, in powder	Half teaspoonful.
Lobelia Herb	A teaspoonful.

Give this as an injection. If the pressure on the womb, the rapid pulse, the dry hot skin, do not disappear, give a lobelia emetic in the usual way, and repeat it if necessary. This treatment is safe, as it is simple. We will give a case that happened in this city some time ago.   A Mrs Parker was confined by a doctor who had been in attendance on a puerperal case.   A few days after, symptoms of the fever began and increased in violence.   Her husband, who was a most devoted nurse, came and consulted us, as the doctor gave little hope of her recovery.   To allay the fever, which was very high, we gave the fever powder (page 298.)   This soon opened the pores and reduced the temperature.   The bowels were relieved by an injection of raspberry leaf and slippery elm tea, and to clear the upper intestines we prescribed the compound leptandrum powder.   This, with the mixture of Coffin's, completed the cure.   The doctor did not forget to summons her husband for five pounds even although the curing was done by others.   If there is swelling and pain in the abdomen, the fomentation of bitter herbs, as in painful menstruation, ought to be given, the digestive food, and a fever diet.

There is another trouble that sometimes follows confinement, called milk leg or phlegmasia dolens.   The leg swells, is painful, stiff, and white.   It is caused by an obstruction of the lymphatic vessels.   Treatment :—Steam with bitter herbs if possible or make a strong decoction of hops, wet cloths in it, wrap round, cover with water-proof cloth to keep in the heat and moisture.   Take the mixture of herbs recommended for inflammation of the womb.   A wine-glassful every two hours to keep up perspiration.   If the fomentation does not relieve after a reasonable time rub in the following liniment :—

Liquid Ammonia..................... One ounce.
Olive Oil .... Two ounces.
Tincture of Camphor .... Half ounce.
Laudanum .... One drachm.
Tincture of Veratrum Viride .... One drachm.

Mix ; anoint, and cover up ; keep the bowels open with the compound mandrake powder ; liver tonic, or pills, and nature will restore.

INFLAMMATION OR GATHERING OF THE BREAST

Is a painful condition that calls for relief. If taken in time it can be aborted by the following means : Put an ounce of strong liquid ammonia in a pint of hot water, as hot as can be applied to the skin. Bathe the breast for 15 minutes, put a wet cloth over it, bathe again in an hour or two if the first does not seem to be enough. It will be well to do it three times to make sure. If this has not the desired effect put on the breast liniment (page 214) ; if it gathers in spite of all, poultice with slippery elm (see page 4) ; take the blood mixture (page 312), with the compound mandrake to keep the bowels free.

CESSATION OF THE MENSES—CHANGE OF LIFE.

In a state of health the menses usually stop with as little disturbance as they begun ; but this is not always the case, as many suffer much at this time of life. The suffering, however, is of a symptomatic kind : headache, backache, weakness, flushings, painful menstruation, &c. These may all be treated and cured under their several heads. Dr. Fox gives a general cure which we have given to many with benefit. It is :—

Peruvian Bark .... One ounce.
Turkey Rhubarb.................. Quarter ounce.
Ipecac. .... Quarter ounce.
Jalap Root .... Quarter ounce.

Put in a jug and pour three gills of boiling water upon them ; stir, let stand, cover, and take a tablespoonful three or four times a day, enough to keep the bowels free. As in most cases we would recommend the course of medicine when the system is not too much run down.

COOKERY FOR THE SICK.

With sickness there is usually an impairment, or loss of appetite, which makes it necessary to prepare the food in such a way, and of such a quality, as will both tempt the appetite and support the strength of the sick one. We need not say that the food ought to be of the best quality, as reason alone will teach that. It is also important (and this is our object in the present chapter) to have it prepared in the best possible manner.

We have already pointed out the digestive food, which is an excellent preparation, not possibly the most palatable, but unsurpassed as a light, nutritious and easily digested food. It can hardly be given amiss in any complaint, but is especially good in troubles of the digestive and urinary organs. Our space will not allow of giving many recipes, nor is it needful to do so, for sickness, like health, is not benefited by a great variety of articles. The diet drinks (page 218) will, we trust, take the place of tea or coffee, unless there be a strong craving for them, then only given sparingly, as it is well known that they possess narcotic properties. We have already spoken of bread—the staff of life. It should be free from adulteration, and made of the unbolted flour, or ground wheat. The only condition when fine flour might be better is in the case of diarrhœa, and even then it is doubtful. Meat, in substance, should not be given where there is acute disease, as inflammation, &c. Pastry is generally unwholesome Ripe fruits are good, and may be taken with safety, in reasonable quantity. Milk is sometimes too rich for delicate stomachs ; if so, let it be skimmed. Goat's milk is believed to be superior to cow's. If it can be had all the better, but this is difficult in places. One of the latter introductions from semi-civilization is a drink called Koumys. It is prepared by adding one teaspoonful of brewer's yeast, and 30 grains of sugar of milk, to a pint of milk, which is slightly warmed, skim and bottle after it has stood six hours. Some makers bottle it at once and tie down the corks. It may be drank the following day in half to cupful doses; is recommended in albuminary or Bright's disease, and other wasting affections. The bill of fare for invalids may be given thus :—

ARTICLES PROHIBITED.	ARTICLES ALLOWED.
Warm Meats of all kinds	Bread made of
Soups (common)	Wheaten Flour
Gravies	Indian Meal
Spices	Rye
Coffee	Good Butter
Green Teas	Potatoes
Salt Fish	Rice
Lobsters	Stewed Fruits
Crabs	Plain Puddings
Fresh Bread	Custard
Pastry	Milk
Mince Pies	Molasses, when they agree
Cake	Cocoa
Ardent Spirits	Weak Black Tea
Malt Liquors	Oysters
Unripe Fruits	Fresh Fish
Pickles	Eggs lightly cooked
Nuts	Well boiled Onions.
Tobacco in every form	
All other kinds of indigestible food.	

In our last number of the *Chicago Medical Times* there is an article on the food for consumptives, which we will quote, as we feel assured its directions, if carried out, will benefit this class of sufferers.

DIET FOR CONSUMPTIVES,

BY JOSEPH ADOLPHUS, M.D., ATLANTA, GA.

A most important question relating to the proper treatment of consumptive patients, is the matter of diet. The older of us can well remember two or three decades ago —yes, even a few years back—when it was claimed that alcohol was a good and desirable remedial agent in this disease. This opinion had for its commendation a certain theory of combustion. It was claimed by the older clinicians that alcohol was readily attacked by the oxygen, and the burning was done in the blood, or just at the threshold of the tissues. Some advanced a step further, and claimed that alcohol becomes part of the organism, or that it was distributed around the tissues, and was thus burned up with the waste of the fats and proteids of the organism, and thus checked the waste the body was so persistently undergoing. The alcohol theory held strong sway, so strong that many of the best men advocated it with earnest endeavour, and put it into practice. The fact is, in some few cases the results were striking, and, indeed, brilliant, and so attention was taken off the vast evil alcohol in large doses was doing to the great number who were falling all around, victims to a gross error.

Then came the next fad, that is, that the consumptive patient must eat plentifully of proteids. This craze got heavy headway under the seemingly wonderful results obtained by Dr. Debove, of France, who stuffed his consumptive patients through the aid of an œsophageal tube when the appetite of the victim was quite or nearly lost. Some of Dr. Debove's cases made wonderful progress— one even recovered—but the fact was, the largest number of patients succumbed to the ordeal, simply because the digestive and assimilative powers of their organism were unable to stand the terrible strain put on them by this surfeiting with rich proteid food.

Then came the doctrine of antiphlogistics and antipyretics in the treatment of consumption. The introduction of antipyrin and antifebrin into medical practice was soon to mark an era in the matter of treatment of phthisis. The fever was made the objective point, and all aim was to keep down the fever with antipyretics. The experiments were numerous, and often as daring and reckless as they were novel. This is one of the weaknesses of allopaths, ever running after new gods, and sacrificing for new idols.

Now all these fads have had their day, yet one must see that they still have their mighty sway, for the dogmas of medicine are ever terrible contrivances in the old school, much after the fashion of the orthodox priests of the recent past, even to the inquisition.

The best diet for the consumptive is one nearly composed of vegetable material of a rich nutritive quality. There is a great deal in good cow's milk, skimmed and unskimmed. A very good aid in the matter of feeding for strength to supply something to burn in the system, is the combination of yolk of egg, two parts; pure glycerine, one part (by weight) An ounce of this combination may be taken in milk.

Recently I had an excellent opportunity of seeing the marvels proper feeding can do in consumption. The case was a lady thirty-six years old. Tubercles, breaking down, expectorations of pus, fever every evening, slight night sweats, complete loss of appetite, emaciating rapidly. I ordered milk, boiled under pressure, that is, a quart bottle is filled with milk, space being left equal to two fluid ounces. The cork was put in tight, and secured by a string tied over it. The bottle was then put into water, and kept boiling for four hours. Beginning with this, she took the quart during the day, and with it the yolk of about two eggs. The doctor who had previously treated her gave her antipyrin to keep down the fever. It was too hot to be controlled this way. The antipyrin was used in six-grain doses, so that the temperature was lowered; but still the fever came on, and she was steadily going down-hill. But little food was taken, and hardly half that digested and assimilated. I found that she digested and assimilated the milk, egg yolk, and glycerine, the fever abated, then ceased; night sweats stopped; her condition was greatly improved in four weeks. I then found that the expectoration was considerably diminished, and there was less cough, better nights' rest, cheerful state of mind, and in ten days more she was eating cracked wheat, rice puddings; an egg or two per day was taken, and in every other way she improved.

I am convinced that proteids are not needed, nor do they answer a good purpose in consumption, and they should be only sparingly used. The cry is that mostly poor people die of consumption. I am sure the statement is correct only in the fact that there are several hundred poor persons to one in good circumstances, and where the ratio of each class is taken, it will be found that as many rich die of consumption as do the poor.

One point may be made out, and that is, people in poor circumstances do not die so fast of wasting diseases as the rich in the same climate, under the same surroundings. Consumptive people must eat more fats, keep in the open air as much as possible, sleep in well ventilated rooms, eat plenty of vegetable food, with fruits, and keep the body warm by wearing flannel next the skin, summer and winter.

In the opening stage of phthisis, I think a rich vegetable diet, plenty of milk and cream, fruit, living in the open air, and filling the lungs to their fullest capacity several times a day, are prime remedial agents.

Were I the victim of consumption, I should go to central Georgia, erect a shanty on a dry knoll in the piny woods, let the cracks take care of themselves; then I would see that I had plenty of woollen cover over me at night. During the day I would roam over the hills, and in good weather sleep out of doors, in a hammock, under the pine trees. Then for my food I would have plenty of first-class hop yeast light bread, which I would not eat until two or three days old, using a very liberal amount of fresh butter and cream. I would have fruits in their season, which I would eat in moderate quantity; in winter, dried fruit should replace the recent. I would eat the yolk of three eggs every day, and, if I felt like it, would devour a well-cooked chicken for dinner. If I had a slight dyspepsia, I would take a few drops of nux and hydrastis.

I have known many cases of consumption to have been cured by this treatment.

Regarding the creosote treatment in consumption, I repeat it has solid merit, and is deserving of further and more extensive trial.

In our treatment of consumption we gave the latest alleged remedy as the inhalation of hot air. Some of our readers would doubtless like to have the directions as to how it is done. The directions are not explicitly given. It seems, however, that the inhalations are usually taken in a hot air room, similar to the Turkish bath. A box may be formed for this purpose, or some other contrivance, which will enable the sufferer to get the hot air into the lungs. We would suggest a pipe, taken out of an oven, at the end of which is a kind of mask to cover the nose and mouth. The object is to get air, the temperature of 160 deg. Fahr. into the lungs.

ISINGLASS JELLY.—

Dissolve an ounce of isinglass in a half pint of water, add two tablespoonfuls of apple jelly, a pint and a half of water, and a quarter of a pound of lump sugar. Gently simmer until the whole are well incorporated, let it cool, and use at any time.

There is much nutrition in this, and in all cachectic and consumptive cases it may be taken with very great advantage.

CARAGEEN MOSS.—

Take a quarter of an ounce of the above moss, steep it for 15 or 20 minutes in cold water, rinse, put it into a pint and a half of new milk, with a few bits of cinnamon stick, a bit of lemon peel, and lump sugar sufficient to suit the taste; gently simmer until the carageen is dissolved, strain through a muslin bag, and let it stand until cold. A small quantity may then be warmed and taken at any time.

This is most excellent in consumptive cases, or where the patient is troubled with an irritable exciting cough, or general weakness of the chest.

MUTTON CUSTARD.—

Take two ounces of fresh mutton suet, shred fine, half a dracham of cinnamon or grated nutmeg, and gently simmer in rather more than a pint of new milk; carefully scum as it rises.

This is highly nutritious, and may be taken in enteric disease, diarrhœa, and consumption, with very great advantage.

JELLY FOR DELICATE PATIENTS.—

Take three ounces of isinglass, two ounces of candied eryngo root, and an ounce each of pearl barley, rice, and conserve of roses; put the whole into two quarts of water, and gently simmer for four or five hours until it is reduced to a pint.

A tablespoonful of this if put into a teacupful of sweetened milk is highly nutritious and useful in cases of atrophy or wasting of the system, weakness of the chest, consumption, &c.

CHOCOLATE FOR INVALIDS.—

Take one square of chocolate (the sixth part of a cake), shave it and boil in a pint of water for five minutes, add a pint of new milk and boil together; after which mix a teaspoonful of arrowroot with a little cold water, add and simmer gently for five minutes longer.

This is a very nutritious beverage, and may be taken by invalids with much benefit.

STRENGTHENING JELLY.—

Take the bones of a knuckle of veal, well scrape all the meat from them, and stew for four or five hours in two quarts of water, let it cool, and skim it clear from all fat and sediment, flavour with a little wine or brandy.

This is highly nutritious, and may be taken by the delicate with advantage at any time.

MEAT JELLY FOR THE DELICATE.—

Take two pounds of lean beef, cut in pieces with a hock of ham about the same weight, a knuckle of veal, and a small quantity of salt and mace, without any other spice, cover the whole with water, and stew for about seven hours, strain, and when cold take off the fat, clear it with whites of eggs, and pass it through a jelly-bag. When prepared it should make about five quarts.

It is highly nutritious, and may be taken cold or warm agreeably with the taste of the patient.

BEEF TEA.—

Take one pound of lean beef, pick all the fat off, cut it into small pieces about the size of nutmegs, or smaller, put into an enamelled saucepan with a quart of water, two cloves, and a half teaspoonful of salt; simmer for three or four hours, and carefully skim as the fat and scum arise.

This is a most excellent nutrient and may be taken *ad libitum* at any time.

SOUP FOR THE CONVALESCENT.—

Put alternate layers of lean beef and turnip, cut small, into a jar, place it in a water bath or slow oven, and let it remain for three hours or more; after which drain, express the liquid, and let it stand until cold; skim the fat carefully off, season, and use as necessary.

This is highly nutritious, and may be used during convalescence with very great advantage.

ANOTHER EXCELLENT SOUP FOR THE CONVALESCENT.—

Take six pounds of shin of beef, an onion cut small, three quarts of water, two teaspoonfuls of salt, and a little pepper; put the whole into a jar, cover, and let it stand all night in a moderately warm oven, strain, skim off the fat, and take with a little crumbed or toasted bread.

This, like the last, may be taken with very great benefit as freely as the system requires it.

ARTIFICIAL WHEY.—

Gently simmer a pint of skim milk, add two glasses of sherry wine, and sufficient lemon juice to turn the milk; set it aside until the curd subsides, strain, and add sugar sufficient to make it pleasant.

A wineglassful three or four times daily may be taken with much benefit in cases of consumption, cough, and weakness of the chest generally.

EGGED WINE.—

Beat up two eggs in a basin, with an ounce and a half of finely-powdered white sugar and a little grated nutmeg; gently simmer a pint of sherry wine and water in equal quantities, stir in the eggs, &c., as it boils, and throw forwards and backwards several times from the saucepan to the jug until it is well incorporated.

This is a very nutritious gentle stimulant, and may be taken with much benefit by invalids at any time.

ROASTED DANDELION.—

This forms a most excellent beverage for invalids, and may be taken with the meals in every condition of the system, whether in health or disease, with the greatest benefit, but more particularly in dyspeptic cases, in convalescence supervening upon diseases of the liver, pancreas, or spleen, or wherever there is a predisposition to these diseases.

DIGESTIVE FOOD.—

Finely-powdered Lump Sugar........ One pound.
Slippery Elm..................... Four ounces.
Cinnamon .... One drachm.

Mix until the whole are well incorporated, and take a teaspoonful in a small teacupful of boiling milk; stir briskly while preparing.

This is most excellent in all cases of disease or debility, whether of adults or children, and may be taken with advantage at any time. It is also excellent for very young children when brought up by the bottle.

FIGS AND MILK.—

Split and gently simmer three or four figs in a half pint of new milk for one hour, and take at any time. The figs may be boiled three or four times over in fresh milk with equal benefit.

This is very beneficial in consumption and diseases of the chest generally.

STEWED APPLES OR APPLE BUTTER.—

Peel a dozen or more of good cooking apples, cut into small pieces, add a little lemon rind and two or three cloves, stew, mash with a spoon into a pulp, and use with the bread instead of butter.

Mixed with new milk, and taken daily, it is exceedingly useful in almost every form of chronic disease.

CRANBERRIES—

Are sometimes stewed for about 20 minutes with little sugar or fine treacle, and a few spoonfuls of water—about three ounces of sugar to a pint of fruit. An excellent strengthening diet may be made by simmering about half a pint each of cranberries, black currants, blackberries, and red raspberries together for about 20 minutes. It may be taken on grist bread, or in any other form according to taste; or may be made into pies or dumpling. The above are all tonic fruits; live upon such as these, and drink pure water, and a professor of medicine will seldom be required.

ENGLISH TEA.—

Take the same weight of raspberry leaves as you would of China tea, and add, if you have any, leaves of black currant or balm. Mix all together, or take them separately, as you like their flavours. Pour hot water upon them, and sweeten as you would the other tea. This is much healthier, and promotes digestion better than the imported tea. Make it weaker or stronger, according to taste

MUTTON CHOP.—

Take a mutton chop, salt it both sides, put it on a gridiron over the fire, turning it over often till about half done ; then put it between two plates in the oven to finish. This is the easiest meat to digest, and by this process the essence is retained, and is much relished by patients recovering from sickness, especially consumptive patients.

RICE.—

This is a very healthy food, made in the usual way, as in puddings, with milk and water, seasoned. It is digested in the shortest possible time (one hour), and as it contains eight-tenths nutritious matter, it is a valuable food for health.

OATMEAL GRUEL.—

Take a tablespoonful of the meal, and salt to suit the taste : stir it slowly in a pint of boiling water, continue the boiling five minutes and skim ; milk may be added, if desirable. This is highly serviceable in dyspepsia and costiveness.

SAGO GRUEL.—

Stir two tablespoonfuls of pearl sago into a pint of water and season with salt to suit the taste ; boil until it is converted into a thickish jelly, which will be in about quarter of an hour ; it may be sweetened if the patient desires. This is soothing in irritation of the bowels and stomach.

SLIPPERY ELM GRUEL.—

Beat a teaspoonful of powdered elm bark into paste with water, adding a small portion of salt, and stir it into a pint of milk just beginning to boil ; take the milk from the fire, and continue the stirring two or three minutes, until the elm is dissolved. This is very useful in diarrhœa and bowel complaints of children ; it affords a nourishing diet for infants weaned from the breast, and renders them healthy and fat. If the infants are very young the milk should be diluted with one-third of water.

TAPIOCA JELLY.—

Pick the tapioca clean, soak it three or four hours in water, spread it on a broad dish; pour additional water till it covers the tapioca an inch in depth; simmer over a slow fire until the jelly is formed. This contains a large amount of nutriment, and is easy of digestion; it may be made with milk, and sweetened with sugar; if milk disagrees with the stomach it can be omitted.

ARROWROOT JELLY.—

This is made by mixing half a teaspoonful of arrowroot with a teacupful of boiling water; season with nutmeg and sugar; this lies lightly on the stomach, and is very good for children. Or boil the arrowroot five minutes, and half a teaspoonful of cream added to a teacupful of the jelly while hot; it is very pleasant to children who have been accustomed to milk.

REVALENTA ARABICA FOOD—

Is produced from the Arabian lentil. It possesses natural restorative properties, and at the same time yields a great amount of nutriment, and may be recommended for persons advanced in age, invalids, and delicate children, and all who suffer from debility, &c. It imparts muscular strength and energy to the most enfeebled constitutions. We sell this article of diet, prepared in Dunedin, at half the price of the imported article, to which it is superior, being newly made.

SELECT MISCELLANEOUS REMEDIES.

We shall begin this division with the contributions of a woman who has had much experience in domestic medicine, as well as a natural taste and strong desire for the healing art.

A FEW HINTS ON SIMPLE HOME TREATMENT.

To those in the country, where medical aid is hard to procure, and especially to my sister women, as being the true ministering angel of the afflicted, these few hints on simple home treatment are respectfully addressed. It may be here mentioned that in our country home we have had ample opportunity of testing the various hints and recipes given, and, although they are few in number, they are given in the hope that, as they are all simple and genuine, they may be the means of helping some poor sufferer, or of enabling some one with a kind heart and willing hands to render the necessary assistance in time of need.

Taking, first, that fell destroyer—fever—it is lamentable to think how many valuable lives are lost yearly, which might be saved by a little simple treatment in the early stages; and even when pretty well advanced fever may be thrown off by getting the patient into a thorough perspiration. This may be done by means of bottles of hot water and plenty of bed-clothes, but a more effectual way is to have three bricks, made hot in the fire, wrapped in cloths wet with vinegar, and placed one at the feet and one at each side; have on as many blankets as can be borne, and administer composition or yarrow tea. Meanwhile cool the fevered brain by having two soft cloths, or towels, and a bucket of the coldest water you can procure; wring one out, and lay it on the forehead, gently pressing it on the heated temples. When it begins to warm, change it for the other one, applied in a similar manner; keep on having one cloth in the water and the other on the head until the heat is subdued. After sweating has been accomplished, be careful not to catch cold, sponge gently with tepid water and vinegar, using cold water to close the pores ; dry thoroughly, and keep warm in bed.

The wet sheet pack may also be administered in the following manner :—Spread a blanket on the bed, over this a mackintosh cloth, or some such thing to exclude the air and prevent evaporation, next wring a sheet out of tepid water, spread this over the mackintosh, have the patient ready immediately the sheet is spread, bring one side round under the arms, the other over the arms. Bring the mackintosh round first from one side then from the other; next bring the blanket round in the same manner ; place over all several pairs of blankets, tuck well in at the sides and about the neck and shoulders. Keep in this for an hour, but do not let the patient sleep. After unpacking bathe or sponge with tepid water. This treatment has a wonderfully soothing effect in cases of feverishness. The chief points to remember are : 1st. Be as expeditious as you possibly can in getting the patient packed and well covered in the sheet. 2nd. Beware of draughts in packing and unpacking. 3rd. Let the sponging and drying be thoroughly and quickly accomplished.

Where the fever is advanced it is well to give a lobelia emetic before sweating.

For inflammations the same sweating course with the emetic and cayenne pepper will produce a good effect.

For female complaints there can be nothing better than the sitz-bath and wet body bandage, which latter is made double, three yards long and twelve inches wide. Wet as much as will cover the top of the stomach, wring it thoroughly, wrap this round the body, the wet first and then the dry. This may be worn at night, or both night and day if thought advisable. This is a potent remedy for chronic indigestion.

For convulsions and nervousness in children place them in a warm bath. It has a soothing effect.

It is a deplorable fact that there is a large amount of suffering in the world which might be averted by a few precautions and a little attention to the ordinary laws of health; seeing that such is the case a few brief hints on various small matters may not be out of place here.

To avoid catching cold never on any account sit or work in a draught. After being heated by walking or working, be careful to cool gradually and not by throwing off clothes or sitting where it is cold.

Be careful not to wear wet clothes, and above all keep the feet dry and warm.

When the air is cold keep the mouth closed and breathe through the nose.

To stop bleeding at the nose place the feet in warm water, apply a cold wet cloth to the spine just at the nap of the neck and give a cup of ginger tea.

For a sore throat try a pinch of salt several times repeated, or a spoonful of tincture of composition. If at night take a hot drink and wrap a wet cloth round the throat with a flannel over it.

To allay sickness take a little tincture of composition with hot water and sugar, or a tea of mint.

TYPHOID FEVER, Prevention and Cure for.—Turpentine 5 to 12 drops on loaf sugar three times a day.

REMEDY FOR THE WHITES.—

Beth Root........................	One ounce.
Unicorn Root	Half ounce.
Peruvian Bark	Half ounce.

All in powder. Pour over them one pint of boiling water, strain, let it get cold, pour off the clear into a large bottle and pour a pint of port wine upon the sediment, shake up, let it stand till clear, pour with the watery infusion, mix the two, bottle and take a wineglassful three times a day.

WORM CANDY.—

Make a strong decoction of sage two parts and wormwood one part. Boil down with sugar till it candies like toffie, pour into greased plates, and give a good piece to a child night and morning. It is said to be infallible.

COMPOSITION POWDER (For colds, indigestion, &c.)—

Bayberry .... Quarter pound.
Balmony .... Two ounces.
Pinus Canadensis .... Two ounces.
Ginger .... Two ounces.
Cloves .... One ounce.
Cayenne Pepper .... Half teaspoonful.

For directions see page 221.

COUGH SYRUP.—

Skunk Cabbage.................... One ounce.
Valerian......................... One ounce.
Liquorice Root................... One ounce.
Raspberry Leaves................. One ounce.
Horehound .... Quarter ounce.
Hyssop .... Quarter ounce.
Lobelia Herb .... Quarter ounce.
Spanish Juice .... One stick.

Add two quarts of water, boil slowly for about one hour, or until reduced to three pints. Stir into this decoction while hot half a pound of sugar, small cup of currant jelly and a teaspoonful of cayenne pepper. Dose: a tablespoonful three times daily ; oftener if required.

FOR HEADACHE.—

Tincture of Ginger................... Half pint.
Salt .... Two ounces.

Shake well together in a bottle. Allow it to settle. For nervous headache a little of the clear poured on the head and gently rubbed in will give instant relief.

TINCTURE OF COMPOSITION.—

Tincture of Ginger .... Half pint.
Composition Powder .... Three teaspoonfuls.

Mix by shaking in a bottle. When the sediment has settled it is ready for use. A spoonful will relieve a sore throat.

STIMULATING LINIMENT.—

Vinegar .... Half pint.
Cayenne Pepper.............. Three dessertspoonfuls.

TEETHING POWDER.—

Podophyllin .... Twenty grains.
Leptandrin....................... Twenty grains.
Ginger .... Ten grains.
Sanguinarin .... Ten grains.
Fine White Sugar................ One and half drs.

Rub up well in a mortar; divide into fifty powders. Dose: One powder at bed-time in a little preserve, or any other simple vehicle.

WORM POWDER.—

Santonin .... Half drachm.
Carolina Pink .... One drachm.
Podophyllin...................... Thirty grains.
Sugar (fine white) .... One drachm.

Triturate as the last, and divide into fifty powders. Dose, one powder in preserve, or any other simple vehicle, night and morning.

The same may be prepared in small cakes or nuts as gingerbread, with the addition of flour and treacle; or as troches or lozenges, with additional sugar and gum tragacynth.

PULMONARY TROCHES OR LOZENGES.—

Sugar (fine white) .... One pound.
Tolu Tincture...................... One ounce.
Antispasmodic Tincture .... Half ounce.
Oil of Peppermint.................. Twenty drops.
Gum Arabic .... Sufficient.

Form the whole into a mass, cut out and prepare in the form of lozenges.

This is a most excellent lozenge, and may be used with advantage in consumption, bronchial disease, coughs, and diseases of the chest generally.

REMEDY FOR POLYPUS.—

Powdered Blood-root .... Half ounce.
Powdered Alum .... Two drachms.
Gallic Acid ....: .... One drachm.

Mix, and use as ordinary snuff; or, where the passage is completely obstructed, take a small camel-hair brush, wet it in cold water, dip it into the powder, and apply five or six times daily.

REMEDY FOR TOOTHACHE THROUGH DECAY.—

Prickly Ash Bark (in powder) ...... Two drachms.
Camphor .... One drachm.
Opium (in powder)................ One drachm.
Oil of Cloves .... Twenty drops.
Galbanum (Gum, in powder) ...... Sufficient.

Add alcohol sufficient to form into a pill mass, and divide into grain-and-half or two-grain pills.

One of these pills placed in the hollow or decayed part of the tooth will afford immediate relief. Keep the pills free from exposure to the air.

REMEDY FOR MENORRHAGIA, OR IMMODERATE MENSTRUATION.—

Beth-root, in powder.............. Half ounce.
Tormentil, in powder.............. Half ounce.
English Rhubarb, in powder ...... Two drachms.

Add sufficient proof spirits of wine to mix, let it stand 24 hours, put into a quart bottle, add a pint and a half of the best port wine, and shake up daily for a week. Dose: a half wineglassful of the liquid only, in an equal quantity of cold water, three or four times a day.

OLD HENRY'S REMEDY FOR CANCER.—

Extract of Poke-root, and ⎫
Extract of Sharp-pointed Dock ⎭ .... Equal parts.

Spread as ointment on white leather, and apply night and morning.

Drink at the same time a small teacupful of the infusion of tag alder.

REMEDY FOR GOUT AND CHRONIC RHEUMATISM.—

Prickly Ash Bark .... One ounce.
Sassafras Bark .... Half ounce.
Betony (Wood).................... One ounce.

Boil the barks gently in two quarts of rain water down to three pints. Throw the whole upon the herb, cover, and when cold express. Dose : a wineglassful three times a day. At bed-time make a teacupful hot, and add a quarter of a teaspoonful (15 grains) of ginger, and sweeten with treacle.

REMEDY FOR OLD ULCERS.—

Prickly Ash Bark .... Two ounces.
Water Dock .... Two ounces.
English Rhubarb Root............. One ounce.

Crush or cut the dried roots small, and gently simmer in five pints of distilled or rain water down to two quarts ; add two ounces of pure spirits of wine. Dose : a wineglassful four times a day.

Wash the ulcers in an infusion of wormwood, sprinkle or cover with powdered prickly ash bark, and cover with cloths, constantly wet with the wormwood infusion until they are healed.

REMEDY FOR SECONDARY SYPHILIS.—

Prickly Ash Bark .... Four ounces.
Sarsaparilla Root (Jamaica) .... Two ounces.
English Rhubarb Root .... One ounce.
Soapwort (root of) .... One ounce.

Bruise or cut the dried roots small, simmer in five pints of rain or distilled water down to two quarts, when cold express Dose : a wineglasssful four times a day.

REMEDY FOR HYSTERIA.—

Mugwort (herb, dry)................ Two ounces.
Balm (herb, dry) .... One ounce.

Infuse in three pints of boiling water, in a covered vessel, let it stand until cold, express and sweeten with lump sugar. Dose : a wineglassful, cold, three times a day.

REMEDY FOR HOARSENESS AND LOSS OF VOICE.—

Horseradish Root (dry, in thin strips,
    or scraped).................... Two ounces.

Simmer with two quarts of rain water, over a slow fire, in a covered vessel, down to three pints ; when cold express, add three pounds of lump sugar. Prepare as a syrup, and take from one to two teaspoonfuls every three or four hours.

OINTMENT FOR SCALDS, BURNS FROM FIRE, AND CHILBLAINS.—

Harts-tongue (dry leaves, powdered).. Four ounces.
Linseed Oil .... Half pint.
Mutton Suet...................... Two ounces.
Beeswax .... Four ounces.

Boil the herb in two quarts of water for one hour, express and evaporate to 'the consistency of treacle ; add the beeswax, linseed oil, and mutton suet, gently simmer, and agitate, or stir, until the whole are well incorporated.

REMEDY FOR REMOVING MUCOUS ACCUMULATIONS AND FILM FROM THE EYES.—

Express Juice of Celandine (Chelidonium majus) and Ground Ivy.... Half ounce.
Bay Salt......................... One drachm.

Strain the juice clear, dissolve the salt, and keep in a cool place.

Gently touch the conjunctiva or surface of the eye with a small camel-hair brush, wet with this twice or three times a day, until the obstruction is removed.

In cases where the deposit or accumulation arises from a strumous taint, alterative medicines should be prescribed internally.

REMEDY FOR ASTHMA OR TIGHTNESS UPON THE CHEST.—

Ground Ivy (herb, dry) .... One ounce.
Angelica Herb (dry) .... One ounce.

Infuse in a quart of boiling water, strain, express, and add four ounces of lump sugar and two ounces of acid tincture of lobelia. Dose : a tablespoonful three times a day, and double the quantity at bed-time.

REMEDY FOR IRRITATION OF THE SKIN AND CUTANEOUS DISEASE.—

Fumitory (dry herb) .... Two ounces.

Infuse in three pints of boiling water, in a covered vessel, express, and add half an ounce of tinc. stillingia, and half ounce of tincture of mandrake. Dose : a tablespoonful three a day.

REMEDY FOR ATROPHY OR WASTING OF THE BODY.—

Eryngo Root, dry and crushed ...... Two ounces.
Comfrey Root, ,, ,, ... One ounce.
Liquorice Root, ,, ,, ... One ounce.
Anise Seed........................ Half ounce.

Gently simmer for one hour in two quarts of boiling water down to three pints, express, add four ounces of lump sugar and one ounce of spirituous lobelia tincture. Dose : from a dessertspoonful to a tablespoonful four times a day, in a wineglasful of new milk.

REMEDY FOR SCROFULA.—

Coltsfoot (leaves, dry).............. One ounce.
Vervain (herb, dry) .... One ounce.
Dog Mercury (herb, dry)............ Half ounce.
Spurge Laurel (leaves, dry) .... Two drachms.

Gently simmer the whole in two quarts of boiling water down to three pints : express, add half ounce of extract of poke root, and an ounce of Spanish juice. Dose : a tablespoonful three and four times a day.

Apply cloths saturated with a decoction of wormwood, hot, at night, and protect the parts with flannel during the day ; or if the glands are likely to suppurate, poultice with powdered white pond-lily.

REMEDY FOR PALPITATION OF THE HEART.—

Motherwort (herb, dry).............. One ounce.
Balm (herb, dry) .... One ounce.

Infuse in three pints of boiling water, in a covered vessel, for one hour, strain, express, add four ounces of lump sugar and one ounce of antispasmodic tincture. Dose: a tablespoonful three times a day.

ERRHINE FOR PAINS OF THE HEAD AND OVER THE EYES.—

Asarabacca (fine powder) .... Half ounce.
Betony,   „   „   .... Two drachms.
Bayberry,   „   „   .... One drachm.

Triturate or rub up fine in a mortar, and use as snuff when required.

NETTLE BEER.—

Nettles .... Two ounces.
Dandelion Root .... Two ounces.
Clivers .... Two ounces.

Boil in one gallon of water, strain, add half a pound of sugar and a tablespoonful of yeast, let it stand in a warm place six hours, bottle, tie the corks, drink as desired.

BEER FOR SKIN DISEASES'.—

Yellow Dock...................... Two ounces.
Clivers .... Two ounces.
Wood Betomy .... One ounce.

Make a gallon the same way as last.

OINTMENT FOR PRICKLY HEAT.—

Salicylic Acid .... Four grains.
Lard .... One ounce.

Mix and rub in after washing with the healing or carbolic soap twice or three times a day.

SYRUP FOR HACKING COUGH.—

Syrup of Ipecac...................... One ounce.
    „   „ Tolu .... One ounce.
Tincture of Wild Cherry .... One ounce.
Balsam of Peru .... One ounce.
Essence of Peppermint .... Quarter ounce.

A teaspoonful every four hours.

CROUP.—

Blood Root, in coarse powder ...... Two ounces.
Vinegar .... One pint.
Water............................. Half pint.

Simmer 10 minutes, strain, add half a pound of honey. Dose:
A teaspoonful.   When recovering use a syrup of golden seal
and burdock.

BLACK SALVE.—

Olive Oil .... One pint.
Common Resin .... Half ounce.
Bees Wax .... Half ounce.
Venice Turpentine.................. Half ounce.
Red Lead .... Two ounces.

Melt over a slow fire till it becomes black; as it cools stir in
half a pound of powdered camphor.   Excellent for old sores,
piles, &c.

SEMINAL WEAKNESS.—

Tincture of St. John's Wort .... Half ounce.
Tincture of Cocoa Leaves .... Half ounce.
Tincture of Damiana................ Half ounce.
Tincture of Cantharides .... Half ounce.
Tincture of Nux Vomica .... Half ounce.

15 to 20 drops in a little water at 3, 6 and 9 o'clock.

ANOTHER FOR THE SAME.—

Damiana Leaves	**Two ounces.**
Unicorn Root	One ounce.
Bayberry Bark	One ounce.
Poplar Bark	One ounce.
Australian Red Gum or Stringy Bark..	One ounce.
Bugle	One ounce.

Simmer in three pints down to a quart. Dose : a wineglassful three times a day.

FOR INTERNAL TUMOURS.—

Fuller's Earth	One ounce.
Water	One quart.

Dose : A wineglassful three times a day.

FOR FŒTID BREATH.—

Take as much powdered gum myrrh as will lie on a sixpence morning and night, or a teaspoonful of the tincture in half a cup of cold water ; drink half and with the rest gargle the throat, wash out the mouth and teeth, or take a teaspoonful of vegetable charcoal in a glass of water every morning, or the following mixture of herbs :—

Rosemary.........................	One ounce.
Wormwood	Half ounce.
Rue	One ounce.
Angelica	One ounce.
Cascara	Half ounce.
Ginger	Half ounce.
Horse Radish	Half ounce.
Calamus	Half ounce.

Boil in three pints of water down to two, strain, and take a wineglassful three times a day.

HAIR RESTORER.—

Milk of Sulphur	Two drachms.
Sugar of Lead....................	One drachm.
Rose Water.....................	Eight ounces.

Rub into the hair one ounce twice a day.

AMBROSIAL HAIR TONIC.—

Gum Benzoin .... **Two drachms.**
Castor Oil .... **Four ounces.**
Spirits .... **One quart.**

Shake and add :—

Oil of Lavender.................. One drachm.
Oil of Bergamot.................. One drachm.
Oil of Cloves .... Thirty drops.
Oil of Lemon .... Thirty drops.
Oil of Rosemary................. Thirty drops.
Oil of Neroli .... Thirty drops.
Tincture of Cantharides .... Half ounce.

Shake well, apply morning and night if required.

TO COLOUR THE HAIR BLACK.—

Take a piece of unslacked lime, the best you can get, pour
sufficient water on it to reduce it to powder ; put to this one
third to a fourth as much litharge as you have of the lime.
Powder very fine, pass through a seive, put sufficient of this
powder into a saucer, pour as much hot water on it as will
form it into a soft paste-like cream. Before going to bed
apply this paste to the hair, covering it from the root, up ; put
over it dark brown paper, and over all a night-cap ; in the
morning shake out the powder, wash with water, and if
desired, a little oil. If not sufficiently black apply again.
This is better than hair dyes.

TO DESTROY LICE AND NITS IN THE HAIR.—

Half an ounce of coculus indicus or fish berries steeped in
a pint of proof spirit one week, wet the the hair and scalp,
taking care not to let it get into the eyes. Label it poison (as
it is), and keep it out of the way.

CURE FOR A WEN.—

Make a strong solution of rock salt, keep a cloth saturated
with it on top of wen till it suppurates, then poultice with
slippery elm till clean, and heal up with the healing ointment.

JUICE OF NETTLES—

Is good for spitting of blood and bronchitis, from a tea- to a tablespoonful three or four tImes a day.

BRIGHT'S DISEASE AND DIABETES.—

Liverwort Leaves	One ounce.
Cascara Segrada	One ounce.
Barbary Bark	One ounce.
Angelica Root	One ounce.
Burnet Herb	One ounce.

In three pints water. Simmer to two pints. A wineglassful three or four times a day.

OIL OF ST. JOHN'S WORT.—

Cover the flowers with olive oil, infuse in the sun several days, paint over sores, inflamed and stiff joints.

CURE FOR DEAFNESS.—

Mullen flowers, fill an open-mouthed bottle, hang it in the sun for a week or more, pour the oil out. Put three drops into the ear night and morning.

GONORRHŒA.—

Fifteen grains of salicylate of soda, three times a day, is given as a sure cure. For the same the oil of sandal-wood, one ounce in six ounces emulsion of gum tragacynth, a teaspoonful three times a day.

Infusion of golden seal makes a good injection after the inflammatory condition of the above is subdued.

LOTION FOR ITCH.—

Take—

Sulphate of Potash	One ounce.
Water	One pint.
Vitriol	Half ounce.

Mix. Apply twice a day after washing with soap.

FOR CONSUMPTION.—

Take a teaspoonful of the juice of horehound every morning in a cupful of milk.

TREATMENT FOR DISEASES OF HORSES AND CATTLE.

Our readers, who are interested in this part of our work, will excuse us for our briefness. To deal fully with the troubles of the above animals would require much more space than is at our disposal. It may be a cause for congratulation that the lower animals are not subject to so many diseases as their lord. There are but a few in the colonies that cause breeders and owners anxiety. It is with them that we intend to deal in the present chapter, and it will be seen from our treatment that our medicines for cattle are about the same as for man. This is so, and it is reasonable, for it is evident to the reflecting that they are built up, so to speak, on the same plan and of the same material. We, with them, are the work of the same Divine mind and power. Doses of medicine for horses and oxen are usually reckoned at eight times the quantity given to man. The difference in the sizes in animals must not be lost sight of, as some are more than twice the size of others. In giving liquid medicine to cattle it is well to give it with a lemonade bottle, as an ordinary one may break in their mouth and cause mischief.

ASTHMA, OR SHORT-WINDEDNESS,

Is a condition that horses sometimes develop. We know of no better remedy than lobelia, in powder. A tablespoonful with one of composition powder may be given once or twice a day. If cough is present, give the cough powder; if it comes on in fits, burn some of the asthma powder under the nose.

GRIPES.

Horses are often subject to this. The treatment that we have known to relieve them is a tablespoonful of composition powder, and a dessert- or half dessert spoonful of cayenne, or substitute the colic powder for the composition, or, if a severe attack, one spoonful of composition and colic powder,

with half a one of cayenne. Give in gruel with lemonade
bottle.

ANOTHER RECIPE FOR GRIPES.

This one we have given several times to an owner, and
it always answers its purpose :—

Spirits of Sweet Nitre	Two ounces.
Laudanum	Quarter ounce.
Castor Oil	One and a half ozs
Oil of Thyme...................	Quarter ounce.
Olive Oil......................	Four ounces.

Give half in gruel, or warm water, as above ; the other half
may be given, if required, in an hour after. As a diuretic, when
the urine is scanty and difficult, give tincture of juniper berries
made with sweet nitre, one ounce three times a day.

LAMENESS.

If noticed at first, bathe with hot water, as hot as the han
can stand, for half an hour, then rub in the following
liniment :—

Oil of Spike	Two ounces.
Liquid Ammonia	Two ounces.
Turpentine....................	Two ounces.
Sweet Oil	One and a half ozs.
Oil of Amber..................	One and a half ozs.
Oil of Thyme..................	One ounce.
Camphor......................	Half ounce.

Measure the oils and liquids, weigh and dissolve the camphor
in the turpentine, shake well before using, and rub in well.
This liniment is also good for sprains in man and beast, or
where an outward application is required for pain or swelling.

There are a good many liniments, each one good in its
way. We can only give a few more.

No. 1.

THE MEXICAN LINIMENT.

Oil of Turpentine	**One ounce.**
Oil of Thyme	One ounce.
Oil of Amber	One ounce.
Black Oil	Half ounce.
Kerosene Oil	One and a half ozs.
Water	Three ounces.
Soap	Half ounce.
Caustic Potash	Twenty grains.

Dissolve the soap and potash in the water hot, then pour in the mixed oil, small parts at a time, till they are all in, then add warm water up to two quarts. If the black oil and the kerosene be omitted, the above is a fair imitation of Elliman's Royal Embrocation, which has a world-wide reputation.

No. 2.

Oil Rosemary	One ounce.
Tincture of Cayenne	Two ounces.
Turpentine	Two ounces.
Camphorated Oil	Two ounces.
Cajeput Oil	One ounce.

Mix, and rub in as others.

No. 3.

BLACK OIL is made with—

Linseed Oil	One pint.
Turpentine	Three pints.
Oil of Vitriol	One ounce.

Mix, shake well, and add three ounces of Barbadoes tar.
Useful for sprains, swellings, &c.

No. 4.

WHITE OIL.—

Spirits of Turpentine	Half pint.
Spirits of Wine	Half pint.
Olive Oil	One pint.
Liquid Ammonia	Four ounces.
Camphor	Four ounces.

Mix for wounds and old sores.

No. 5.

HOOF OIL.—

Oil of Tar............................ Half pint.
Whale Oil........................... Half pint.

For greasy heels make the following ointment :—

Linseed Oil .... Two ounces.
Beeswax.......................... Two ounces.
Gum Frankincense .... Two ounces.
Black Pitch .... Quarter ounce.

If there is swelling, poultice with slippery elm, wash with Castile soap, dry and melt, and apply the ointment ; cover the sores.   It will also be well to give an occasional dose of the following

CATTLE POWDER.

White Mustard Seeds, bruised........ Two ounces.
Fenugreek Seeds .... Two ounces.
Gentian Powder.................... One ounce.
Ginger .... Two ounces.
Cayenne Pepper .... One ounce.

Give one ounce. If very bad the dose may be doubled. Cover up all night, and rub well down in the morning.

CONDITION POWDER.

Elecampane Root.................. Four ounces.
Flax Seed .... Four ounces.
Fenugreek Seed .... Four ounces.
Juniper Berries .... Four ounces.
Resin............................ Four ounces.
Poplar Bark .... Four ounces.
Mustard.......................... Four ounces.
Bran .... Four ounces.
Liquorice Root................... Three ounces.
Ginger Root...................... Three ounces.
Washing Soda .... Three ounces.
Salt .... Three ounces.
Sulphur .... Three ounces.
Sulphate of Iron .... Three ounces.

CONDITION POWDER—*Continued*

> Carbonate of Soda .... Two ounces.
> Gentian Root .... Two ounces.
> Black Sulphurate of Antimony ...... One ounce.
> Saltpetre .... One ounce.
> Coriander Seeds .... One ounce.
> Valerian Root .... One ounce.
> Blood Root .... Half ounce.
> Lobelia .... Half ounce.
> Mandrake .... Half ounce.
> Burnt Alum .... Half ounce.

All in powder, mix.

DOSE FOR HORSES.

One tablespoonful with each feed. They need not stop work, but should have extra care in the stable. For acute attacks double doses may be given. Cattle need one and a half tablespoonfuls, sheep and hogs one at night. Some of our readers may think this a terrible mixture ; so we should have thought, and would not have given it if we had not known of its virtue. This is an American mixture which we have sold for some time and found it really good. We retail it at 1s 6d per pound. To get the things and mix them yourself will cost about 1s. We have them in stock. The following is a simpler one :—

> Flowers of Sulphur .... Half pound.
> Powdered Liquorice .... Half pound.
> Fenugreek .... Half pound.
> Gentian .... Half pound
> Sassafras......................... Half pound.
> Saltpetre......................... Half pound.

Dose :—Same as last.

FOR COWS' TEATS WHEN FESTERING.

Wash with the healing soap, dry, and cover with a soft rag on which is spread the marshmallow ointment. As this ointment is of such a nature that it can be eaten there is no fear of it injuring the milk

TO KILL LICE AND FLEAS ON HORSES, CATTLE, DOGS, &c.

Equal parts of powdered quassia chips and aloes, dust it into their coats at night and currycomb or brush off in the morning.   Repeat two or three times.

TO KEEP OFF FLIES.

Oil or Tar	Two ounces.
Oil of Pennyroyal..................	Two ounces.
Oil of Hemlock	One ounce.
Carbolic Acid	One ounce.
Linseed Oil	Two ounces.

Mix, and rub over the hair.

LAXATIVE MIXTURE FOR THE BOWELS.

Aloes, powdered	Two ounces.
Mandrake, powdered	Four ounces.
Senna, powdered	Four ounces.
Cayenne.........................	One ounce.

Mix, and give a tablespoonful in gruel or water the first thing in the morning or last at night.

FOR THE SCOUR.

Give a heaped tablespoonful of the following powder two or three times a day :—

Bistort Root	Two ounces.
Cranesbill	Two ounces.
Tormentil	Two ounces.
Cayenne.........................	One ounce.

Mix.

Milk Fever and Pleuro-Pneumonia are contributed by a stock owner.

MILK FEVER.

The greatest scourge to which dairy cows are subject is undoubtedly milk fever, and the time they are most liable to take it is when the grass is getting hard, or from Christmas on to harvest.   It is a disease that is much easier prevented than cured.   When cows are approaching calving attention should be given to them to see that their bowels are kept open.   If

inclined to be costive administer half a bottle of linseed oil,
with a dessert spoonful of cayenne pepper ; infuse the pepper
in a little boiling water and mix it with the oil.   If the udder
is heavy, draw the milk off a day or two before calving.   The
first symptoms appear immediately after calving and are :
stoppage of the flow of milk, suspended rumination, and
staggering.   Various remedies are applied, but except they
are prompt and thorough there is very little hope of a cure
after it has fairly set in.   After a long experience with cattle
the only remedy that we have found effectual is the
following :—

Have ready a sheet, two or three blankets, or bags opened
out lengthways, and a horsecover.   Soak the sheet in water,
wring it out, and pass it under the cow, being careful to cover
all the stomach ; bring it up each side, overlap on the back ;
now take your blankets or open sacks, pass these round over
the sheet one after the other, fix on each one with a nail or
two in the form of pins, see that the wet sheet is all covered ;
next place the large cover of the back and fix it underneath.
You cannot be too careful in covering all the wet sheet, this
careful covering is to raise a heat and make the animal sweat.
When the covers are fixed give the animal one pound of salts
and two dessertspoonfuls of cayenne pepper, also give
injections of warm water and soap every half hour.   In two
hours from packing the covers may be removed and the
animal well rubbed down, packing being repeated if
necessary.

PLEURO-PNEUMONIA.

This is one of the most virulent animal diseases of
modern times, for it is only within the memory of living men
that such a disease came under observation.   Introduced from
Ireland to England by half-starved cattle, it spread rapidly
over the country.   Since then the animal loss from this disease
exceeds perhaps any estimate that has been made.   Town
dairies suffered severely, in some cases entire stocks were
swept away.   In rural districts sometimes the disease would

be found on one farm while others in the same neighbourhood were free. Those who have studied the disease have no difficulty in detecting the symptoms, which are in the early stage a slight cough, laboured breathing, dry hide, watery eyes and hot muzzle ; in milk cows stoppage of the lacteal flow. These signs sometimes disappear for a time, returning with increased force, breathing becomes more laboured, cough more painful, the animal moves unwillingly, the appetite is impaired, and rumination ceases. In the last stage respiration is short and painful, the cough more painful and deep, the eyes become glassy, and the animal dies from suffocation. Many remedies have been tried, the most efficacious being the vapour bath and cayenne pepper freely administered. The best way to vapour-bath a cow is by means of a large box (such as those in use for shipping horses), with a tight-fitting door. Shut the animal in the box, keep the head out, have the box perforated below, introduce steam by means of a tube from a boiler. As this cannot always be managed the next best remedy is the wet sheet packed as described for milk fever. Give cayenne pepper and pleurisy powder freely, and nourishing feed

CLEANING COWS AFTER CALVING.

Drench with a teaspoonful of cayenne pepper and two tablespoonfuls of composition ; mix with water, and give in a lemonade bottle.

To Heal Wounds in Horses and Cattle.—

Wash with a decoction of marigolds, and apply the healing ointment, or—

Vaseline.......................... One ounce.
Carbolic Acid .... Half drachm.

Mix, and rub in. Here is another remedy, which may be called

THE SMOKE CURE.

For painful wounds nothing can be more beneficial than smoke. A short article on this useful remedy appeared in the " Health Column " of the *Otago Witness* of May 11th, 1888, in which old leather, woollen rags, and brown sugar were named as producers of healing smoke. An easy way of applying smoke to wounds in animals is by means of a bee-smoker. Charge the smoker with woollen rags and brown paper, light it and let the stream of smoke play on the wound. A horse's knee that was very badly broken was cured in little more than a fortnight by means of smoke and Friar's balsam. The mode of treatment was as follows :—

Smoke was applied to the wound, as above, with the bee-smoker, for half an hour at a time ; after which it was gently touched with a feather dipped in Friar's balsam. This treatment was repeated thrice daily for three days, after that twice a-day for two weeks, when a complete cure had been effected.

WORM POWDER.—

Areca Nut	Two ounces.
Worm Seed	Two ounces.
Powdered Senna	Two ounces.
Aloes	One ounce.
Cayenne	One ounce.

Mix, and give a heaped tablespoonful in water with a suitable bottle.

COUGH POWDER.—

Lobelia	Two ounces.
Skunk Cabbage	Two ounces.
Marshmallow Root	Two ounces.
Cayenne	One ounce.

Give as last, three times a day. These powders may be made into balls, with gum and water, or treacle.

ANOTHER SCOUR MIXTURE.—

Take a handful of the Koromiko leaves, chopped up among the feed, or a strong decoction of stringy bark, wattle, or lawyer scrub.

WARTS

On horses can be cured by painting them over with tar or strong acetic acid. Take care that the acid does not get on to the sound flesh.

FOOT-ROT IN SHEEP.

No. 1.

Scrape and wash off the decayed parts of the hoof, then paint with the following mixture :—

Fluid Extract of Blood-root .... Four ounces.
Strong Tincture of Myrrh .... Two ounces.

Paint over sores, and cover with black salve.

No. 2.

Butter of Antimony .... One ounce.
Tincture of Myrrh.................. Two ounces.

No. 3.

Carbolic........................... Two ounces.
Sulphate of Copper .... One ounce.
Glycerine .... Two ounces.

Use same as No. 1.

OINTMENT FOR SCAB IN SHEEP.—

Lard .... One pound.
Blood-root........................, Four ounces
Sulphur .... Four ounces.
Turpentine .... Four ounces.

Mix, and rub well into the parts.

To KILL LICE, TICK, MAGGOTS, &C.

Staphisagria Seeds .... Four ounces.
Quassia Chips .... Four ounces.

Boil in a gallon of water, or take Coculus Indicis, one ounce to a pint of methylated spirits. Rub well into the roots of hair.

NATIVE MEDICINAL PLANTS.

We are sorry that so little attention has been given to this class of plants. This is no doubt due to the fact that there is such an endless variety of others imported growing wild and cultivated. We have collected all the information we could concerning those that the Maoris have been using for generations, and are indebted to our manager, Mr. King, of Auckland for the following descriptive notes, which he gathered for our work.

FLAX (PHORMIUM TENAX.)
(Native name, HARA-KEKE OR KORARI.)

The fresh root is pounded and the juice used as a lotion to kill ringworm, also by natives to prevent galling of the skin of infants. It is taken internally to stop bleeding of the bowels and dysentery. The pulp of the bruised root it is tied tightly over wounds to stop bleeding. Mixed with equal proportions of the Kohia berry it is taken internally for flatulency. The gum found in the folds of the leaf near the root is put into water and applied to burns, scalds, and old sores, with good results. The roots roasted on a wood fire and beaten into a pulp are used warm as a poultice for abscesses or swollen limbs or joints.

HI NAU (ELAEORCARPUS HINAU.)

This produces a berry about half an inch long, oblong in shape, and of a dusky olive colour. The berry is covered with a thin but tough rind, and between it and the kernel is a soft, flour-like meal of an olive colour. This is prepared for food by steeping some months in water and then dried in the sun. It is too oily for European palates. The bark yields a brown dye.

KARAKA (CORYNOCARPUS LÆVIGATA.)

The berry of this tree, after an elaborate process of preparation, is eaten. The kernel, however, contains a virulently poisonous alkaloid which produces the most violent convulsions, and leaves the patient's body, when death does not ensue, in the most fearful state of incurable distortion. It is said to twist the head round.

KARE-AO (Rhipogonum Parviflorum), Supple Jack.

Decoction of the roots good in rheumatism, bowel complaints, also for fever and general debility, and for skin diseases, &c.

KAWA KAWA (Macropiper Excelsum) PEPPER TREE.

Ornamental shrub, very aromatic, diuretic. The leaves are chewed for toothache, or reduced to a pulp in hot water and applied to the face when swelled) ; also to any part of the body for rheumatic pains. Decoction of leaves and young twigs macerated in hot water is good for pains in the stomach; drank hot and continued for several days for gonorrhœa.

KORO-MIKO (Veronica).

Astringent, for dysentery, &c. The decoction is good for ulcers, and for venereal disease.

KOHE-KOHE (Dysoxylum Spectabile.)

A few leaves macerated in hot water, forming a very weak decoction, taken by women who have lost their children, to stop the secretion of their milk. The decoction must be weak, and not taken more than once a day. Invalids take it as a tonic to strengthen the stomach and allay irritating cough.

KO-HIA (Passiflora Tetrandra) a Climbing Plant.

The seeds are bruised into a pulp, and treated in a Maori oven, then pressed, yielding a clear oil, which is used as a salve for obstinate old wounds and sore breasts. The oil is called " Hinu Kohia."

KOPA-KOPA (Common Plantain.)

Boiled leaves applied to ulcers. The upper side of the leaf draws. When it begins to heal, the under side is laid on.

MANUKA (Leptospermum Scoparium.)

Infusion of leaves taken to allay fever. A white coloured gum, of sweet taste, which exudes from the tree, is given to suckling infants when costive, and for coughs in adults.

RATA BARK (Metrosideros Robusta)

Is steeped in water, and used as a lotion for ringworm and venereal, when bark of the Puka-tea is taken inwardly.

PUKA-TEA (Atherosperma N. Zealandiæ).

The bark is removed; the outer rind being scraped off, steeped in water, and used as a lotion for obstinate running sores and scrofula. Decoction of bark, taken inwardly for venereal, and used as a lotion

HOROPITO (Drimys Axillaris.)

The bark is a pungent aromatic, the stimulating tonic and astringent properties of which are little inferior to "Winter's Bark," (Drimys Winteri.)

It is closely allied to sarsaparilla, and popular repute makes it quite equal to the smilax family, in anti-scorbutic and alterative properties.

POHUTU KAWA (Metrosideros Tomentosa).

The "Christmas Tree," so called from its brilliant display of scarlet flowers at Christmas season. The bark is rich in tannin, and is valuable in dysentery.

TAREKAHA (Phyllocladus Trichomanoides.)

The "Celery Pine," growing to 60 feet in height. The bark yields a large percentage of tannin, and is consequently much used in New Zealand tanneries. It is second only to the celebrated "Divi Divi" in the yield of tannic acid; in dysentery, an astringent of much value. A red dye is obtained by the Natives from the bark.

TU PAKIHI TUTU (Coriaria Ruscifolia)—"The Toot.'

The seeds are extremely poisonous, causing severe colic and convulsions. Nevertheless, the juice of the berry is innocuous, being fermented and drank by the Natives as a relish and laxative. If we may judge from the tetanic spasms of those who have been poisoned by "Tute," it is not improbable that the active principle is closely allied to strychnine.

THE COTTON PLANT,

Found growing on the ranges of Otago, are long leaves about six inches; same shape as flax; green on the upper side, white under. It has been found a good substitute for tobacco, and for relieving asthma.

THE SPEAR GRASS.

We should judge from its taste that it is a diuretic. It is certainly not poisonous, as the wild pigs feed on it It may be used as a diuretic when nothing of the nature can be had.

IRISH MOSS.

A moss equal to the above is found on the rocks along the coasts of New Zealand.

CONCLUDING REMARKS.

We feel as if a few words of apology were needful, for notwithstanding our care, several mistakes have been overlooked in revising; fortunately, these are not such as will lead to any danger. Several words are misspelled, but not in such a way as to confound them with others. We find, however, that there is considerable difference in spelling amongst botanical writers. We feel also that we might be charged with the twofold aspect of sin, for some things we have omitted that we ought to have put in and others are in that some may think ought not; but we trust our readers will excuse imperfections when they reflect we were subject, while writing, to constant interruption consequent, on managing our extensive business. Our work has now gone forth with the hope that it will do good in removing pain and sickness, and enabling some to live longer the life which God has given us.

J. NEIL, 74 George Street, Dunedin

∽DR. NEIL'S∽
FAMILY MEDICINE CHEST.

There can be no two opinions as to the advisability of having the above, especially to those living in the country where it may be impossible to get anything needed in time to cope with sudden attacks of sickness, and even in the city and suburbs illness often comes on during the night, when it is difficult, if even possible, to get what is needed in time to be of service. The following medicines, which will be found in OUR FAMILY CHEST, are such as ought to be kept at hand in every household. Our own experience, and that of other herbalists, confirms this. Each tin or bottle will have full printed directions for use.

1. ASTHMA POWDERS. — Full Directions on Tin.

2. ANTI-SPASMODIC TINCTURE. —For all kinds of Fits, Fainting, etc.

3. CHOLERA DROPS. — For Inward Pains, Cramps, Diarrhœa, etc. Directions on Bottle. A most valuable Medicine.

4. COMPOSITION POWDER.—For Colds, Chills, and to Equalize the Circulation.

5. STOMACH BITTERS. — Quick Remedy for Indigestion.

6. BILIOUS POWDER.

7. CAYENNE PEPPER.— Invaluble for Fomentations.

8 DIGESTIVE FOOD.

9. SLIPPERY ELM POWDER.

10. HEALING OINTMENT.

11. BLOOD STAUNCHER.

12. SOOTHING SYRUP.

13. FEVER POWDERS.

14. PAINCURER.

15. DIURETIC DROPS.

16. DANDELION PILLS.

17. TR. GUM MYRRH.

18. COUGH SYRUP.

19. LOBELIA EMETIC POWDER.

20. ADHESIVE PLASTER.

These articles will be found described in the Book. See Index.

The Retail value of these medicines are £1. We will give in the chest with them, which is worth 5/-, for the 20/-

APPENDIX.

In our list of illustrations of the plants we find that a few are not described. As we know this would annoy some of our readers, we will now give a description of them.

CALAMINT (THYMUM CALAMINTHA.)

This plant belongs to the mint family, and like the other mints it is aromatic, stimulant, carminative, and diaphoretic. It is good in headaches, brain inflammation, windy colic, and flatulence. Infuse one ounce to the pint of water, sweeten, and drink in wine-glass doses every hour; this will bring out a perspiration. It is also recommended for gravel and female obstructions.

BROOKLIME (VERONICA BECABUNGA).

According to Dr. Robinson this herb is not only medicinal but a good article of diet. It has a hot, pungent taste, and may be eaten as water cress. As a medicine it is antiscorbutic, diuretic, and has the property of breaking and dissolving stone, hence it is good for difficulty of urine, gravel, and purifying the blood. Decoction : one ounce to the pint of water, and a wineglassful three or four times a day.

ERYNGO ROOT OR SEA-HOLLY (ERYNGION CAMPESTRE).

This plant grows by the sea-shore, but is sometimes cultivated for its medicinal qualities. It is highly reputed for its strengthening and fattening the system. In our select remedies is one for atrophy or wasting of the body (page 476), in which this root is the chief ingredient. Dr. Robinson says it is good for strengthening the procreative faculties, removing obstructions from liver and spleen. The roots bruised and applied to thorns that cannot be extracted will draw them out and heal up the wound. It is also, he says, good for jaundice, &c.

EYEBRIGHT (EUPHRASIA OFFICINALIS).

This little plant is undoubtedly good for strengthening the eyesight. If those coming to be about forty and feeling the eyes failing them were to use this plant they might do without "specs" for a few years longer. The juice dropped into the eyes relieves inflammation. We usually recommend our customers to use the infusion as a lotion, at the same time drinking a wineglassful three times a day. Infusion : One ounce to a pint of water.

FIGWORT (SCROPHULARIA).

This is said to be the best remedy for scrofula and swelling of the glands. The root mashed and applied as a poultice to external piles is a good remedy. An ointment may be made of the leaves for ulcers and sores. The herb is a good general blood purifier. Infusion : one ounce to pint of water. Decoction : 2 ozs. to the pint. A wineglassful of the former. Tablespoonful of the latter.

SOAPWORT (SAPONARIA OFFICINALIS).

Its properties are similar to the above in purifying the blood. It is affirmed to surpass sarsaparilla, guaiacum, especially for venereal affections ; being diuretic it is good for dropsy. The decoction of the root, two ounces to a pint of water. Dose : from half to a wineglassful. The decoction, when shaken, generates a foam similar to soapy water, hence its name soapwort.

HOPS (HUMULUS LUPULUS).

The virtues of the hop are so well known that we need only say that as a tonic and nervine it is a good medicine. The simplest way to extract its virtues is by infusion. One ounce to a quart of water, and half a teacupful taken three times a day will prove its virtue, which is similar to camomile.

FLUELLIN (ANTIRHINON ELATINE).

This is a very common herb in Europe, where it is well known as possessing good blood-cleansing properties. Dr. Fox gives a remarkable case cured by it of an eating ulcer of the nose. The herb was drank in decoction, and the juice applied to the sore. It also makes a good healing ointment, prepared in the usual way.

ST. JOHN'S WORT (Hypericum Perforatum).

This is a small shrub, found growing in all parts. The small yellow flowers are followed by berries of a dark-brownish-purple like the juniper. Its principal property is expectorant. Dr. Skelton recommends it for whooping and other coughs. We can endorse his good opinion of it, having used it frequently. It makes a good wound salve, chopped up and simmered in lard or vaseline. A decoction of the flowers is highly recommended for retention of urine. The persistent use of the herb decoction will, it is affirmed, cure sciatica and epilepsy.

GROUND PINE (Ajuga Chamœpitys).

This is a small plant, growing from four to six inches. It is a good diuretic and cleanser of the liver and spleen, also an excellent herb for female obstruction. It is best to take it in powder, as it is resinous and does not yield its virtues to water readily. Dose of the powder: a teaspoonful three or four times a day. Dr. Robinson recommends a mixture composed of the Dandelion root and agrimony for liver complaint and obstruction.

PLANTAIN (Plantago Major).

Commonly called healing leaves, and well do they deserve this name. Bound over a fresh cut or bruise they generally produce healing by the first intentions. As an internal medicine it is cooling, diuretic, alterative, and slightly astringent. The decoction of the roots makes a blood purifer, while the bruised leaves heal old sores. A gentleman in this city was cured of an inflamed ulcer on the leg by binding on the leaves, after trying various ointments, &c. It is found growing by the roadside almost everywhere.

ELDER BARK.

The regular doctors have found out the virtues of this tree, and testify that it is a genuine remedy for dropsy. A decoction of the bark is given in tablespoonful doses four to six times a day.

SANTILENA, OR GROUND CYPRESS.

This is an herb of great value. It is strongly recommended by Professor Kirk, of Edinburgh, in his papers on health, for worms; it is also good for indigestion. An ounce to the pint decoction is taken in tablespoonful doses three or four times a day. Price 6d per ounce, post free.

NOTE.—All herbs are sent post free at 6d per ounce.

———

We will now give some new remedies which, we feel assured, will benefit those of our readers who may suffer from any of the troubles they are intended for :

ASTHMA.

A new treatment for this distressing complaint consists in the injection of 1-50th of a grain of nitro-glycerine into the skin about the chest or arm. This can only be done by those experienced in the use of the hypdermic syringe.

BILIOUSNESS.

The Bilious and Aperient Powder we have found is a good remedy. Prepared thus :—Alex senna 2oz., jalap 1oz., mandrake ½oz., cloves ¼oz., carbonate of soda ¼oz., mint ¼oz., all in fine powder. Mix and take from a half to a teaspoonful in sweetened water. First thing in the morning is the best time to take it.

BURNS.

In addition to what will be found on page 423, the application of glycerine has been tried with success. It soon eases the pain and removes the discolouration. We had occasion to use it ourselves and found it justify what we have stated. Apply it at once if at hand, if not use cold water.

If the parts are scalded under the clothes do not take time to remove them, but pour the water over the parts.till patient can stand getting them off. As a soothing ointment when the pain is intense, after the water or glycerine has been used, mix 1oz. vaseline with 10 grains of morphia, spread thinly on cloths.

BLEEDING FROM THE NOSE.

When other means failed in three cases it was stopped almost immediately by applying a blister over the liver. This remedy was suggested by one of the founders of medicine, Galen, the Greek philosopher. This bleeding is also stopped by immersing the feet and hands in water as hot as can be borne.

BED-WETTING.

The cause of this trouble is said to be the sensitiveness of the neck of the bladder. In addition to remedies, page 385, raise the foot of the bed by putting a brick under the foot posts. This will keep the urine from the neck.

CONSUMPTION.

A new and favourite remedy for consumption is creosote, administered in drops; three to five are given in emulsion. It is, however, difficult to retain it on the stomach, and is likely to cause its disagreeable fumes to come up. When this is the case it may be given as an enema into the bowels. In this way fuller doses may be given, which will be absorbed into the system. Five drops three times a day will be the largest dose that can be given with safety. The creosote made from the beech tree is by far the best.

CARBUNCLE.

Three to five drops of pure carbolic acid put into the centre of it will relieve pain and hasten the cure.

DIPHTHERIA.

The vapour of the blue gum is said by one Australian doctor to be a specific for the above. Keep the room charged with the vapour and fill under the bed with the leaves and branches. The vapour may be kept up by means of an atomiser, which we can supply for 5s. A spoonful of the oil put into a tin and hung over a lamp will do. A case is recorded of a boy two years of age when past hope being cured by the green fluid extract being sprayed into the throat.

DISINFECTANTS.

One pound of crude carbolic acid mixed with 10 to 20 lbs. of slacked lime is both a cheap and good one.

An American journal gives another still cheaper. Dissolve one teaspoonful of nitrate of lead in one pint of boiling water, then dissolve two heaped teaspoonfuls of common salt in eight quarts of water, warmed. When both solutions are quite cold mix them together and the disinfectant is ready for use. In summer time it should be sprinkled freely where there are any unwholesome smells. As these are only helps in preventing sickness their power will be of little avail unless cleanliness is also carried out.

SPIRITS—DRINKING HABIT.

A simple cure is said to consist of eating as many apples as the stomach can bear. Continue the eating till all taste for the liquor is gone.

EPILEPSY.

The latest remedy found for these fits is a simple one—Borax. The dose is small, 10 grains three times a day, gradually increased to sixty. Dissolve in hot water, sweetened with glycerine or syrup

HAY FEVER.

Equal parts of menthol and carbonate of ammonia in a Preston salts bottle, inhaled as smelling salts, is a good means of relieving, and as affirmed, curing the above trouble.

LIVER ENGORGEMENT.

Symptoms: dull heavy pain on right side, yellowness of skin, constipation, &c. The following is a favourite American remedy :—Soda bi-carbonate 2 drams, leptandrin 1 dram, podophyllin 2 grains ; mix well, and divide into 60 powders. Take one in water every four hours.

MEGRIM OR EARACHE.

An American doctor speaks well of common salt as a remedy for the above. It is taken in half to a teaspoonful in water when the attack threatens.

MOTHER'S MARKS.

A new method for their removal. Paint round the mark for half an inch with collodion, then paint the mark with a four per cent. solution of corrosive sublimate ; cover this with a layer of the collodion, and remove the mark in a week, then heal with herbal ointment.

NEURALGIA.

In addition to remedy page 394, menthol internally in five grain doses three times a day and a solution in chloroform painted on the surface over the pain.

LA GRIPPE OR INFLUENZA.

This is a new form of disease, having some symptoms common to influenza, which it is also called. It seems to be a universal disease, said to have originated in China. It has appeared in all parts of the earth. The symptoms by which it is distinguished are many and variable ; pain in the muscles and joints, depression, and general debility. The remedy which we think will benefit all cases is, first, a good course of medicine (see page 255), or if difficult and cannot be had, the yarrow cure, page 79. If the pains in the muscles are severe take the treatment for rheumatism, page 392 ; when the severer symptoms are subdued a tonic of gold thread and composition, page 118. When it affects chiefly the chest use the remedies for bronchitis, page 406 ; or the balm of gilead and yarrow combined will cure. While we are writing, this complaint (having more of the influenza symptoms) is very severe in Australasia. A

Melbourne doctor claims that he has discovered a specific, which is, small doses of the perchloride of mercury or corrosive sublimate, the 30th to the 50th of a grain dose distilled in water. As this is a very dangerous drug, and distilling is not generally done in private houses, it would be advisable to get this remedy put up at a chemist's. It seems that this infectious trouble is caused by climatic influence and will generally run its short course. All that can be done is to assist nature to throw it off. This we are certain the botanic medicine we have given will do. Use composition powder as a preventative.

PILES.

There are many remedies for this painful affection. In addition to treatment, page 379, the following may be tried : Gum frankincense. Put a few embers in a chamber-pot or other vessel, sprinkle a few pieces of the gum on the red embers, and sit over the vessel so as to get the smoke on to the piles, for 10 or 15 minutes night and morning, or at night alone. This remedy is highly spoken of. Another simple cure is to spread some fat on a piece of brass till it is green, then apply night and morning. Our own pile ointment and powder have wrought many cures.

PLEURISY.

Ten grains muriate of ammonia, every two hours in a wine-glass of water. Infusion of pleurisy root is a more effective remedy than the water.

PNEUMONIA OR INFLAMMATION OF THE LUNGS.

One ounce powdered pleurisy root infused in a pint of boiling water. One tablespoonful of the clear infusion with 10 drops of the compound tincture of myrrh every 15 minutes is a treatment that cannot be surpassed. Few will suffer long under it. Compound tincture of myrrh is given on page 185.

PARALYSIS.

Paralysis, when accompanied with wasting of the muscles, caused by a want of phosphorus in the system, was cured by the taking of one 80th of a grain in a teaspoonful of oil of sweet almonds. The patient was a girl 10 years of age. For an adult the dose is the 30th of a grain. To prepare it properly is the work of a chemist, as the drug is dangerous and must be weighed in grain scales.

RHEUMATISM.

The oil of winter green has been found useful for this complaint. It is taken internally, six drops on sugar three or four times a day; and mixed with an equal part of olive oil. It is rubbed into the affected parts for five minutes, and the surface rubbed covered with cotton wool.

Eucalyptus oil is also good, used in the same way, or boil the blue gum leaves and lay them over the painful parts.

SWELLINGS, &c.

Iodine, which is generally used for treating them, is much improved by mixing with equal parts of glycerine. It softens and penetrates much better than the iodine alone.

SORE THROAT.

In addition to our general treatment, page 332, two new remedies are recently introduced. 1st. The vapour of turpentine—a teaspoonful is put into a cup of hot water and the steam inhaled for five minutes. 2nd. A four per cent. solution of cocoaine spread into or painted with a throat brush will usually give almost immediate relief.

A FOUR DOLLAR CURE FOR INDIGESTION, WORMS, CONSTIPATION, &c.

An American man of medical pursuits sells a secret for the above sum. Everyone who pays for it has to sign a bond that he will not divulge it. The cure is simplicity itself. To inject into the bowels three pints of hot water as hot as can be borne every night until cured. We know a gentleman who tried it and declares it a good thing.

TAPE WORM.

Eat the whole of the inside of an ordinary sized cocoanut, grated fine, at bed time. If the bowels don't move early a dose of castor oil or the bilious powder may be taken, when the worm will soon be expelled.

2. One drop of croton dissolved in 30 drops of chloroform, and one ounce of glycerine given at night on an empty stomach, followed in the morning by a bilious powder.

SCIATICA.

Chloroform and menthol. A strip of cloth saturated in above solution and laid along the line of pain, covered with oiled silk or rubber cloth, will soon give relief.

SPRAINS.

Immerse part in hot salt water. Keep up the heat for half an hour by putting the basin or bucket on hot bricks. Wipe dry, and put on a plaster bandage, which is prepared. Then get a 3 in. strip of cheese-cloth from 6 to 9 ft. long, rub into it dry plaster of Paris, roll it up, put a piece of flannel next the skin, keep out creases; now dip your rolled bandage in warm water and roll it round the part. In a short time it will form a splint which may be kept on till all pain and swelling are removed.

VOMITING.

This is often an indication of early pregnancy, in some cases continuing till the patient is exhausted. Nothing will lie on the stomach. The cause is that the womb, which, so to speak, is drawing the chief forces of life to itself is in its first position. The pelvis or lowest part of the abdomen or belly, after quickening, rises out of this position, when the vomiting usually ceases, as the sickness is caused by pressure or dragging on the nerves. The simplest way to obtain relief is to elevate the lower part of the body. This may be done by putting one, two, or three pillows under the hips, or assuming the knee-chest position, that is, lying on the knees and chest. If one way fails try the other. For a simple cure nothing surpasses an infusion of peach bark. Get a few of the last year's growth of shoots, smash them so as to loosen the bark, which strip off, fill a jug with them, cover with boiling water, infuse one hour, then give a dessertspoonful every half hour till vomiting is stopped. We have a tincture of the bark, dose half a teaspoonful, or the dry bark 4d per ounce. We can strongly recommend our digestive food for ordinary cases of vomiting, as it lies on the stomach when nothing else will.

PAINS IN THE OVARIES.

Many females are troubled with these pains. The location is above the groins or bottom of the belly. Five grains of salicine three or four times is strongly recommended; taken with a little water or in any simple liquid. In addition the seat of pain may be painted over with the magic liniment.

BRIGHT'S DISEASE.

A complete cure of the chronic form of this disease was obtained by seven drops of the fluid extract of Canadian hemp (apocynum) three times a day, the dose slightly increased so as not to cause vomiting or purging.

ANTIPYRINE.

This is a new remedy, resembling quinine. Is has been found very valuable for headaches and for reducing the temperature in fevers, which it does, keeping it down for several hours. The dose is from five to twenty grains. For a severe headache eight grains in water usually gives relief.

THE MICROBE KILLER.

For curing all disease by killing the germs. That it cures all we know is not true, still those who want a microbe killer can make one for about 1s. a gallon. Take six to eight ounces sulphorous acid, put in one gallon of distilled or rain water, dose a wineglass three times a day; or one ounce solution permanganate of potash in a gallon, same dose, is good and cheap.

OUR SPECIAL PREPARATIONS

As we have given a little over the number of pages we promised, and there are a few left to make a complete print-ing, we intend to devote them to giving a description and prices, &c., of our manufactured medicines. By experience we know that most people will not take the trouble to make things from the raw material when they can get them directly to hand. There is some reason more than simply to save trouble, for experience teaches those in constant practice how to do things in the best way; and further, our appliances are adapted to the work required. In fixing our prices, we have not followed the common custom of puttir.g a fancy price on our goods because they are medicines, thinking, as some affirm, that if you do not charge high prices, people will not think them any good. Our prices we have made to harmonise with the cost of the material used, time of making, &c., and they are such, we think, that no reasonable economist can charge us with extortion. We can assure our readers we shall see to it that we make them up to the standard of first-class medicines. We shall begin with our justly celebrated

READY-RELIEF ASTHMA POWDER.

Having given its name, we will follow out the Scriptural injunction—" Let another praise Thee." We have only space for one testimonial.

To Mr J. Neill.

Dear Sir,—I learn that you are about to publish a Book on the Botanic System of Medicine. I would like to testify to the great benefit I have received from your Medicine, especially your Ready Relief Asthma Powder. You have well named it Ready Relief, for so it is to me. I have been troubled for several years, and have tried almost everything, but I can solemnly say that nothing has done me anything like the amount of good that your Powder has. It ought to be well known, as it is a blessing to those suffering from Asthma.—I am gratefully yours,

J.W., TIMARU.

BALM OF GILEAD.

It is now about ten years since we first introduced this preparation. Our reason for making it was to furnish in one bottle a medicine that would cure both coughs and colds. To do this we made a careful selection of the most noted herbs for chest and throat affection. Our selection has been very successful, as may be judged from the fact of having sold over 10,000 bottles with very little advertising. The balm is not unpleasant to take, and, if taken as directed on the bottle, gives ready relief at first, and usually cures before the bottle is done. 2/6, 12 ounce bottle; 5 for 10/. We have no room for testimonials.

COMPOSITION POWDER.

This powder is now a household word in thousands, if not millions, of homes through all parts of the civilised world. Our readers will find its component parts on page 6. Suffice it to say, it ought not to be left out of any house. as it is the stitch in time that saves lives. It is, single ounce, 6d ; 4 ounces, 1/6 ; 8 ounces, 2/6, and 4/- per lb.

COUGH POWDER

Is a good mixture of herbal powders for dry hacking coughs. It promotes expectoration. Same price as composition.

COUGH PILLS

Are also a good mixture of highly concentrated medicines for relieving coughs, tightness on the chest, and kindred troubles, 1s, 3 dozen box ; 3 boxes for 2s 6d.

BOTANIC COUGH SYRUP,

A pleasant and effective mixture of Horehound, Lobelia, Skunk Cabbage, Elecampane, Comfrey, &c. This syrup has been a blessing to parents and children. We have also got a blessing from grateful customers for the good is has accomplished. 1s, 4 oz. bottle. Three in one at 2s 6d will last some families all winter.

DIURETIC POWDER AND PILLS,

For difficulty with urine, pains in the back and bladder, gravel, &c. These medicines have been highly extolled for the above purposes. Powder, same price as composition powder. Pills, 1s a box ; 3 for 2s 6d.

DANDELION COFFEE.

While in training in Glasgow in 1872, we anticipated that when we introduced this preparation in New Zealand (the land where we had resided for ten years, and to which we were about to return), that it would be a great success. We have not been disappointed, having, during the last 14 years, manufactured many tons of the root into the healthful diet drink. It has been a source of revenue to the settlers and others, who previously contemptuously cast away the roots, which now bring them over £1 for a bagful. The Dandelion Coffee has sold so well, that our trouble now is that we cannot get enough of roots. It is good for people with weak stomachs, sluggish livers, and nervous temperaments ; a fine substitute for the ordinary coffee or tea, The price is most reasonable : 2s a pound ; ½lb tin, 1s.

DANDELION PILLS.

To use what some might say was a boasting and questionable statement, these pills have beat Holloway's hollow, and knocked Cockle's into a cocked hat, for the simple reason that the above-named pills are composed chiefly of aloes, jalap, &c.—old drugs that have been eclipsed in these later days of progress. Our dandelion pills contain four of the most valuable medicines, viz., podophyllin, leptandrin, euonymin, and hydrastin, that are worth about as much per ounce as the old drugs are per pound, and yet let it be noticed that ours are only half the price considering the number and size.

Again, we pearl-coat ours. They are about three grains, and four dozen in a box for 1s, three for 2s 6d. Good for indigestion, biliousness, the liver and bowels. As a family medicine they are highly prized, not only in the Colonies, but they have been sent for from the Old Country.

COMPOUND RHUBARB PILLS.

A mild aperient and stomach correcting pill. We make them from Dr. Coffin's recipe, which has stood the test of 50 years. Same price as the dandelion.

DIGESTIVE FOOD.

For invalids, babies, and persons of weak digestion, who often vomit their food. This is really a good food and medicine combined. When nothing else has staid on the stomach this has. Most reasonable price 1s per half pound tin, three for 2s 6d.

EAR DROPS,

For temporary deafness, caused from accumulation of wax, colds, &c. A gentleman who complained of deafness used one bottle. He told us that he could hear too well now, for it seemed to him that he had nails in his boots. Even cases of permanent deafness have been greatly relieved by these drops. 1s a bottle.

EYE WASH AND EYE OINTMENT.

This delicate organ is liable to inflammation of a mild or severe form. In our treatment of inflammation, page (331). will be found directions how to deal with the severe attacks The drops and ointment are for the milder form, and they will be found really good, as many have testified. Popular price, 1s.

FEMALE CORRECTIVE POWDER AND PILLS.

For suppression of and difficult menstruation these have a good reputation, as they generally accomplish the purpose intended. Powder, 1s 6d per quarter tin or box; pills, 1s a box; three for 2s 6d.

FEMALE RESTORATIVE POWDER.

Good for excessive menstruation, leucorrhœa, and as a general tonic. Highly prized both in England and the colonies. 1s 6d per tin.

GOUT MIXTURE.

The best combination we know of for the above trouble. Price 2s 6d; liniment for the same, 1s 6d.

GOLDEN PILLS.

Good for purifying the stomach, bowels, pains in the back, &c. 1s per box.

GONORRHŒA.

This complaint, though generally the result of wrong-doing, needs to be cured. We have a first-class treatment for it comprising mixture, injection and syrup, 5s.

HEADACHE PILLS.

A long established well-tried remedy for headaches. 1s a box, in constant sale.

HERBAL BEER EXTRACT.

This is likely to become one of the most popular domestic drinks in New Zealand, and no wonder, when a shilling bottle makes 4 gallons of healthful, refreshing, and pleasant beer. In summer time it will take the place of tea and coffee.

MOTHER'S FRIEND—SOOTHING SYRUP,

Free from the shadow of poison, prepared from simples, such as best rhubarb, cinnamon, ant-acids, &c. Some time ago we sent to England to Dr. Coffin for some of his soothing syrup. We got 2 ounce bottles, which cost 1/6. The lady, at whose request we sent for it, afterwards was persuaded to try our own. When she had given it a fair trial with Coffin's, she said she preferred ours. 3 ounce bottles, 1/.

NEURALGIC MIXTURE.

This is another of few positive cures ; it is almost unfailing. We have experienced its curative effects ourselves, and have been pleased to see the relief it has given to others. 2/6 per bottle.

PAIN KILLER AND PAIN CURER.

We have been making these two for the last 12 years with gratifying success. The first giving relief in rheumatic pains, or pains of any kind. Toothache, chilblains, &c., are generally relieved with it at once. The curer is either taken internally or applied externally. It is preferred by many to the Perry Davis. 1/- per bottle.

IRISH MOSS.

As most people are putting up this mixture, we have also a mixture which is similar to the botanic cough syrup, with the Irish Moss and a little chlorodyne added. 1/-, a 4 ounce bottle makes it the cheapest in the market. It is said to stop the cough very soon.

LIVER TONIC.

This is one of our most successful mixtures. There is hardly a person that takes it without benefit. Indigestion, liver trouble, yellowness of the skin, &c., all yield to it. 1/6 and 2/6 ; 5 large bottles for 10/.

LIVERWORT—KIDNEY CURE.

The great American kidney cure, at 5/- a bottle, cannot excel this at 2/6. We have customers who have tried both and give ours the palm. Difficulty of urine, and pains in the back, yield to this mixture.

HOP BITTERS

Are getting out of date now. This is no doubt due to the fact that the original make is composed mostly of whisky. Our make is medicinal, being double the strength and half the cost; 2/6 a reputed quart. We have sold thousands of this good tonic and stimulant.

PERFUMERY.

We are now making a large quantity of the various kinds. Our lavender water is only 6d per ounce, and is preferred to the imported kinds at double that price.

RHEUMATIC CURE.

We can promise immediate relief, if not permanent cure with this mixture. 2s 6d.

PILLS FOR ALL COMPLAINTS.

1s a box; 3 for 2s 6d.

QUINSY EMBOCATION.

This is an outward application which has earned a good reputation in sore throats, painful swellings of any kind. 1s.

STOMACH TONIC, STOMACH BITTERS, SPICED BITTERS.

Are all well proved remedies for indigestion. 1s 6d per tin or bottle.

WHOOPING COUGH, SYRUP AND LINIMENT,

Generally efficacious in removing this distressing complaint. Syrup, 2s; liniment, 1s.

ROSEMARY TRICOPHEROUS

This is fast taking the place of the American article. It is the same size bottle, at 1s. We are assured by a gentleman that it began to tell on his bald pate after a month's use. Pleasantly perfumed.

HEALING MEDICATED SOAP.

We specially prepare this, which is one of the best toilet soaps It softens and whitens the skin better than any we have ever seen. Besides its healing quality, it is sweetly scented. 6d per cake.

CHOLERA DROPS.

As we have spoken of this mixture before, we need only say that it will not disappoint anyone with diarrhœa. 1s per bottle.

OINTMENTS.

We make the following kinds : Healing, Itch, Marshmallow, Sulphur, Zinc, Carbolic, and Pile, &c., in 6d and 1s boxes.

WORM POWDERS, 1s per dozen.   PILLS, 1s per box. CAKES, 2d each.

These preparations we will send by parcel post, postage free, if 5s. worth is ordered, (with stamps or the amount in any way) securely packed and promptly sent to any address. Should any person wish to ask our advice, or wish anything explained in the Book, an addressed and stamped envelope will meet with our immediate attention. In writing for advice, please be particular in giving your age, symptoms, how long ill, &c., as lucidly as possible.   Our terms are for one month's treatment £1. This will include medicine and postage. When persons cannot afford this, a week's or a fortnight's will be sent. As we are constantly receiving goods from England, Germany, and America, anything in the shape of Medicine or Medical Books we will get for our patrons.

Our Branch Establishments are under the management of experienced men, who were all trained under our personal care. They will send you anything you want, and treat you carefully.   The addresses are : Tay-street, Invercargill ; Main South Road, Timaru ; and Wellesley-street, Auckland.

INDEX.